Nursing the Highly Dependent Child or Infant

NURSING THE HIGHLY DEPENDENT CHILD OR INFANT

A manual of care

Edited by

Michaela Dixon
Clinical Development Nurse – Lecturer/Practitioner
School of Health and Social Care
Faculty of Health and Life Sciences
University of the West of England
Bristol

Doreen Crawford
Senior Lecturer in Children's Nursing
School of Nursing and Midwifery
Faculty of Health and Life Sciences
De Montfort University
Leicester

Debra Teasdale
Head of Department – Health, Wellbeing and the Family
Canterbury Christ Church University
Canterbury
Kent

Jan Murphy
Clinical Development Sister
Paediatric Intensive Care Unit
Birmingham Children's Hospital NHS Foundation Trust
Birmingham

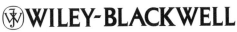
WILEY-BLACKWELL
A John Wiley & Sons, Ltd., Publication

This edition first published 2009
© 2009 Blackwell Publishing Ltd

Blackwell Publishing was acquired by John Wiley & Sons in February 2007. Blackwell's publishing programme has been merged with Wiley's global Scientific, Technical, and Medical business to form Wiley-Blackwell.

Registered office
John Wiley & Sons Ltd, The Atrium, Southern Gate, Chichester, West Sussex, PO19 8SQ, United Kingdom

Editorial offices
9600 Garsington Road, Oxford, OX4 2DQ, United Kingdom
2121 State Avenue, Ames, Iowa 50014-8300, USA

For details of our global editorial offices, for customer services and for information about how to apply for permission to reuse the copyright material in this book please see our website at www.wiley.com/wiley-blackwell.

Library of Congress Cataloging-in-Publication Data
Nursing the highly dependent child or infant: a manual of care / edited by Michaela
Dixon [et al.].
     p. ; cm.
   Includes bibliographical references and index.
   ISBN: 978-1-4051-5176-4 (pbk. : alk. paper) 1. pediatric nursing—Handbooks, manuals, etc.
2. Pediatric intensive care—Handbooks, manuals, etc. 3. Intensive care nursing—Handbooks, manuals, etc. I. Dixon, Michaela
   [DNLM: 1. Pediatric Nursing. 2. Subacute care—methods. WY 159 N9749 2009]

RJ245.N87 2009
618.92′00231—dc22

                                                                    2008028174

A catalogue record for this book is available from the British Library.

Set in 10/12.5 pt Sabon by Newgen Imaging Systems Pvt Ltd, Chennai, India
Printed in Singapore by Fabulous Printers Pte Ltd

1 2009

CONTENTS

LIST OF CONTRIBUTORS

Katie Anderson
Staff Nurse
Neonatal Unit
University Hospitals of Leicester NHS Trust
Leicester

Sandra Batcheler
Sister
Paediatric Intensive Care Unit
Bristol Royal Hospital for Children
Bristol

Tina Clegg
Service Manager
Specialist Children's Play Consultant
University Hospital of Leicester NHS Trust
Leicester

Jill Cochrane
Clinical Educator
Paediatric Intensive Care Unit
Royal Liverpool Children's Hospital
Liverpool

Doreen Crawford
Senior Lecturer in Children's Nursing
School of Nursing and Midwifery
De Montfort University
Leicester

Michaela Dixon
Clinical Development Nurse – Lecturer/
    Practitioner
School of Health and Social Care
Faculty of Health and Life Sciences
University of the West of England
Stapleton
Bristol

Graham Gordon
Principal Specialist Nurse
The Liver Unit
Birmingham Children's Hospital NHS
    Foundation Trust
Birmingham

Caroline Haines
Consultant Nurse in Paediatric Intensive and
    High Dependency Care
Paediatric Intensive Care Unit
Bristol Royal Hospital for Children
Bristol

Felix Hay
Staff Nurse
Emergency Department
University Hospitals of Leicester NHS Trust
Leicester

Jane Leaver
Lecturer/Practitioner
Birmingham City University
Birmingham

Janet Murphy
Clinical Development Sister
Paediatric Intensive Care Unit
Birmingham Children's Hospital NHS
    Foundation Trust
Birmingham

Marian Perrott
Sister
Outreach Service
Bristol Royal Hospital for Children
Bristol

Sarah Roberts
Clinical Nurse Specialist in Children's Pain
University Hospitals of Leicester NHS Trust
Leicester

Karen Selwood
Advanced Nurse Practitioner
Paediatric Oncology Unit
Royal Liverpool Children's Hospital NHS Trust
Liverpool

Kathryn Summers
Senior Lecturer and Professional Lead
  for Children's Nursing
Department of Health, Wellbeing and the Family
Canterbury Christ Church University
Canterbury

Debra Teasdale
Head of Department – Health, Wellbeing and
  the Family
Canterbury Christ Church University
Canterbury
Kent

Clare Thomas
Lead Nurse for Burns
Birmingham Children's Hospital NHS
  Foundation Trust
Birmingham

Colin M. Way
Nurse Consultant
Children's High Dependency Care
Paediatric Intensive Care Unit
St George's Hospital
London

Gill West
Lecturer
Department of Health, Welbeing and
  the Family
Faculty of Health and Social Care
Canterbury Christ Church University
Canterbury
Kent

Michelle Wright
Advanced Nurse Practitioner
Paediatric Oncology Unit
Royal Liverpool Children's Hospital NHS Trust
Liverpool

Chapter 1

INTRODUCTION TO PAEDIATRIC HIGH DEPENDENCY CARE

Colin M. Way and Doreen Crawford

Introduction

The care of critically ill children has received some attention over the past 10 years, and many of the recommendations from reports relating to the provision of paediatric intensive care (PIC) have been implemented (Department of Health (DH) 1997a, 1997b). However, paediatric high dependency care (HDC) is only just beginning to emerge as a speciality in its own right, with a distinct body of knowledge, clinical skills and its own organisational and educational concerns. With the increase in the dependency of children admitted to hospital over the last 5 years (Haines 2005), there is now an urgency to review the provision and development of paediatric HDC within the United Kingdom in much the same way as PIC services have been reviewed.

This chapter explores HDC definitions and current models of care, reviews current standards for the development of high dependency (HD) services and explores the concept of 'critical care without walls'. Also considered will be the ethos behind the development and growth of the early warning scoring systems and the utilisation of outreach services. There will be some consideration of the holistic nature of HDC of children and, in order to ensure the quality of care provision, an appraisal of the educational and support needs of staff that care for these children and their families.

High dependency care – an elusive concept

Wright (2006) points out that HDC is not a new concept because, as individuals become sicker and more dependent, a higher level of care and attention is required. HDC has been recognised informally for many years. HDC remains an elusive concept in terms of its nature and degree of patient dependency and the preventative and therapeutic services provided within it. HDC has come a long way since Nightingale's description of it in 1852 (Jennet 1990) as a valuable area where post-operative and other patients requiring close attention can be watched. Despite this vision the lack of formalised and nationally agreed admission and discharge criteria for HDC has resulted in a diversity of therapeutic and preventative treatments offered in HDC units which differ between hospitals (McDonald 1999). One of the key issues is the criteria used to define HDC.

In some hospitals HDC is defined by levels of technology and treatment; however, in order to provide these dynamic forms of treatment in a safe environment, human resource issues need to be considered (Baur 2001). Sheppard and Wright (2000) believe that although 2:1 nursing care ought to be the minimum aim for staffing in HD units, there is not a linear relationship between levels of patient anxiety and severity of illness. Should managers aim to resource HD units at 1:1

just like intensive care? This approach recognises that HD can be defined in relation to a number of different but interrelated factors:

- The physiological stability/instability of the child
- The level of observation or therapeutic intervention required; and/or
- The acuity of the child in relation to patient dependency and nursing workload

Within the last 5 years there has been a political drive to develop paediatric HD services within some acute hospitals across the UK (DH 2006). However, significant work still needs to be undertaken to determine the focus of HDC and how it should be delivered. PIC nursing can now defend its staffing levels by arguing that 1:1 nursing care is essential for the safe delivery of, e.g. invasive positive pressure ventilation (DH 1997a). If the defining attribute of critical care nursing in the PIC environment is determined by the technological level of nursing care, then what defines HDC? If health-care personnel are to offer a service that is fair and equitable to all children and adolescents then close consideration of the meaning of HDC is required.

What is HDC?

A common understanding of HDC is the provision of a service that is suitable for those patients who are too sick for the general wards but not unwell enough to merit admission to an intensive care unit. An alternative interpretation may include care for patients who are no longer receiving intensive therapy but still require close observation/ monitoring. However, this assumes that HDC is uniform throughout the UK. Sheppard and Wright (2000) believe that HD will not be uniform throughout the UK as wards and intensive care units differ from hospital to hospital and that it would be wrong to be overly prescriptive or restrictive. Accordingly one might infer that HDC is whatever one considers it to be.

In 1996, a report of the National Confidential Enquiry which examined adult peri-operative deaths (Royal College of Anaesthetists and Royal College of Surgeons 1996) concluded that there was an inadequate provision of HDC units across the country and that this impacted on performing major surgery on patients who were physiologically compromised as there were insufficient facilities to recover them post-operatively. Although HDC, in this case, was considered an extension of the operating theatre recovery room, its value was recognised. The document 'Guidelines on Admission to and Discharge from ICU and HDU' (DH 1996), although designed for adults, identified four main categories of patient for whom HDC was appropriate. These are:

- Patients who require single organ support
- Patients who require more detailed observation/ monitoring
- Patients who no longer require intensive care but are not well enough for the general ward
- Post-operative patients who require close monitoring for more than a few hours

If these categories are accepted, HD units could be perceived as extensions of the intensive care unit. These guidelines are open to interpretation. The medical interpretation of a patient's needs varies and frequently differs from that of nurses in relation to calculating the patient's actual dependency scores. Single organ support is vague; it could mean the administration of low-grade oxygen to promote tissue oxygenation or it could mean the administration of inotropes to prevent blood pressure from falling. The ramifications of each of these treatments significantly affect the ability of the nursing staff in HD units to deliver safe care in the face of strict resource constraints.

These issues are reflected in 'A Bridge to the Future' (DH 1997b) and the Bristol Royal Infirmary Inquiry (Kennedy 2001) in which PIC provision and care was the subject of national debate following a series of incidents. The enquiries following each incident outlined problems inherent within the NHS, and in particular 'A Bridge to the Future' focused upon the ability of PIC services to cope with peaks in demand (DH 1997a).

Three levels of intensive care are defined but HDC is only ascribed one. Level 1 care (HDC) is described as 'care provided to a child who may require closer observation and monitoring than is usually available on an ordinary children's ward', although much of this care is already provided, with higher staffing levels than usual, in such locations. Examples of the type of observations undertaken and the medical conditions involved include:

- Continuous monitoring of the heart rate
- Non-invasive blood pressure monitoring
- The child requiring single organ support
- Moderately severe croup
- Suspected intestinal obstruction
- Suspected poisoning

Doman *et al.* (2004) argue that this definition is too vague and leads to confusion as to which children meet the criteria for this level of intervention, so there is difficulty in obtaining accurate information about the numbers of children requiring HDC. Indeed accurate auditing of numbers of HD admissions and where these children are located has become the 'Holy Grail' of health professionals particularly since the introduction of payment by results, health care resource groups and the NHS financial restraints which potentially impinge on staffing levels. This is pertinent considering Doman and Browning's (2001) concerns that children with HD needs are still being nursed on general wards without an increase in staffing levels. With this fixation on hospitals and acute settings, can these definitions be applied to support the care planning of stable but highly dependent children with a myriad of complex needs to return them to the community ?

Day (2005) suggests that the DH definition is flexible enough to encompass all children with HD needs, but five sub-categories within the level 1

Table 1.1 Breakdown of level 1 definitions.

Sub-divisions	Descriptor
Level 1a	Children who trigger an early warning scoring system and clinical condition and demonstrate a trend of deterioration
Level 1b	Children who trigger an early warning scoring system but demonstrate a trend of improvement
Level 1c	Children who require more frequent observations than every 60 minutes who have undergone an elective procedure, e.g. liver biopsy
Level 1d	Children requiring long-term ventilation
Level 1e	Children who are time-consuming in terms of manpower

definition are required to ensure effective and appropriate location of care, care delivery and funding. This breakdown is certainly sufficiently flexible to consider community care (see Table 1.1).

Despite attempts at defining HDC, it can be argued that current descriptions remain superficial and offer little practical assistance to nursing staff that are managing and delivering HDC on a daily basis. The DH in their report 'High Dependency Care for Children – Report of an Expert Advisory Group for the Department of Health' (DH 2001) commented on the lack of clarity with the previous definition of HDC (DH 1997a) and attempted to identify children in need of HDC in acute and speciality hospitals. This attempt used illness classifications to identify children in need of HDC and made specific reference to diabetic ketoacidosis (Chapter 7), meningococcal septicaemia (Chapters 4 and 6) and bacterial meningitis (DH 2001). However, it cannot be assumed that children requiring HDC do so as a result of the classification of their illness. Although illness classification may identify children who require HDC during their hospital stay it cannot provide information on the duration of the HDC need. Such detailed information is required for service planning. A child may be admitted and discharged with the same diagnosis yet move between all three levels of care. Without a clear definition it becomes impossible to determine the number of these children and the duration of time that they receive HDC. Because of this lack of clarity there has been a move over the last 5 years to look at other ways of capturing the exact nature of HDC by developing patient acuity and dependency scoring tools and HDC measurement tools.

Tools to measure work load and dependency

The Yorkshire HDC measurement tool

This tool was developed following a large regional research study which audited nursing and medical staffing and ward activity within 36 paediatric ward areas from 10 hospital trusts across West, North and East Yorkshire over a 7 month period in 2005 (Rushforth 2006). The patient activity proformas returned ($n = 24\,540$) helped inform the development of the tool. Work to validate the tool is ongoing. The measurement tool is designed for staff to mark the appropriate boxes for interventions performed for a child every 12 hours during a patient episode of care and should be completed retrospectively at the end of a shift. There are 36 interventions which are divided into three groups A, B or C with a score assigned to each (see Table 1.2).

The total score for the child is calculated by adding up all the individual scores for all the

Table 1.2 Yorkshire HDC measurement tool, partial exemplar.

Group	Intervention	Score
A	External ventricular device or cardiopulmonary resuscitation	6 points
B	Use of airway adjunct, sedation during/after a procedure	4 points
C	Airway suction greater than once an hour, hourly urine measurement	2 points

boxes ticked – a child is categorised as HD with a score of 6 or above. Personal experience suggests that this tool is simple and easy to use, requires a relatively simple database and, with further development, can provide consistent measurement of HDC across a variety of ward environments. This tool does exactly what it set out to do, which is to identify children within the ward environment that have HDC needs. What it does not do is attribute a nurse/patient dependency ratio to the score calculated. However, a label of HD assumes a requirement for staffing levels above that which would normally be required on a children's ward.

The Great Ormond Street paediatric dependency and acuity scoring tool

This tool which has been developed over the last 3 years uses a wider range of interventions in order to identify a wider range of dependency levels (Great Ormond Street Hospital 2005a, 2005b). The tool consists of the following:

- A data collection tool consisting of 47 elements of care which are based on DH (2001) criteria has been refined and added to during the pilot phase of the project and through consensus opinion of experts. These elements have been organised into nine colour-coded categories to ease data collection.
- Patient dependency levels have been defined and, through consensus, opinions assigned to each of the 47 elements of care. These dependency levels are based on recommendations from the Royal College of Nursing and the Department of Health (DH 1997b; RCN 2003). There are five levels: 1 = ward intensive care, 2 = HDC, 3 = normal ward dependency (children over 2 years), 4 = normal ward care (children under 2 years), 5 = bed empty.
- A detailed Microsoft® Excel database has been developed to allow (with the appropriate scanning hardware and software) the data from the completed data collection forms to be scanned in directly.

Data is collected on all children every 12 hours and this enables a more detailed picture of the dependency of all children from normal dependency though to intensive care to be captured. Additionally, Excel automatically calculates patient numbers in each dependency level as data are entered and determines the number of nursing staff required to care for them. Potentially this is a powerful workforce planning tool, but the current data set is complex. It would need modification for successful use in district general hospital (DGH) settings and consideration must be given to the need for additional manpower and finance in order to utilise the tool. It would appear that the development of such tools is highly dependent on what it is hoped that the tool will achieve and on the local context.

Ball *et al.* (2004) is critical of the concepts of patient dependency and nursing workload because they fail to address the knowledge, skills and experience of nurses and consequently could not acknowledge the risk presented by critically ill patients. Although dependency tools help to measure workload and dependency in terms of nursing numbers required, they do not address the element of risk associated with the care and management of the critically ill by nurses (Garfield *et al.* 2000; Adomat and Hicks 2003). For example, although a ward may have sufficient numbers of staff to care for the acuity of the children, if these nurses do not have the experience, knowledge and skills to care for a child, for instance, with a chest drain then that child could be at risk of having suboptimal care. Experience, education and training of professionals is fundamental to good outcomes in caring for children with HD needs. This is reflected in the practical nature and content of this book.

Provision of HDC

Following the reorganisation of PIC services and publication of guidelines for the HDC of children (DH 1997a, 2001) there has been increased interest in setting up designated areas to care for children with HDC needs within DGH's and specialist children's units and hospitals. This type of model has definite benefits because it:

- Ensures children with similar HD needs are based in one discrete geographical area
- Allows scarce manpower, expertise and equipment to be used cost effectively
- Promotes the development of staff with good HD skills and knowledge

Children attend a wide range of departments and geographical areas within the acute hospital setting and theoretically any one child could unexpectedly deteriorate and become highly dependent and possibly require transfer to an internal/external HD or critical care facility. HDC can occur in many different areas within the acute hospital setting, be they formally established for this purpose or otherwise (Wright 2006). Additionally, with the increasing dependency and complexity of children admitted to hospital over the past 5 years (Haines 2005) and the increased demands placed on staff caring for the acutely unwell child in ward environments there is an urgent need to develop a more holistic model for providing HDC which does not just look at the physical environment or equipment needs.

Organisational model of HDC

There is a need for a model of HDC that transcends purely the physical environment (Thorne and Hackwood 2002; Richardson *et al.* 2003; Day *et al.* 2005). This model would ensure that every child, wherever he or she was geographically, would have access to a high quality service which would provide him or her with HDC. The model would require the following components:

- A designated area for delivering HDC which is appropriately staffed and equipped. Alternatively an area that allows assessment and stabilisation of a critically ill child prior to transfer or retrieval to an HD or critical care facility

- Provision of education, training and skill development for staff that have contact with children who have HDC needs
- Utilisation of a recognised tool or system to detect the deteriorating child (early warning scoring tools)
- Provision of an outreach service or access to a designated team of professionals expert in the stabilisation of the critically ill child
- Development of locally agreed admission and transfer policies and access either internally or externally to an HD or intensive care facility
- A system that is sufficiently flexible to ensure continuity of HDC, to allow stable, highly dependent children with complex needs to return to the community, live at home, experience education and enjoy good quality life
- The ability to carry out regular research and audit of services and collect data on patient activity and outcomes

The physical environment and continuum of care

HDC should not be seen as a completely segregated or isolated facility but rather as a continuum of care for children. An important function of HDC is to provide a 'step up' facility (i.e. for patients who become too sick for a general ward, yet are not sick enough for intensive care) and a 'step down' facility (i.e. for children who progress to the point where intensive care is no longer required but they are still too sick for a general ward). Children may also need to be admitted directly to HDC from the community if they have open access and it is appropriate.

At the time when the Department of Health was very much 'hands on', the expert advisory group for paediatric HDC (DH 2001) stipulated that all hospitals providing care for children (including those only providing dental or surgical care either as an elective, day case or emergency patient) should have arrangements in place for HDC. These arrangements should include 24 hours availability of medical staff (with the appropriate

competency in advanced paediatric life support). The physical layout of HD facilities will, as stated in the report, vary according to ward design, size and layout and whether the facility is in a DGH or children's hospital with specialist PIC/HDC facilities (DH 2001). Additionally the need for HDC may at times arise, suddenly and unpredictably, within a variety of locations, e.g. a paediatric ward within a DGH or specialist children's hospital, theatre recovery or an emergency department. As a consequence, there are a variety of models for the provision of HDC. These include the following:

- A designated area in a DGH (e.g. emergency department, paediatric ward or theatre recovery), which is able to provide resuscitation and stabilisation facilities prior to transfer of the child to a designated HD or intensive care facility
- A designated HD unit attached to a paediatric ward within a DGH
- A stand-alone HDC unit which is separate to the PIC unit or a combined PIC/HDC unit within a children's hospital

Because of the number of models that spread across a wide geographical area with different working environments, it is difficult to be too prescriptive about design and equipping of the facilities. However, it is essential that all hospitals caring for children should have a designated lead clinician for HDC who is responsible for overseeing the establishment and running of the service. This person should also lead a multidisciplinary users group, because the clinical issues relating to HDC will be different from hospital to hospital, and inform the individual design of the HD facility. The Department of Health (2001) stipulated that HD facilities should include the following:

- Availability of appropriate facilities
- Provision of appropriate equipment and drugs
- Availability of trained and suitably skilled staff

- Development of protocols for the management of common conditions
- Agreed arrangements for transfer to a PIC unit
- Procedures to be followed in the event of bed/staff/equipment shortage
- Close liaison with the relevant PIC unit, and with other departments within the hospital (especially the emergency department and intensive care)
- Training and audit
- Provision of adequate support and accommodation for parents

The current DH position is one of setting policy direction and commissioning. Local providers are responsible for determining how policy is implemented.

Recommended minimum equipment

The expert working group for HDC recommends the following minimum equipment for an HD area:

- Piped medical gases – oxygen and air – and vacuum
- Multi-module monitor (compatible with ICU/theatres) providing, ECG/respiration monitor with apnoea alarm, invasive pressure monitoring, pulse oximetry, non-invasive blood pressure with a variety of cuffs, end tidal CO_2 and temperature monitoring
- Hand ventilation circuit
- Syringe pumps
- Infusion pumps
- Suction units
- Oxygen analyser
- Defibrillator
- Resuscitation trolley
- Head box for oxygen administration
- Easy access to continuous positive airway pressure (CPAP) driver and anaesthetic machine

Within the DGH, easy access to a ventilator is essential to facilitate the initiation of level 2 intensive care and stabilisation of a child requiring level 2 care and a stock of disposables, not usually available, i.e.

- Central venous pressure lines
- Arterial lines
- Chest drains
- Circuits for ventilator and CPAP driver
- Cricothyroidotomy set

A fully equipped transport box should be available, containing everything needed to transfer a sick intubated child safely. Although practice will usually involve the PIC service retrieval team, this will still be needed as a reserve option.

Lastly, a list of available drugs should be agreed with colleagues.

Outreach and paediatric early warning scoring systems

Several adult studies (Franklin and Mathew 1994; Rich 1999) have demonstrated that patients in hospital exhibit premonitory signs of cardiac arrest, which may be observed by nursing and medical staff but are frequently not acted upon. Similar findings have been observed in relation to deterioration in patients' conditions prior to admission to adult intensive care units (McQuillan *et al.* 1998; Goldhill *et al.* 1999a), with the suggestion that early recognition and treatment of these signs may prevent the necessity for some intensive care admissions. This situation has been attributed in part to suboptimal care owing to the lack of knowledge regarding the significance of findings relating to dysfunction of airway, breathing and circulation, causing them to be missed, misinterpreted or mismanaged (McQuillan *et al.* 1998). Several strategies for reducing the occurrence of suboptimal care have been proposed, which focus on the identification of patients at risk of critical illness and the provision of some form of critical care outreach service to provide expert advice in the management of these patients (Lee *et al*. 1995; Audit Commission 1999; Goldhill *et al*. 1999b; DH 2000).

During the last 5 years there has been an increase in the paediatric literature supporting the use of outreach and early warning scoring systems and a corresponding development of paediatric early warning scoring tools and outreach services (Tume and Bullock 2004; Monaghan 2005; Haines *et al*. 2006). Although there appears to be a consensus that outreach and early warning scores can contribute to improving outcomes and quality of care, Tume and Bullock (2004) are cautious, suggesting that, rather than just adapting adult tools, the profession needs to utilise primary audit and research data in order to develop valid and reliable tools. It would be true to say that currently there is no national co-ordination for developing these tools and, rather than concentrating on researching a few tools, there appears to be a desire to develop tools in isolation.

Track and trigger

Early warning scoring systems are based upon the allocation of points to physiological observations, the calculation of a total score and the designation of an agreed calling trigger level. Some early warning systems use calling or referral criteria, based upon routine observations, which are activated when one or more variables reach an extreme value outside the normal range (DH and Modernization Agency 2003). The use of physiological track and trigger warning tools therefore seeks to enhance equity and quality of care by giving:

- Timely recognition of all children with potential or established critical illness irrespective of their location
- Timely attendance to all such children, once identified, by those possessing appropriate skills, knowledge and experience

Table 1.3 Physiological track and trigger warning systems classification (DH 2003).

'Single parameter' systems
Tracking: periodic observation of selected basic vital signs
Trigger: one or more extreme observational values

'Multiple parameter' systems
Tracking: periodic observation of selected basic vital signs
Trigger: two or more extreme observational values

'Aggregate weighted scoring' systems
Tracking: periodic observation of selected basic vital signs and the assignment of weighted scores to physiological values, with calculation of a total score
Trigger: achieving a previously agreed trigger threshold with the total score

---

The aim of an early warning scoring system is to provide staff with an aggregate physiological score generated from baseline recordings of vital signs. The more the child deviates from the normal parameters, the higher the scores. Clinical deterioration is subsequently detected and medical intervention can be implemented at an early stage in the child's illness. Many physiological tracking and triggering systems have been developed and modified to enable early recognition and treatment of acutely ill patients. Table 1.3 outlines the classification of these systems.

Examples of paediatric early warning scoring tools

Currently, the only published paediatric early warning scoring tool that has undergone rigorous research is the Bristol Royal Hospital tool (Haines *et al*. 2006). This tool is a single parameter system and is illustrated in Chapter 3. An earlier tool which was developed at the Royal Brighton Children's Hospital (Monaghan 2005) is an aggregated weighted scoring system (see Table 1.4).

With this tool, children are scored in relation to three parameters every time a set of observations are recorded; i.e. behaviour, cardiovascular

Table 1.4 Brighton paediatric early warning (PEW) score.

Score	0	1	2	3
Behaviour	Playing/ appropriate behaviour	Sleeping	Irritable	Lethargic/confused Reduced response to pain
Cardiovascular	Pink or capillary refill 1–2 seconds	Pale or capillary refill 3 seconds	Grey or capillary refill 4 seconds Tachycardia of 20 above normal rate	Grey and mottled or capillary refill 5 seconds or above Tachycardia of 30 above normal rate or bradycardia
Respiratory	Within normal parameters, no recession or tracheal tug	Rate of 10 breaths above mean, using accessory muscles, 30% + oxygen or 4+ L/min	Rate of 20 breaths above mean, recessing, tracheal tug, 40% + oxygen or 6+ L/min	30 above or 5 below mean, with sternal recession, tracheal tug or grunting, 50% + oxygen or 8+ L/min

and respiratory. They can score 0, 1, 2 or 3 for each parameter depending on how ill they are. Each box describes the parameters a child needs to be observed for in order to receive that score; e.g. under behaviour, if the child is irritable, he/she would score 2. The child only has to manifest one of the observations in a box and the highest score taken. So, e.g. a child who is pale and tachycardic with a rate of 20 heart beats above his/her normal rate would score 2, not 1. The three scores are then added together and this represents the child's PEW score. Additionally, the scoring system allows two discretionary points each for back to back nebulisers and persistent vomiting following surgery. The tool also provides a table of normal physiological parameters.

Clearly, the two early warning scoring systems that have been outlined are very different in their approach, which is a consequence of the development drivers. The Brighton tool developed out of an audit which looked at the recording of patient observations within an environment where observations were taken and recorded by health care assistants and qualified nurses. The Bristol tool (see Chapter 3) looked at identifying clinical and physiological triggers in children and

was developed within a large tertiary children's hospital with a large PICU. These two tools are being utilised in a number of units within the UK, following minor adaptations to suit individual environments.

However, any type of physiological tracking and triggering tool should be accompanied by an algorithm to ensure an early and appropriate response either from the medical team or from the outreach team on duty. The content of the algorithm should reflect the environment, staff skill mix and local clinical policies within each hospital and be agreed at Trust level. However, a basic principle of all algorithms is that any actions should be unambiguous. Such actions will depend on the availability and nature of a critical care outreach programme or reflect other systems that are in place to assist with a child who is unwell or deteriorating. At the Bristol Royal Children's Hospital, when a child triggers the algorithm staff must call the outreach team. With the Brighton tool, if a child triggers a response a variety of actions are implemented, depending on the score. These range from increasing the frequency of the observations, calling out the doctor or outreach service to assess and treat, or putting out a cardiac arrest call.

Stop and think

While early warning scoring systems are useful tools for proactively detecting children who are deteriorating, it is essential that there is:

(a) A system in place that ensures proactive assessment and treatment of these children
(b) A package of education that develops health care professionals' skills in recognising the deteriorating child
(c) A system that provides support for parents
(d) Good communication systems between tertiary children's and DGHs that allow proactive transfer of sick children.

These tools are only part of a 'package of care'. The literature states that seriously ill patients may be identified by the clinical signs of life-threatening dysfunctions of the airway, breathing or circulation. However, these signs may be missed, misinterpreted or mismanaged because of a lack of knowledge and a failure to appreciate the urgency (McQuillan *et al*. 1998). Therefore, the ability to provide a holistic quality package of care to acutely ill children within ward areas and HD units requires the additional support of outreach services, educational packages and systems of audit and research.

Discussion points

Physiological track and trigger warning systems *are not*:
• A substitute for good clinical judgement
• Predictors of the inevitable development of critical illness
• Predictors of overall outcome from critical illness
• Comprehensive clinical assessment tools
• Indicators for immediate admission to the PICU or HDU
Physiological track and trigger warning systems *are*:
• Aids to good clinical judgement
• 'Red flag' markers of potential or established critical illness
• Generally sensitive depending on their complexity

• Aids to effective communication in care of the critically ill and a means of securing appropriate help for sick children
• Indicators of physiological competence
• Indicators of physiological trends
• Valuable even in the absence of a formal critical care outreach service

Outreach services

The establishment of a critical care outreach team has been regarded as an effective way in which patient care on the ward can be improved (DH 2000). The philosophy behind outreach is the use of expert health professionals who are able to move between different ward areas and departments within a hospital and empower nursing staff to care for children with critical care needs (Day *et al*. 2005). Currently, a wide variety of level and type of outreach service is delivered because the service is dependent on the level of funding and staff resources available for critical care within individual trusts. Some services are run by a team of nurses qualified in critical or HDC and others by a mix of medical, nursing and physiotherapy personnel.

Although outreach services are being developed across the UK – in the guise of nurse-led outreach services, hospital at night services or site practitioners – only one published article has attempted to articulate a model for paediatric HDC and share the experience of setting up an outreach service (Day *et al*. 2005). What this model clearly states is that any outreach service requires clear aims and objectives and an agreed operational structure on which to base the outreach service. This is imperative in order that staff know how and when they can access the service, e.g. is it available 24/7 or is it a Monday to Friday 9 to 5 service. As a gold standard an outreach service should be able to provide the following:

• An outreach service that is provided by a team of expert nurses who are qualified in providing high dependency/critical care nursing (either through attendance at a recognised university-based course or through in-house competency-based education)

- Ongoing competency-based training for ward staff which includes recognition of the acutely ill child, clinical assessment and when to call for assistance
- Effective systems that allow ward staff to refer children and follow-up children and their parents discharged from intensive care or HDC
- Facilitation of timely admission to intensive care or HDC
- Development of guidelines relating to clinical issues in HDC, e.g. care of the child with a chest drain
- A team of nurses who have the time to support their colleagues by working fluidly across boundaries as role models in clinical practice

Top tip

Development of an outreach service requires formulation of a robust and detailed business plan.
    Pre-implementation audits and questionnaires should be undertaken to ascertain the need for such a service and to allow evaluation of the service once implemented.

The holistic approach to HDC

Boundaries between complex needs, continuing care and acute/critical care are increasingly fluid, and acute ward areas are frequently required to care for critically ill children (Haines *et al.* 2006). Treatments that were traditionally only utilised on intensive care units, e.g. nasal CPAP, are now being carried out at home or provided on wards and in HD areas either to manage episodes of critical illness or to support the respiratory needs of otherwise stable children.

HDC in the community

Advances in neonatal and PIC with supportive technology and pharmacology have reduced mortality but have created a new morbidity, with a growing number of children who are medically stable but require periods of technological support. Children should not spend their entire childhood in a hospital. Regardless of location, hospital is an unsuitable environment for a developing child and an inappropriate use of resources. Community HDC care can be facilitated with appropriate support and careful planning, using the appropriate resources such as the national need assessment tool (NHS 2004). This tool was modified from the original Bradford scale and is currently used by a variety of hospitals that discharge complex needs children into the community (Bradford Community Children's Team 2002). By using such assessment methods, even long-term ventilation for children in the home is feasible (Jardine and Wallis 1998). This would allow for more normal development and for children to maximise their educational opportunities. It would also decrease their risk of a hospital-acquired infection and permit other members of the family to function as near normal as possible. As networking expands and the distance to appropriate paediatric facilities becomes greater, families will have to travel further to visit stable children in HDC. As the number of acute beds comes under pressure, individually commissioned packages of care to support children at home will be an increasingly popular solution (RCN 2007).

There is considerable interest in promoting the provision of HDC in the community for children who would benefit from such a provision. The ethos of the National Service Framework (NSF 2004) is that children need appropriate care. Families need a seamless, child- and family-centred service that addresses all types of need, provides continuity across all transitions in the child's family life and is not limited by separate agency roles. Noyes and Lewis (2005) and McConkey *et al.* (2007) indicated that a child requiring HDC and complex care has many diverse needs; one agency cannot provide such services in isolation and a multi-agency plan would best meet the family's needs. This should be backed up with open access to a hospital for emergency treatment and management. To ensure continuity of care, communication is of principal importance. Some form of patient/parent-held record to detail the child's requirements which would accompany the usual childhood record book would be required.

The responsibilities that these parents take on and the skills that they have to master must not be underestimated (Glendinning and Kirk 2000). The need for organisation and provision of respite care to allow parents and carers to have a break is an important point and these services are being developed and expanded. With a carefully tailored assessment, a child and family could be supported by using a package comprising a combination of state, voluntary and private providers of care.

Staff educated and prepared

There remains a shortage of HD skilled and specialist children's nurses to service the needs of these HD children and their families and recruitment has been problematic. This has delayed discharge in many cases (Edwards *et al.* 2004) and as these children are stable it will probably not be possible or appropriate to use qualified in-service staff to provide care for HD children in the community. Health care workers have been prepared to perform the day-to-day routine care required (McConkey *et al.* 2007). These skills should not be unrecognised and there are programmes and qualifications available which prepare and acknowledge areas of personal development and which can build a platform for a potential career in health care (Skills for Health 2007).

Educational developments are not restricted to preparing staff to work in the community. There are ongoing requirements for HD staff in hospitals and staff on general wards to maintain their skills level. Staff working in these areas need to have access to ongoing education and support, as research suggests that acute ward staff caring for these patients often feel ill-prepared to do so. This can lead to increased anxiety and stress (Doman *et al.* 2004). Concerns regarding the clinical practice abilities of newly registered diploma nurses have been expressed and the increasing theory/practice gap continues to be highlighted as an urgent issue. Experience and the ability to apply theory to practice are essential to provide effective care for highly dependent children in acute ward areas, and clinical-based practitioners have been identified as the most important role models to help learners translate theory into practice (Gibson 1997).

Conclusion

The ability to define HDC may appear to be elusive, but our ability to provide it must not be. It remains essential that the profession continues to develop tools that help to identify the increasing numbers of children who require HDC. Paediatric HDC has become a speciality within itself and it is imperative that adequate resources and forward planning are provided in much the same way as in PIC. This chapter has outlined the important elements of the infrastructure required to ensure services that are fit for purpose and able to provide quality evidence-based care. The following chapters will discuss the underpinning nursing skills and knowledge required to support this.

Chapter 2
PHYSIOLOGICAL MONITORING

Debra Teasdale

Introduction

All qualified nurses are able to assess and monitor the health and wellbeing of children. They evaluate a myriad of intermittent clinical observations to establish normality or reveal/monitor changes. These clinical observations provide a snapshot picture of the child's condition at any given time and are repeated at intervals depending on the child's clinical status. The more unstable the child, the more frequently the observations need to take place. This reflects the level of dependency.

However, the unpredictability of the timeframe, the multiple parameters that require observation and the swift spiral effect of deterioration in the sick child present challenges to the most dedicated and competent nurse, since the information provided by snapshot observations is limited in depth. Alongside this is a shift in practice to the centralisation of paediatric intensive care services into tertiary units. Now a complex situation exists:

- Referrals may bypass the general paediatric ward completely.
- Stabilisation and transfer from paediatric wards can occur quickly, so limiting opportunity to build up experience and knowledge
- Pressures on PICU beds may prevent immediate transfer from the district hospital environment, so the general ward becomes a holding area for new patients or a high dependency (HD) recuperation area for recovering patients.

For some nurses, within the district/general hospital settings, this intermittent short-term but pressurised exposure to highly dependent patients is an uncomfortable experience. However, when dealing with highly dependent children, they need to be conversant with monitoring techniques beyond those normally employed. Constant physiological monitoring is essential. The assumption throughout this chapter will be that the nurse has a broad understanding of the paediatric pathologies involved, allowing the technical skills required in the application and use of the equipment to dominate.

Why 'different' monitoring is required

Manually performed clinical observation skills remain a primary feature of physiological monitoring, but intermittent observations may result in a time lag between deterioration and detection. The correct use of technology to support constant physiological monitoring allows rapid detection of a change in the clinical picture. Earlier identification of deterioration should allow earlier initiation of treatments and, in some cases, the technology may provide documentary evidence which will inform/speed transfer to specialist settings.

This chapter aims to provide nurses working in a generalist setting, whose remit extends to providing HD care on an intermittent or transitory basis, with a working and safe knowledge of the correct application and use of technology to aid physiological monitoring. Key clinical observations will be identified and the use of supporting technologies discussed. Cross references to other chapters are included as physiological monitoring underpins most aspects of nursing care. However, before any monitoring can commence, preparation is required.

General preparation

Efficient delivery of HD care can be greatly enhanced by adequate preparation of both equipment and staff. As part of the induction to a ward area the competence of staff in the use of local equipment must be established. As new equipment becomes available and using it is added to the repertoire of nursing skills, additional training will be required for all the staff who may need to use it. *This is a joint responsibility* – since employers must provide this and nurses must actively seek out training for any deficits expected within their area of practice (NMC 2008). As equipment may be used intermittently it is good practice to ensure that instruction manuals are accessible, that training updates are organised and that a mechanism for technical support is established. Often advice on physiological monitoring can be sought from local NICU or ITU staff.

Familiarity with the HD area

Being familiar with the location of equipment and where specialist supplies are to be found reduces stress for the staff involved. Often, in general paediatric wards, a dedicated area is assigned to HD care, which should be cleaned and checked on a daily basis both when vacant and when in use.

The use of checklists – devised via multidisciplinary consultation – act both to ensure that all needs are catered for and as an educational tool for staff and students. A comprehensive example of equipment included can be found in Appendix 1. This was derived from West Midlands Strategic Commissioning Group Standards for the Care of Critically Ill and Critically Injured Children (NHS 2004). Equipment should only be used if it is serviceable.

Whenever possible disposable probes should be used; however, non-disposable probes, leads and transducers need to be identified as such (i.e. labelled on the item) and stored to prevent damage, since they are costly to replace. Generally, after decontamination, loosely wrapping into a bundle and storing in individual plastic bags will prevent damage and keep items clean and ready for use. Effective storage should divide items and indicate links between the contents and equipment – use a designated area, e.g. a drawer or small box for each type of lead for each piece of equipment. To raise the profile of the cost of equipment and help prevent waste, an indication of the cost of each piece acts a prompt towards effective, efficient care and use.

Temperature monitoring

Thermal control within the body exists within narrow parameters to ensure the efficiency of the homeostatic process which sustains life. The effect of body temperature outside normal range needs to be acknowledged, since physiological change in one parameter affects others.

An elevated temperature raises the oxygen requirement of the body as the metabolic rate increases. At tissue level the demand for oxygen is greater, so oxygen bound to haemoglobin will be released more easily. However, if the cause of the hyperthermia is linked to respiratory compromise or the metabolic demand for oxygen is exceeded, the oxygen levels within the blood will be insufficient and anaerobic cellular respiration will occur, increasing the acid load within the local bloodstream. Conversely, when the core temperature is lowered, the haemoglobin molecule is more reluctant to release oxygen to tissues. Once again anaerobic cellular respiration will occur, increasing the acid load within the blood. If either situation is not reversed, buffering mechanisms to counteract the rising acid load within the blood become overwhelmed, pH alters and metabolic imbalance occurs within the body. Without treatment this cycle extends from cells to tissue to the organs that comprise the body's systems. Once systems malfunction there is increased likelihood of failure and death.

When measuring temperature, an approximation of the core temperature is obtained. This is defined as the temperature of blood within the pulmonary artery (Bartlett, cited in Carroll 2000). Current technology uses non-invasive methods to determine 'normal' temperature, which alters with age, time of day (increases in the afternoon), gender (increases during ovulation) and exercise. Key to any temperature monitoring is an appreciation that there is variation in normal temperature between body sites when compared to each other and to the absolute core temperature (MHRA 04144 2005). These differences are known as physiological 'offsets' and have been studied in a limited fashion in teenagers and young adults, but little information is available in younger children. A range rather than a discrete value is used.

Skin temperature reflects the local peripheral temperature and as such is lower, with the normal range set between 36 and 36.5°C. Physiological changes in temperature, blood pressure (BP) and general oxygen status will alter blood flow to the skin, causing changes in skin temperature. In addition, the method employed, the efficiency of the operator and the co-operativeness of the child may impact on the result. As a consequence, on most ward areas, the method of temperature measurement used is dictated according to the child's age or clinical condition.

Axillary route

Indications
- Infants <1 year
- Immuno-suppressed child
- Unconscious child
- Seizure-prone child
- Child with an anatomical anomaly which prevents other methods being used
- Child with ear infection

Equipment
Generally this is achieved by using an electronic thermometer in the axilla which measures core temperature derived from heat from the underlying brachial artery. Some electronic thermometers offer a choice of probes – check the manufacturer's instructions to determine if these are calibrated differently – e.g. red = core, blue = peripheral. Choose accordingly.

Method
- Single use disposable protective sheaths reduce the risk of cross infection; however, thorough cleaning of the underlying equipment prior to and after use is still required
- Turn the thermometer on and ensure the self check is error free
- Place the probe into the axilla and then press the child's arm closely to the side of the body
- Follow the instructions from the manufacturer. Normally a beep or tone sounds when the reading has stabilised
- Read, record measurement, site and equipment. Implement action as appropriate.

Caution
Correct placement allows measurements that are ~0.6 degree lower than oral temperature; however, this gap widens with increasing pyrexia so this route is not as accurate as others for identifying fever (London et al. 2006).

Tympanic route

Indications
For infants less than 1 year old or children. However, if an ear infection is suspected, use the axillary method instead to prevent further discomfort.

Equipment
The commonest equipment used is the tympanic thermometer, which is a quick, convenient method of temperature assessment. The tympanic membrane derives its blood supply

from vessels which supply the hypothalamus, so reflecting core temperature within the brain.

Method

- Discuss the need with the child/parents and gain consent
- Check equipment self check is error free. If the equipment is moving from a cold to hot environment a period of acclimatisation (~15 minutes) is required to reduce errors (Mackechnie and Simpson 2006)
- Accurate tympanic measurement of temperature relies on a clear view of the tympanic membrane, so inspect/clean the equipment lens cap and review the ear for obstructions, e.g. wax/dirt/Lego and so on, and remove where possible
- Poor measurement procedure significantly alters results. Enhance measurement efficiency as follows.

For younger children 1–3 years old:

- Place supine on a flat safe surface. Move the head to one side so easy access to one ear is established.
- Gently pull the pinna of the ear backwards and down.

For children over 3 years old:

- Position the child on the parent's or assistant's lap with the head secure.
- Gently pull the pinna backwards and up.

Top tip

For the right ear hold the thermometer in your right hand.

For the left ear hold the thermometer in your left hand.

- Approach from the back of the ear and guide the thermometer tip into the ear canal, pointing anteriorly towards the tympanic membrane.
- Advance the probe into the ear until a seal is formed. Turn on the scanner and leave *in situ* according to the manufacturer's instructions.
- Read and record measurement, site and equipment. Implement action as appropriate.

Caution

Some manufacturers calibrate tympanic thermometers to reflect physiological offset. Temperature measurements may be a reflection of the local tympanic membrane, i.e. local core temperature or, if the software has a conversion algorithm, the calculated value may reflect oral temperature (MHRA 04144 2005), so the index of suspicion should be alerted at a lower temperature. At ward level it is prudent to ensure that all equipment is set to measure the same outcome to ensure consistent responses.

Continuous temperature monitoring

Intermittent monitoring of temperature remains the mainstay of information gathering. However, continuous temperature monitoring is an option that is sometimes not considered due to unfamiliarity with equipment.

Continuous monitoring in open cots/beds

Many ECG/cardio-respiratory monitors allow temperature monitoring either via a single port (allowing constant monitoring of 'core' temperature) or occasionally via two temperature ports (allowing core–toe monitoring). Free-standing temperature monitors are occasionally available.

Continuous monitoring in incubators or in open heated cots

Design improvements allow incubators and open heated cots to monitor temperature, via either a single or double port. Generally all that is required for monitoring the temperature is to place the probe(s) onto the infant as described below and an electronic readout will be generated.

The heating mechanism on the incubator/open heated cot can be set to AIR MODE; this allows the incubator thermostat to drive the heater to keep air temperature within the incubator at a designated set temperature. The separate infant temperature reading reflects the infant's temperature.

An alternative is the SERVO or BABY mode, where the infant becomes the 'thermostat'. The infant probe links to the heat source and the set temperature will drive external heat generation until the infant and set temperatures are equal. Although the infant temperature display will provide information on the infant's temperature, 'SERVO' is *not* a monitoring mode. It is a heating mode for cold infants. Problems can occur if the probe becomes dislodged, causing the infant to overheat.

Single probe monitoring – core monitoring. A probe on the abdomen or axilla reflects the child's core temperature. Monitoring thermal wellbeing in this way allows swift adjustment of the local environment. It can also justify the use of or allow monitoring of the effects of antipyretic therapy.

Double probe monitoring – core–toe monitoring. To increase information for decision making, two probes can be used – generally denoted as T1 (core temperature from abdominal placement) and T2 (peripheral temperature from placement on the sole of the foot or hand).

Minimal gap between the two readings indicates thermal stability since it reflects differences in local vasoconstriction/dilation. Normally this central–peripheral (core–toe) gap should be less than 2°C.

In addition to thermal stability, core–toe monitoring is used in conjunction with capillary refill time (CRT) as a marker of cardiovascular wellbeing.

The assumption is that hypovolaemia/reduced cardiac output will result in less heat loss via the peripheries, so the core–toe gap widens (Rutter 2000).

> **Pause for thought**
>
> This theoretical assumption has yet to be proven and so interpretation requires additional information from CVP and BP monitoring

Equipment
- Temperature probe
- Compatible monitoring device – as described above
- Disposable proprietary temperature probe fixation pads

Method
- Discuss the need for and method of continuous temperature measurement with the child and parents, and gain consent. In addition, confirm the presence/absence of any plaster allergy.
- Check the equipment (incubator/ECG/monitor/temperature monitor) in use on the child for number of ports and select compatible temperature probes.
- Prior to applying the probes to the child, check that the probes are working by connecting to the already functioning monitoring equipment – a new parameter will be displayed on the screen which will reflect the local environmental temperature surrounding the probe end.
- If required prepare the skin, gently cleansing the area with soap and warm water, followed by drying.
- To monitor core temperature place the end of the probe flat against the skin on the abdomen over the liver. Avoid direct placement over bony prominences. The end of the probe may be cylindrical or disc shaped. For discs, the monitoring side is generally shiny, but check the manufacturer's instructions.
- Secure with a proprietary temperature probe adhesive fixation pad directly across the probe.

- If necessary place a small piece of tape ~3 cm below the probe end across the probe lead, to angle and secure the lead away from the child and assist in preventing dislodgment.
- To monitor peripheral temperature place the end of the second probe flat against the skin on the sole of the foot. Secure as above, but since this position is more likely to dislodge due to movement, secure further by wrapping a thin crepe or self-sealing bandage around the foot.
- Position the leads away from the child's body to prevent any adverse pressure or tourniquet injury.
- Set alarm limits for T1 and T2 and set T1–T2 gap on the monitor at the extremes of the normal range. The alarm parameter for T1–T2 gap should be set at >2°C.
- Temperature probes take time to settle – accurate readings are obtainable with correct placement after 10 minutes in most cases.
- Probe position should be altered every 4 hours, or more frequently in the malnourished child. Check digits for swelling/discolouration if the probes are secured with bandages (MHRA 2001).
- Document T1, T2 and T1–T2 gap as requested – normally hourly. Use Table 2.1 as a guide to interpret findings.

Bedside cardiac-respiratory monitoring

Many HD children will require continuous cardiac or cardio-respiratory monitoring using machinery which provides a continuous representation of the electrical activity of the heart and an indication of breathing activity. Continuous monitoring is useful to support the normal clinical observation of the heart and respiratory system (e.g. direct assessment and auscultation) – but should never replace these.

Respiration

A resource for the assessment of respiratory function is described in Chapter 3, but attention is required when placing ECG leads in position on the child's chest to ensure an adequate and accurate respiratory waveform (see 'Application' section later).

Heart rate

Evaluation of the heart rate involves the palpation of an artery usually compressed against a solid structure to elicit the pulse. This is counted to assess changes in rate, rhythm and pulse

Table 2.1 Possible causes of temperature variations.

Core temperature (axilla)	Peripheral temperature (toe)	Probable cause
Normal (→ high)	High	Environmental overheating likely
High	Low	Sign of febrile illness, abnormal pathology
High or normal	Low	If CRT >2–3 seconds this may indicate reduced cardiac output/hypovolaemia
Normal (→ low)	Low	Excess heat loss – possibly environmental, but could be result of abnormal pathology

Note: When temperature parameters move outside the accepted range always look for logical explanations first.

Check the position and security of probes – when probes are under pressure, i.e. laid upon, the temperature will increase and when probes are insecure temperature will generally decrease.

When the child has been disturbed, uncovered or handled the core–toe gap will increase temporarily – so it is important to record interventions that have occurred alongside temperature changes.

volume; for further consideration of these refer to Chapter 4. An alternative method is auscultation of the heart rate using a stethoscope. In the child, the normal process of inspiration and expiration can alter the heart rate by up to 30 beats/minutes, so assessment should occur over a 1-minute period (Blows 2004); however, in initial resuscitation situations this may not be practical.

The child's age, co-operation and clinical condition will dictate the most appropriate route for intermittent clinical assessment. However, in general, infants are best assessed via auscultation over the apex of the heart, using a paediatric stethoscope. The apex is located more centrally in the infant, moving laterally with increasing age. Accurate assessment of heart rate in toddlers can be achieved by palpation using the brachial or temporal pulses, although the co-operative toddler may allow radial assessment as with older, and more accepting, children (Hockenberry 2003; Blows 2004).

> ### Stop and think
>
> Palpation of the carotid arteries is not advised due to interference in the cerebral blood flow.

Heart rates differ depending on age and activity state. When possible assessment should occur during sleep or a quiet state. A heart rate within normal limits is known as sinus rhythm and is controlled by the sino-atrial node. Normal ranges are detailed in Chapter 4.

When using a stethoscope, the rate auscultated (apex) should be similar to the pulse rate felt digitally. Variations indicate potential pathology. When an apex is higher than a peripheral pulse it suggests that an abnormality of ventricular function may be present, since some pulsations would appear to be weaker than others and are not transmitted into the systemic circulation.

> ### Stop and think
>
> The apex beat can be higher than the peripheral pulse *but* this situation can never reverse. If findings suggest this, there is inaccuracy in the recording of the peripheral pulse.

Heart rhythm

The rhythm of the heart reflects the cycle of contraction and relaxation of the differing heart chambers and should be felt as a regular interval pattern between pulsatile beats. On auscultation a regular 'lub-dub' sound pattern should be heard. The 'lub' is the closure and vibration of the cusps of the atrioventricular valves, whilst the dub is the closure and vibration of valve cusps in the semi-lunar valves. Additional noises prior, between or after heart sounds are generally abnormal. These 'murmurs' can be suggestive of turbulent blood flow within the heart, which may result from a benign or pathological. This should always be assessed by a paediatrician. Differences in rhythm patterns may occur due to alterations or obstruction or abnormality of the electrical conduction system.

Pulse volume (the bounce of the pulse on palpation) reflects the difference in systolic and diastolic BP and may alter for a variety of reasons, e.g. anaemia or congenital cardiac defects. This parameter cannot be assessed by auscultation. Alterations in rate, rhythm and volume are more difficult to detect by intermittent manual palpation of arterial pulses if the child is peripherally shut down, so in HD care, continuous monitoring by ECG supplies additional and complementary information. More information on abnormalities of rhythm can be found in Chapter 4.

Most ECG/cardiac monitors are able to supply information about the child's respiratory rate in addition to heart rate and rhythm. However, if the monitor is used or applied incorrectly the consequences may be dire – misinterpretation of arrhythmias, mistaken diagnosis, wasted investigation (Jevon and Ewans 2005). Additionally there will be increased anxiety for the child, parents and staff.

Indications for use of cardio-respiratory/ECG monitoring

- General surveillance of heart rate and rhythm in sick child
- Monitoring of the apnoea and bradycardia sequence. For example in gastro-oesophageal reflux (GOR) or acute life-threatening events (ALTE)
- Evaluation of temporary pacing
- Evaluation of effects of response to drugs, e.g. overdose of prescribed medication
- Pre- and post-operative assessment

Equipment
- Cardiorespiratory monitor/ECG
- ECG lead compatible to machine
- ECG electrode – size depends on age, but pack of three must be 'in date' and moist to touch on the patient side

Application of continuous bedside ECG monitoring
- Discuss the need for and method of continuous monitoring of the heart rate with the child and parents, and gain consent. Ensure privacy by drawing blinds/curtains.
- Check the operation of the ECG or cardiorespiratory monitor for use on the child. Select the correct lead and electrode size.
- If required, remove the clothing from the upper body. Inspect the child's chest. If required prepare the skin, gently cleansing the area with soap and warm water, followed by drying. Occasionally hirsute adolescents require the removal of body hair; however, this should be avoided if possible.
- Position the three electrodes on the skin of the chest; one on each shoulder (or under each clavicle) and the third below the diaphragm

to minimise muscular interference and allow access to the chest in the event of the need for defibrillation (Jevon 2004). To optimise the trace, electrodes should remain moist – generally replacement is required every 48 hours (Perez, cited in Jevon 2004).

- Attach the electrode leads to the main ECG lead from the monitor. The lead connections are generally colour coded – the electrode on the left shoulder attaches to the yellow port, on the right shoulder to the red port and the third electrode (placed below the diaphragm) attaches to the green port.
- Turn on the electrical supply to the monitor. Following the warm-up, check the monitor calibration if required.
- From the lead options select 'II'.
- Lead II is the dominant lead. Set the alarms – generally at the limits for the age range (see Chapters 3 and 4).
- Trail the leads away from the child without applying any tension to the electrodes. This enhances child safety, reduces the risk of pressure effects from the leads and prevents any disconnection or peeling of electrodes away from the skin.
- Observe the quality of the trace as shown in the following section.

Troubleshooting ECG monitoring
Flat line or poor quality trace:

- Complex size too small
  - Adjust size/gain, reposition electrodes, change to lead II
  - Poor connection
  - Check electrode connections to leads, check lead connection in monitor
- Electrode contact poor
  - Check moisture/date of electrodes, remove loose skin/hairs under contact site
  - Apply small amount of Hydrogel® under electrode
  - Prevent drying out by changing electrodes every 48 hours (Perez 1996b)

Interference/artefact (fuzzy trace) or wandering trace:

- Poor electrode contact
  - Follow above directions
  - Electrical interference from patient movement or local electric infusion pumps
  - Move electrodes over bone rather than muscle (normally the reverse applies).
  - Ensure the lower electrode is placed well below the lower ribs to prevent respiratory interference

Incorrect heart rate display:

- Complex too small – rate low
  - Increase size/gain
  - Check Lead II selected
- Complex too large – rate high
  - Observe for T wave size and for artefact which will lead to elevated rates due to increased pick up of 'complex'
  - Alter lead selection until normal complex seen
  - Decrease size/gain.

Adapted and extended from Jevons and Ewans (2005) and Laight *et al.* (2005).

If there is any doubt about the accuracy of the rate seen on the trace, auscultate the apex of the heart and make direct comparison to the heart rate on the monitor. The troubleshooting guide shown below will assist.

Top tip

Good practitioners perform this check for accuracy on handover, prior to episodes of care-giving and following any apparent deviations in the child's condition.

Assessment of the PQRST complex is a useful nursing skill to aid early referral for further medical assessment and investigation. In the main the focus should be maintained on observing the trace for alterations from the norm in rate or rhythm – see Chapter 4 for more detail.

Troubleshooting rate/rhythm

The ECG monitor will determine the rate according to the number of complexes measured on the continuous waveform. Inaccuracies can occur when:

- Complexes are too large, being double counted as part of the results
- Complexes are too small so are not picked up at all
- Lead II is not selected for measurement and electrodes are incorrectly positioned or linked to the incorrect lead

Hiccoughs can be seen as electrical disturbances and can be observed visually occurring simultaneously with alterations on the ECG complex; however, 'ectopic' beats may also occur. These may increase the heart rate and be benign or pathological – assume the latter until proven otherwise.

Due to the faster rates in children, alterations to rate, rhythm and complex appearance are often difficult to assess. Further investigation by 12 lead ECG is warranted.

The 12 lead ECG

The normal electrical activity of the heart results in changes to an electrical field which is represented graphically as the complete PQRST complex. The distances between and height of parts of the complex are known to alter with age; however, during normal continuous monitoring it can be difficult to be sure of any potential changes. When abnormalities are suspected the heart can be viewed using the 12 lead ECG to create a three-dimensional electrical picture of the heart – potentially providing a wealth of information in a short time span (Zeigler 2001). At birth the newborn heart has an enlarged right ventricle (due to fetal circulatory routes) which creates a very different ECG from that of the adult. By 3–4 years of age, right ventricular dominance has been replaced by left ventricular dominance – the ECG becomes similar to the adult.

Indications for use

- To determine the presence of cardiac anomalies of function and structure
- To correlate and accurately assess abnormal observations found during continuous ECG/cardio-pulmonary monitoring. The detailed analysis allows assessment of a strip of PQRST complexes from multiple electronic angles to determine the presence and location of any problem

Equipment

- Portable 12 lead ECG monitor with leads
- Lead adapters as required (machine dependent)
- ECG electrodes appropriate to infant/child size

Method

Preparation

- ECG quality depends on the expertise of the operator (Zeigler 2001) so ideally this procedure should be performed by an ECG technician proficient in the use and recording of the ECG. However, this service is rarely available on a 24 hour basis so local staff should be trained in the technique (SCTS 2005).
- Discuss the need for and method of obtaining the 12 lead ECG with the child and parents, gaining consent and checking the child's ID. Ensure privacy by drawing blinds/curtains.
- Remove the clothing from the upper body. Inspect the child's chest. If required prepare the skin (as in ECG monitoring). Occasionally gentle abrasion of the skin surface may be required; however, care must be taken not to damage skin.
- The appearance of an ECG can vary according to the body position so ideally the child should adopt a supine position and be entirely still for the recording (SCTS 2005). However, practically, this is often not possible, with the child becoming upset. The child can sit up if this prevents restlessness (SCTS 2005). If necessary parents can hold the child to assist in maintaining calm and preventing movement during the recording (Zeigler 2001).

Electrode location

- It is usually easier to apply the electrodes to the skin, then attach the leads. Leads are generally colour coded to assist identification. The colours stated here are those conforming to the IEC (European) recommendations. Some leads will require adapters or clips for infants. Ensure that these are available before starting.

Top tip

To assist correct attachment, it is useful to keep a diagram tied to the machine showing correct positions for the colour-coded leads.

Different size electrodes should be available as standard. Some will require adapters to allow attachment to the machine.

Ensure that the ECG machine is plugged in at all times so battery life is maximised.

- Limb electrodes/leads should always be placed slightly proximal to the ankle and wrist to ensure consistency between recordings (SCTS 2005) – see Table 2.2. When the limbs are by the side the electrode tabs should point towards the midriff. Deviations from normal placement, e.g. due to the presence of IV lines, should be recorded.

Table 2.2 Limb lead placement guide.

Lead/electrode	Code	Position
Right arm lead	RA – red	Right forearm, proximal to wrist
Left arm lead	LA – yellow	Left forearm, proximal to wrist
Left leg lead	LL – green	Left lower leg, proximal to ankle
Right leg lead	RL – black	Right lower leg, proximal to ankle

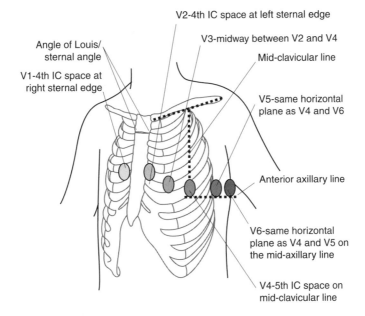

V2-4th IC space at left sternal edge

V3-midway between V2 and V4

Mid-clavicular line

Angle of Louis/ sternal angle

V1-4th IC space at right sternal edge

V5-same horizontal plane as V4 and V6

Anterior axillary line

V6-same horizontal plane as V4 and V5 on the mid-axillary line

V4-5th IC space on mid-clavicular line

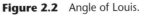

Figure 2.1 Correct lead placement. Adapted from SCTS (2005).

- Precordial/chest leads must be correctly placed. Research suggests that V1 and V2 are often placed too high, with V5 and V6 too low (Wenger and Kliefield cited in SCTS 2005). Figure 2.1 shows the correct placement.

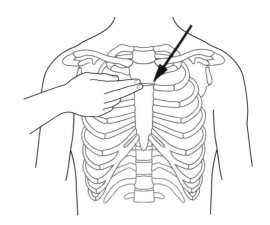

Figure 2.2 Angle of Louis.

> **Top tip**
>
> To assist positioning electrode correctly ensure that rib spaces are palpated, using as a reference point the anatomical landmark of the sternal angle (angle of Louis) (see Figure 2.2). Sliding the finger down laterally from this point will reveal the second intercostal space.

- Once landmarks are located spaces should then be counted down to the fourth intercostal space. V1 should be located on the sternal edge on the child's right side. Repeat the same for correct placement on the left side of V2. Subsequent electrodes should be placed in order (Table 2.3), ensuring that positions are correct.

- Occasionally different configurations for precordial leads may be requested, e.g. V3R (mirror image of V3 on right side of the chest), V4R (mirror image of V4 on right side of chest) and V7 (posterior axillary line at same level as V4).
- For adolescent females, V4, V5 and V6 are conventionally placed under breast tissue to reduce signal interference.

Table 2.3 Correct placement of chest leads.

Lead	Position
V1 (C1)	Fourth intercostal space at right sternal edge
V2 (C2)	Fourth intercostal space at left sternal edge
V4 (C4)	Fifth intercostal space in the mid-clavicular line
V3 (C3)	Midway between V2 and V4
V5 (C5)	Left anterior axillary line, same horizontal level as V4
V6 (C6)	Left mid-axillary line, same level as V4 and V5

Recording

- With electrodes secure and fastened to the appropriate leads, input patient ID number and name.
- Recording quality and thus accuracy of interpretation are maximised when the child is still, relaxed and calm. Clenched and/or moving fingers will reduce quality – gently stroking the back of the fingers should encourage hand relaxation.
- Normally the default settings on the machine are 25 mm/s with a gain of 10 mm/mV. Press the 'start' or 'auto' button on the machine to initiate automatic ECG recording of a rhythm strip and 12 lead ECG.
- If technically good, record the position of the patient and any deviations in lead placement on the graph.
- Technically poor ECG recordings should be repeated after reviewing the troubleshooting in the section below.

Troubleshooting

- Muscle interference evident on recording:
  - Reassure parent and child, and take actions required to calm infant/child.
  - If interference remains on repeated recording with an apparently relaxed child, switch on the filter button and repeat the recording.
  - Document this setting on the recording.

- Initial QRS complexes are so large they overlap:
  - Repeat recording using 5 mm/mV gain.
  - Document setting on recording.
- High heart rates prevent accurate assessment of complexes:
  - Increase the speed from 25 to 50 mm/s.
  - Document on recording.
- If an irregular rhythm is seen, an additional 10-seconds rhythm strip should be recorded. Any obvious changes that might require urgent attention should be identified and medical assistance immediately sought; however, ECG interpretation in the infant and child is age dependent and generally the remit of the medical team.

Blood pressure monitoring

Blood pressure (BP) is 'the force per unit area exerted on a vessel wall by the contained blood' – the systemic pressure in large arteries near the heart is principally controlled by the cardiac output (i.e. stroke volume × rate) and the peripheral resistance and blood flow.

This pressure peaks (systolic pressure) when the ventricles contract and blood is expelled into the aorta. Diastolic pressure reflects the lowest pressure in the system when the valves in the origins of the aorta and pulmonary arteries close to prevent backflow into the heart. Systemic arterial vessel walls contract to force blood forward. As the pressure within the aorta fluctuates it is the mean arterial pressure that propels blood to the tissues (Marieb 2003). BP provides an indication of how effective physiological processes are within the body. An adequate BP underpins the transport systems in the body since fluids will only move under pressure. BP is essential to ensure that all the organs and tissues of the body are appropriately perfused, allowing nutrients to be delivered to cells and waste products to be taken away for disposal. In HD care BP monitoring is standard.

Non-invasive BP monitoring

Different modes of non-invasive BP (NIBP) monitoring are available – the principal types are:

- Auscultatory monitors, e.g. sphygmomanometers
- Oscillometric methods, e.g. Dinamap®

Recent recommendations suggest that both approaches have value within the clinical environment (MHRA 2005b), with standard paediatric texts providing a good appreciation of different techniques. However, the use of mercury sphygmomanometers is likely to decline in response to legislation on hazardous substances within the workplace (Commission of the European Communities 2005).

In practice, NIBP monitoring remains problematic, with research suggesting that the precision of the results is questionable due to inaccuracy in application, poor technique (Gillum 1995; Arafat and Matteo 1999) or variations due to calibration drift (Severn and Coleman 2005 in Mackechnie and Simpson 2006). Reviews of this area suggest factors that commonly alter BP measurements – see Table 2.4.

Commonplace disparity in practice, particularly in how to determine cuff size and the method of application (Arafat and Matteo 1999), can be minimised by defining a standard approach – although which is best remains questionable. Some texts suggest using a cuff width that equates to 40% of the arm circumference and covers 80–100% of the upper arm length; however, this latter figure varies (cited in Arafat and Matteo 1999). This may reflect the differing growth velocities and anatomical findings within children, so further research is required. If the arms are not available for NIBP

Table 2.4 Factors affecting NIBP measurement accuracy.

Problem	Result	Recommendation
Cuff too narrow	Overestimate	Standard method of determining cuff size should be employed by whole team
Cuff too large	Underestimate	
Poor bell seal on auscultation	Korotovs sounds not clearly heard	Use diaphragm to auscultate sounds in small children
Recent exercise/activity	Overestimate	Prior to BP measurement: No eating/drinking for 30 minutes; rest quietly with uncrossed legs for 5 minutes
Forearm higher than heart	Underestimate	Right arm pressure is generally 5 mmHg > than left – always try to use right arm
Forearm lower than heart	Overestimate	For children >3 years keep forearm at heart level. Measure sitting up
		For children <3 years consistent measurement whilst supine is acceptable
White coat syndrome	Overestimate	Although established as a factor in adults, it is unclear if this is the case in children
Environmental factors		
Season/temperature	As temperature falls, BP rises	Keep temperature of ward environment constant
Time of day	BP falls during sleep, peaks late morning and late afternoon	Record sleep state
Calibration drift	Over-/underestimate	Check service date and only use if current

Adapted from Gillum (1995) and Blows (2005).

monitoring EG where multiple IV sites are in use or if an arterial line is sited, it is common paediatric practice to utilise the calf (Summers 2007). Records need to indicate the site and cuff size used.

Whilst a manual sphygmomanometric determination of BP is time consuming, oscillometric methods provide an automated, non-invasive, rapid measurement of BP and were originally introduced into operating theatre and critical care units where high levels of precision and accuracy at end points were not required. With appropriate alarm settings, oscillometric monitoring alerts the team to significant changes in both systolic and diastolic pressures (MHRA 2005b). Inaccuracy at end points presents problems when monitoring the BP of the HD/critically ill child since hypotension and hypertension can have wide-ranging systemic consequences. To accurately determine systolic and diastolic end points and thus prevent and/or manage the effects of hypo- and hypertension, invasive monitoring of BP is seen as the 'gold standard'.

Invasive arterial BP monitoring (IABPM)

This is achieved using the pressure measurement generated by the flow of blood at the tip of an arterial catheter. The pressure measurement is picked up by a transducer, which is attached to the monitor, producing a dynamic BP waveform with numerical data (heart rate, systolic, diastolic and mean BP) on the screen as shown in Figure 2.3.

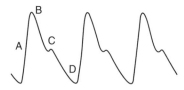

Figure 2.3   Arterial pressure waveform.

Each part of the wave represents different parts of the cardiac cycle:

A = ventricular contraction, i.e. QRS phase
B = peak systolic pressure
C = diacrotic notch, i.e. closing of the aortic valve as the heart empties
D = diastole or relaxation phase (McGhee and Bridges 2002; Smith *et al.* 2004).

In paediatrics the arterial catheter may be centrally placed, e.g. femoral or umbilical (neonate), or peripherally placed, e.g. radial or auxiliary. Brachial arteries should be avoided if other options are available as this is an end artery; moreover, ulnar, posterior tibial and dorsalis pedis should be used with caution due to an increased risk of digital ischaemia (GOSH 2005).

However, the smaller vessel size and distance from the heart will 'dampen' the signal, providing an accurate mean BP only. IABPM is uncommon within HD care. However, it may occur when critically ill neonates are admitted onto paediatric units where medical staff have a significant background of neonatal experience or at the request of a PICU transfer team prior to their arrival to assist in accurate assessment of the clinical condition.

In addition, many critically ill children require frequent blood gas analysis, so insertion of an arterial line provides an opportunity for IABP to be continuously displayed on physiological monitors, adding to data that inform decision making.

Indications for use

These will mirror the indications for use of an arterial line:
• Cardiovascular instability and/or respiratory compromise
• Pre-/post-surgical assessment
• Patient requiring regular arterial blood gas (ABG) analysis
• Child receiving continuous infusion of inotropic/vasoactive drugs

Equipment

- Patent arterial catheter plus three-way tap with trickle infusion of HepSal® (0.5 IU/mL)
- Physiological monitor with IABPM capacity
- Non-disposable compatible pressure lead
- Disposable pressure transducer monitoring kit
- Syringe driver or pressure infuser bag
- Normal saline or heparinised saline (1–5 IU/ml – locally determined)
- Arterial infusion line, e.g. Lector®-catheter or equivalent low-compliance IA line
- Alcowipe® or local equivalent to 'clean' end of infusion lines
- All equipment/lines used within arterial lines must be of the luer-lock variety to minimise the risk of disconnection

Top tip

Wherever possible this type of monitoring should be commenced upon insertion of the arterial line. A child with an IA line *in situ* requires 1:1 nursing and should not be left unattended.

Method

- If the situation permits, discuss the need for monitoring with the child and parents.
- Strict aseptic procedures apply due to the proximity of the access point. Check and prepare the prescribed fluids, then either draw up 40 ml into a syringe or set up a prepared bag in the pressure infuser bag, inflating the bag to 200–300 mmHg. This needs to be labeled and documented according to the local protocol.
- Prepare the infusion line by attaching the IA line to the disposable pressure transducer line. This disposable pressure line will contain a three-way tap immediately proximal to the transducer for calibration purposes.
- Attach the completed IA circuit to the fluid source (either syringe or pressure infuser) and prime with fluid, ensuring that the line and

all three-way taps are free of air bubbles, so reducing inaccuracies in measurement (McGee and Bridges 2002), collecting the fluid in a gallipot/bowl to prevent spillage. Most transducer systems have a flush mechanism prior to the transducer which needs to be depressed to allow priming to occur.

Top tip

Holding the transducer kit vertically allows air to flow upwards easily, so preventing air bubbles occurring in the transducer dome. Whilst opening three-way taps sequentially to the atmosphere allows any trapped air to flow out, remember to close them afterwards!

In addition, a number of systems have open-ended caps on all ports to allow air expulsion without opening the circuit – however, once complete these open-ended caps must be replaced with the accompanying closed-head caps to reduce infection risk (Garretson 2005).

- The syringe should be placed into the syringe driver and set to run at the prescribed rate (1–3 mL/h dependent on fluid Rx). The pressure infuser should be hung on an infusion stand close to the bed – inflation pressure should exceed arterial pressure, i.e. >150–200 mmHg (GOSH 2005).
- Connect the non-disposable BP pressure lead to the already functioning monitor – a display area for BP monitoring should be seen. Connect the opposite end of the non-disposable BP monitoring lead to the disposable pressure transducer within the IA lead; the attachment varies – some are circular structures which require gentle twisting together to fix and lock, or the lead end may simply insert into a small socket on the disposable pressure transducer.
- Check the arterial catheter is correctly dressed, i.e. it is visible through a clear adhesive dressing and firmly fixed into position – if

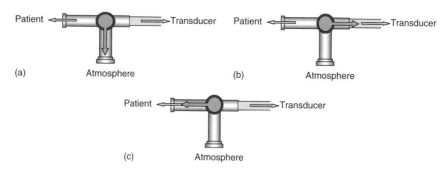

Figure 2.4 Three-way tap sequences. Adapted from Garretson (2005).

sutures are in place ensure they are secure. Turn the three-way tap at the end of the arterial catheter to position 'off to the child' to prevent exsanguinations.

> **Top tip**
>
> Ask a colleague to assist. That way the end of the IA line remains sterile.
>
> To prevent confusion refer to Figure 2.4 to ensure that three-way taps are correctly turned at each point.

- Clean the end of the arterial line (e.g. use Alcowipe® wrap or local equivalent), then connect the prepared and primed IA infusion line to the end of the arterial line. Once connection is complete and the luer-lock secured, the three-way tap proximal to the arterial catheter may be turned 'on to the child', so allowing the infusate to flow (position (a) in Figure 2.4). Commence the infusion at the prescribed rate.
- Position the IA line so the transducer is on the bed/cot mattress, level with the heart/mid-axillary line (Imperial Perez and McRae 2002), ensuring that the line remains unkinked and untrapped. The transducer must remain in this position for all measurement events to allow comparison. The child should remain flat or with the head tilted to a maximum of 45 degrees to maintain accuracy of readings (GOSH 2005).
- To allow accurate monitoring the transducer must be calibrated to zero pressure. This is performed as follows:
  ○ Cancel monitor alarms temporarily and stop infusion flow into arterial catheter by closing three-way taps (position (c) in Figure 2.4).
  ○ Open the transducer three-way tap to air (position (b) in Figure 2.4).
  ○ Press zero key on monitor and allow calibration to complete – visually the waveform will fall to zero.
  ○ Close transducer tap to air, allowing infusate to flow forward (position (a) in Figure 2.4).
  ○ Open arterial catheter three-way tap to allow continuous flow of fluid to the arterial catheter and child (position '(a' in Figure 2.4)).
- A waveform should be evident on the screen; set the waveform scale so the entire pressure wave is visible and input appropriate limits.
- Record zero calibration on nursing documentation. Repeat calibrations should be performed and documented each time the circuit is accessed, when erroneous results are found or at the handover of responsibility at shift/allocation changes to ensure accuracy of results. Refer to Table 2.5 for advice to resolve problems with the trace.
- Observe, record and report deviations from normal as with any other infusion; however, pay particular attention to avoid complications specific to arterial lines, e.g.

Table 2.5   Troubleshooting for IABP lines.

Potential problem	Action
Flat or damped trace – this can occur suddenly and may reflect a change in the child's condition, so check the child first. Then use the following as a guide	
Monitoring equipment	
Transducer positioned too high	Reposition so level with the heart/mid-axillary line; re-zero after altering position of child
Incorrect scale options	Try smaller scale
IA line patency	
Three-way taps incorrectly positioned	Realign to allow forward flow
IV clamps applied	Remove clamps
Tubing kinked, compressed	Unkink, decompress
Blood/clots present in IA line	Call for medical assistance; clots require aspiration and then the IA line to be flushed
Arterial catheter site occlusion	
Overtight splint straps/bandages	Release pressure and re-strap
Arterial spasm – blanched tissue which is not reperfusing	Call for medical assistance; catheter may require urgent removal
Arterial disconnection	
Unsecure/loose three-way taps	Refasten – ensure luer lock
Complete disconnection	Apply immediate pressure to the site and call for medical assistance
Fluids	
An empty infusion bag/syringe can result in back flow and a reduced trace	Renew prescribed fluids urgently
Large fluid loss such as internal haemorrhage	Urgent medical review
Drugs/treatment	
Inadvertent bolus of vasodilator	Urgent medical review
Side effect of recent drug administration	Urgent medical review
Elevated trace – this can occur suddenly and may reflect a change in the child's condition, so check the child first. Then use the following as a guide	
Monitoring equipment	
Transducer positioned too low	Reposition so level with the heart/mid-axillary line; re-zero after altering position of child
Fluids	
Accidental rapid fluid bolus due to equipment fault/human error	Reduce high infusion rate; take equipment out of service; report via clinical incidence process
Drugs/treatment	
Inadvertent bolus of vasoconstrictor drug	Urgent medical review
Side effect of recent drug administration	Medical review
Sedation wearing off	Administer more sedation PRN (prescription required as needed)
Child in pain/discomfort	Remove discomfort (e.g. wet bed); treat pain

Adapted from Garretson (2005).

arterial thrombosis, air emboli, infection, exsanguinations.

- Any swelling or bruising must be recorded to allow adequate assessment of the colour of surrounding digits or limbs which may become affected by arterial spasm and loss of perfusion. Arterial spasms can occur spontaneously; however, they are more common after blood sampling from the IA line – if this does not rapidly resolve, i.e. return to normal pink and warm skin, immediate action is required by the medical team.
- Dressings over arterial sites should be changed according to local protocol. Lines should be distinct – label as ARTERIAL.

Stop and think

Incorrect opening of the three-way taps within the IBP circuit will compromise the child and the accuracy of the measurements. Ideally two staff should be present when the arterial line is accessed to prevent accidental opening of the circuit which could allow exsanguination or contamination of the transducer/line with blood.

Central venous pressure (CVP) monitoring

CVP monitoring is a key physiological indicator in the peri-operative management of the child undergoing cardiovascular surgery as it provides an indicator of the child's haemodynamic state. As such, CV lines are a common feature on PICUs; however, they may also be found in HD areas.

Indications for CV monitoring include:

- Pressure measurement
- Drug and fluid therapy

CV lines are also present with many children who require long-term trans-parenteral nutrition (PN). Whatever the indication, strict aseptic technique is required in management. As this is a central access device, the infection risks are increased.

Method

Traditionally, CVP measurement involved manual measurement of pressure in a column of fluid using a manometer, held at the level of the heart to determine the value. However, with the advent of pressure monitoring within standard ECG monitors, in general the same technology can be applied as used in the monitoring of IBP via arterial lines, though several differences are apparent:

- There is no need for a pressure infuser bag on the fluid as the intravenous solution is entering a low pressure system – a normal infusion via syringe or pump will suffice.
- The infusate does not require heparinisation.
- The access point is the end of a catheter inserted into a large vein. The internal tip of the catheter should ideally sit at the junction of the superior vena cava and the right atrium and be firmly secured to prevent further advancement. This may have negative or fatal consequences if the catheter tip becomes inserted within the internal tissue of the heart (MHRA 2001 DA4).
- The resulting trace shown on the monitor will be a softly undulating waveform (Cole 2007).

Top tip

Observe the ECG trace for signs of ectopic beats at any time during and following the insertion and monitoring of the CVP catheter – this is an indicator that the catheter tip is tickling the cardiac tissue and requires adjustment.

The position of the catheter tip should be determined by ultrasound scan (USS) and/or chest X-ray prior to any large volume fluid infusion commencement. Once position is confirmed the same set-up procedure is employed as with IABP monitoring.

The displayed results are single values only and reflect the pressure of the blood returning to the right side of the heart – normally between 0 and 5 mmHg. Low CVP readings can indicate hypovolaemia and high levels are associated with fluid overload. Consensus on normal values is difficult to determine; it could be argued that it is the trend of the measurement that needs monitoring as much as the specific numeric value. In addition to Table 2.5, Cole (2007) identifies common causes of raised and lowered CVP measurements which need to be considered against serial changes in CVP measurement. These are shown in the considerations section.

There is some evidence that the dangers of this route in terms of catheter misplacement/movement may be overcome in the future by the use of peripheral venous pressure (PVP) measurements, since PVP showed good agreement with CVP in the perioperative period for children undergoing elective major non-cardiac surgery. Both Tobias and Johnson (2003) and Anter and Bondock (2004) found that changes in PVP reflect changes in CVP, regardless of catheter size or position, although the values were not absolute.

Stop and think

Traditionally methods of haemodynamic assessment included the use of capillary refill times and core–toe temperature gaps. However, these parameters need to be used with caution as other medications (e.g. vasodilators following cardiac surgery) will reduce their predictive value.

Physiologically the presence of a CVP line allows easy access to the child's venous blood supply, i.e. it offers a painless access route for routine bloods for investigations. However, sampling should occur from a three-way tap in close proximity to the child (i.e. before the transducer can be reached by back flow) and be slow, and the line should be flushed to remove any blood remnants. If blood gases are required as well then single access via the arterial route is preferable.

Considerations for interpreting raised and lowered CVP measurements
Falling CVP:

- Fluid loss by haemorrhage, vomiting, burns, ketoacidosis
- Inappropriate use of diuretics
- Systemic vasodilatation due to medication, sepsis, neurogenic shock

Elevating CVP:

- CVP catheter occlusion; kinked catheter, occluded line, either mechanical or due to a clot resulting from inadequate flushing or interruption in flow.
- Fluid overload
- Systemic vasoconstriction from medication
- Heart failure or pulmonary emboli
- Increased intrathoracic pressure – the introduction of CPAP or increased pressure for those receiving artificial ventilation support can affect this.

Modified from Cole (2007).

Pulse oximetry monitoring

The gold standard measurement for oxygen status is still intermittent arterial blood sampling, but many clinicians would agree that the advent of pulse oximetry has revolutionised the clinical setting. This continuous, simple and non-invasive monitoring method can generally indicate the adequacy of oxygenation within the patient's body. Within research, although the actual impact of pulse oximetry in terms of patient outcomes has yet to be tested, it is clear that:

- It can reduce arterial blood sampling (Salyer 2003).
- It removes the subjectivity of observer bias in determining oxygen status (Jevon 2004).
- It provides an earlier indication of hypoxia than possible from visual observation alone

(cyanosis will only start to be visible when SpO$_2$ <80% Giuiliano and Higgins 2005).

Initially used in anaesthetics, its use has spread to intensive care, high dependency and, more recently, the general paediatric environment. Mower *et al.* (cited in Tume and Bullock 2004) suggested that this has become commonly known as the fifth paediatric vital sign. However, there remains continuing evidence that nursing and medical teams often fail to understand the basic principles and limitations and often misinterpret readings (Howel 2002; Tume and Bullock 2004).

Understanding measurements

Oxygen is inspired during respiration, flows down to the alveoli of the lungs and diffuses across the alveolar walls into the underlying pulmonary vascular bed. From here it is transported around the body:

- Either dissolved in plasma; this accounts for 1–2% of oxygen transported

- Or attached to haemoglobin found in the erythrocyte; this accounts for 98–99% of oxygen transported (Chandler 2000).

Traditionally, blood gas analysis measured the oxygen dissolved in the plasma in the form of a partial pressure unit (kPa or mmHg) – since each molecule of oxygen carried within the blood contributes to the pressure effect. Pulse oximetry measures the amount of oxygen carried by the haemoglobin molecules, describing it in terms of 'percentage saturation' or SpO$_2$ values. There is a relationship between the partial pressure and oxygen saturation which is demonstrated by the oxyhaemoglobin dissociation curve (ODC) – see Figure 2.5.

When levels of oxygen are adequate within the plasma (PaO$_2$) there is usually an increased amount of oxygen bound to haemoglobin; conversely, when plasma levels are low, less oxygen will be bound to the haemoglobin – this provides indicators of change in oxygen status. However, the relationship between the two measurements can be altered by external factors which shift the position of the curve on the ODC graph. A shift

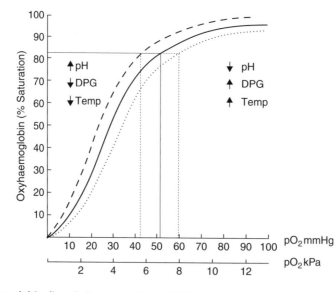

Figure 2.5 Oxyhaemoglobin dissociation curve. (*Note*: DPG – diphosphoglycerate now more often referred to as BPG – 2,3-biphosphoglycerate, a substance found in the red blood cells.)

to the left will result in an increase in saturation against a standard kPa value, whilst a shift to the right will result in a reduction in the saturation against a standard value.

> **Pause for thought**
>
> Changes in saturations can only provide guidance and should be followed up with additional blood gas determinations to determine the dissolved component.

Oxygen needs to be delivered to all cells to allow aerobic cellular respiration, promoting effective function. When blood oxygen levels become too low (hypoxaemia), delivery of oxygen to tissues is reduced. Low levels of oxygen in the tissues (hypoxia) results in anaerobic respiration (energy created without oxygen) within cells, which is inefficient and produces toxic acid by-products. If this situation continues, the increasing acid load and lack of oxygen causes cellular malfunction. The resulting damage may be transient (producing minor and temporary alterations in function) or permanent (resulting in significant and irreversible pathology/loss of function or death).

The risk is heightened in children due to lower pulmonary reserves which can lead to a rapid decompensation and deterioration (Chandler 2000). So ensuring that adequate oxygen is delivered to the body's organs/tissues/cells is paramount, and monitoring allows for early warnings of potential deterioration.

In children and adults, mechanisms generally limit damage caused by hyperoxia; however, this can become important when a neonate is receiving supplementary oxygen therapy. For some neonates (particularly with early stage bronchopulmonary dysplasia), hyperoxia releases excessive oxygen free radicals which act as destructive agents within many organ systems, prolonging recovery times. For neonates with duct-dependent cardiac anomalies, elevation of blood oxygen levels can promote closure of the ductus arteriosus (DA), causing crisis. Monitoring can assist in limiting saturations to a prescribed level.

As the majority of oxygen is carried by haemoglobin to be delivered to the cells and tissues, at this level, three main factors will affect the efficiency of the delivery process:

- Tissue perfusion
- The amount of haemoglobin
- The saturation of haemoglobin by oxygen

Assessment of organ perfusion requires pressure and fluid balance monitoring, whilst haemoglobin concentration can be determined by laboratory analysis. However, pulse oximeter monitoring will provide a 'hands off' continuous indication of the saturation of haemoglobin – allowing swift and timely interventions to prevent deterioration.

How pulse oximetry works

The application of a pulse oximeter probe to either side of a digit or appendage works on the basis that the probe has two surfaces/sides; one side is a light-emitting diode (LED) which emits light at 660- and 940-nm wavelengths across the tissue bed. The second side of the probe located underneath the digit/appendage uses a photodetector to measure the amount of light transmitted across the tissue bed. The saturation of the haemoglobin is calculated against the light absorbed by the two different wavelengths since the absorption of each alters as blood pulses through the tissue bed. This reflects changes in the levels of oxygenated and deoxygenated blood. The software algorithm within the monitor removes the non-pulsatile component/background artefact, then processes the measured changes in light absorption to produce numerical values for the heart rate, and local arterial oxygen saturation (SpO_2).

Advances in technology have enhanced the removal of motion artefact and improved the clinical performance of new generation monitors (Giuliano and Higgins 2005). However, the key to successful monitoring remains the presence of an adequately perfused tissue bed, a pulsatile flow and correct direct alignment of the two probe ends either side of the digit/appendage.

Using pulse oximetry

Indications for continuous pulse oximetry are any neonate, infant or child who is:

- Receiving supplemental oxygen or respiratory support, e.g. NCPAP or IPPV (LeGrand and Peters 1999; Salyer 2003)
- Undergoing procedures where respiratory depressant is being used, e.g. CT/MRI scanning (RCPCH 1999 in Chandler 2000)
- Experiencing respiratory difficulties but particularly if less than 3 months of age due to bronchiolitis (Perlstein *et al.* 1999)
- During ward-based resuscitation and potentially in delivery room resuscitation (Kopotic and Linder 2002)
- Receiving patient-controlled analgesia (Salyer 2003)
- In the immediate post-operative period, and for 12–24 hours post-operatively for some (Salyer 2003)
- Undergoing triage in a paediatric ambulatory care unit, minor injuries unit or emergency care department

Additional indications may include:

- Where there is concern regarding GOR or ALTE
- To assist in the diagnosis of cardiac anomalies (two monitors required – probes placed on right hand and on either foot)

Equipment
- Pulse oximeter and connecting lead
- Measurement probe – size specific to manufacturer's recommendations
- Designated supportive wrap
- Tape (see comments below)

Method
- Whenever possible discuss the need for the monitoring with parents/child to gain their consent.
- Choose an appropriate probe for the monitor and for the size of the child – see manufacturer's instructions. Adult rubber probes have been found to operate successfully; however, they should not be used since they operate on a higher intensity light which increases the risk of thermal injury (Moyles 1999). Using the wrong probes with equipment also increases this risk (Chandler 2002).
- Attach the probe to the monitor lead, attach monitor lead to machine and turn on the monitor to check function. Keep the monitor on mains function wherever possible to ensure that the battery pack is fully charged, should it be required during transfer. Confirm that the light-emitting diode in the probe is working. Temporarily silence alarms to prevent noise pollution.
- Prepare the patient – explain or demonstrate to the child (or parent) how the probe will fit onto the finger/toe and so on to reassure them that it is pain free. Choose a site that allows adequate observation with minimal disturbance if possible.
- Prevent any increase in the non-pulsatile component of the readings, which will alter the result, by:
  o Observing areas for adequate perfusion (neonates often have cold and poorly perfused peripheries; choose the opposite side)
  o Cleaning area with soap and warm water to remove debris/dirt
  o Removing nail varnish if using fingers/toes
- Positioning the probe:
  o Place probe in position: for neonates place on the outer aspect of the hand or foot below the digits; for younger children place on the finger or big toe or on the outer aspect of the palm; for older children a self-adhesive finger probe can be used on the finger or big toe.
  o The light-emitting diode must face the skin on the upper surface directing the beam

down to the photo-detector on the under surface. Direct alignment of the beam with the receiver through the digit/appendage is crucial to efficient monitoring.

o Manufacturers generally provide a support wrap which prevents disconnection from the skin, prevents harm when the limb is moved onto other surfaces, assists maintenance of correct position and excludes additional light. However, care should be taken to ensure this is not secured too tightly. Securing the probe in place with tape is not considered good practice unless recommended specifically by the manufacturers (MHRA [SN08] 2001); however, securing the supporting lead into position with a small piece of tape on the limb may assist in preventing artefact caused by movement (Chandler 2000).

- Commence monitoring, switching alarms back on and ensuring that the volume is appropriate for the environment of care. Set heart rate alarm limits appropriate for age and observe the plethysmographic waveform or pulse strength indicators to ensure that the readings produced are reliable.

- Large waveforms and high pulse strengths indicate that readings are *reliable*. Flat or unequal waveforms or low pulse strengths mean that the displayed results are *unreliable*. Accuracy can be checked by comparison of the readings with manual radial pulse assessment.

- Saturation limits also need to be set; however, these will vary according to the clinical condition. In general, setting a lower limit of 92% is considered acceptable as tissue perfusion is adequate up to this point (Horne and Derrico 1999). An upper limit of 95% for the neonate/child receiving oxygen may assist in the prevention of hyperoxia, but a full assessment should be made and the saturation levels should be dictated by the medical needs or local protocols.

- Observations of HR and SpO_2 should be documented hourly, but emergency situations may warrant more frequent records. In addition,

Good practice

Alarm settings need to be re-established every time monitoring is recommenced.

In addition it is recommended that the alarm limits are formally established at handover.

the position of the probe, the position of the patient and your responses to hypoxia and hyperoxia should be clearly demonstrated within the documentation.

- Effective monitoring can be disrupted by a wide variety of factors – see Table 2.6. Correct alignment of the probe and adequate perfusion at the probe site are vital. Monitoring should include observation of the site to prevent ischaemic injury. Rotating the site of the probe between the feet and hands or different fingers will prevent local pressure buildup that may affect perfusion. The maximum time for leaving probes in place is 4 hours; however, more frequent rotation should occur when skin integrity is suspect, the circulation is compromised or on manufacturer's recommendations (MHRA [SN08] 2001). After each move the probes should be refastened as above.

Stop and think

It is important to note that pulse oximetry provides limited information about overall respiratory status. Most significantly elevation of pCO_2 is not detected by pulse oximetry so the nurse *must* link together other clinical observations to assist in detecting this event – an elevation of respiratory rate with deeper breathing should trigger a consultation from physicians for an assessment of pCO_2.

Pulse oximeters all have default settings to ensure safety. However, if the default settings have not been altered from 'adult' to 'child' or 'neonate' when the machines were turned off and then restarted, all alarms will revert to these defaults. If alarms are not promptly individualised there is a risk of hypoxia and bradycardia being undetected.

Table 2.6 Factors that have an impact on pulse oximetry monitoring.

Factors	Recognised effects	Action
Restriction in blood and lymphatic flow to the local area caused by excessive tightness in supportive wrap or increased fluid shift in unwell infant	Oedema, swelling, cyanosis distal to probe placement site	Remove probe. Resite. Increase frequency of rotations. Avoid use of wrap
Probe surfaces dirty or broken	Low/poor quality readings	Replace probe if broken. Clean away debris (caution if blood)
Excessive ambient light, phototherapy, infrared heaters, diathermy	Poor quality trace	Cover probe area with protective shield to reduce light load
Low peripheral perfusion/peripheral vasoconstriction	Loss of signal or false low reading	Move to another site, e.g. right arm, which will reflect central SpO_2 more accurately
Motion artefact – general movement, shivering, fitting	Noisy signals/poor quality signal	Aim to use newer monitor with 'fuzzy logic' software to eliminate artefact
Black, blue or green nail polish (NB: unpolished acrylic nails have no effect)	False low	Remove nail polish
Different makes of pulse oximeter	Provide marginally different SpO_2 results due to measurements of either functional or fractional oxygen saturation	Theoretically little difference but practically reduce conflict by consistency in purchasing, i.e. single model for each area. Newer models potentially offer improved clinical performance
High blood levels of carbon monoxide Smoke inhalation from fire Smoking within 4 hours of monitoring	False high readings	Check with physicians regarding appropriate lower limits
In an anaemic child with HCT <10%	False high readings	Always observe clinical status; if pale request check Hb
Dysrhythmias, e.g. atrial fibrillation causing irregular perfusion and rates	Unreliable low readings	Check and record apex radial deficit. Alert medical team
Use of intravenous dyes during CT/MRI scanning	False low readings	Check half life of dye and during interim use clinical observations
Haemoglobinopathies – e.g. sickle cell disease	High/low reading	State diagnosis when checking with physicians
High levels of methaemoglobinaemia	False low readings	Use arterial blood gas to guide care, discuss and set acceptable limits with clinicians
Level of hypoxia	Most pulse oximeters are reliable in the 90% region. Reliability rapidly declines with increasing hypoxia	Significant falls in saturation require physicians to undertake ABG sampling

Compiled from LeGrand and Peters (1999), Moyles (1999), Chandler (2000), Giuliano and Higgins (2003), Salyer (2003).

Blood gas analysis

The previous section briefly discussed the relationship between oxygen saturation (SpO$_2$) and dissolved plasma oxygen (pO$_2$), which is illustrated by the oxyhaemoglobin dissociation curve (Figure 2.5). Looking at this diagram it becomes clear that on the upper section of the bold curve, small alterations in PaO$_2$ result in steady incremental drops in SaO$_2$. However, on the steep section of the curve, significant changes in the PaO$_2$ can occur for quite small changes of SpO$_2$. Clinically this means that measurements of oxygen saturation (SpO$_2$) below 93% can quickly result in tissue hypoxia – however, the severity of the hypoxaemia can only be determined by direct arterial blood gas analysis which measures the following five parameters:

(1) pH (the acid/base concentration within the blood)
(2) PaO$_2$ (the dissolved oxygen in plasma)
(3) PaCO$_2$ (the dissolved carbon dioxide in the blood)
(4) Bicarbonate (one of the blood buffer systems)
(5) Base excess (calculated value relating to the availability of buffers)

The body will only function effectively if the right internal environment is established and maintained. One crucial factor is the maintenance of a stable acid–base balance – or pH – within the blood.

Maintaining normal pH

Normal body function constantly produces acid as a by-product so this needs to be controlled. In normal aerobic cellular respiration the main form of acid produced is carbon dioxide, whilst in anaerobic respiration metabolic acids are produced. The presence of these acids lowers blood pH and cellular processes become less efficient. In the healthy body this increased acid load is controlled in the short term by a reservoir of buffer agents (including bicarbonate, protein and other systems). These buffering agents act like sponges within the bloodstream, removing the increased acid load from the blood by converting the acids temporarily into another chemical compound. This shifts the blood pH back into a normal range. The buffers transport the acids to either the respiratory system (primarily CO$_2$) or the renal system (the only route for metabolic acids) for excretion. Since the amount of 'buffers' within the bloodstream is limited and acid excretion relies on adequate ventilation and in the longer term a functional renal system, acid-base disturbances are common in sick children.

Deviations from normal pH

Respiratory acidosis: a fall in pH directly related to an increase in CO$_2$ in the bloodstream. This occurs when the CO$_2$ being produced by cellular activity is unable to be excreted by the lungs. There are two key elements that may cause this – ventilation of the alveoli and perfusion of the pulmonary vascular bed – and inadequacy in either or both will prevent CO$_2$ excretion (Table 2.7).

Respiratory alkalosis: a rise in pH directly related to a fall in CO$_2$ in the bloodstream, as demonstrated in Table 2.8.

Metabolic acidosis: a fall in pH attributed to an increase in metabolic acids or a fall in bicarbonate (base), as demonstrated in Table 2.9.

Metabolic alkalosis: a rise in pH due to either loss of acid or increase in bicarbonate load, as shown in Table 2.10.

However, it is common to review the ABG measurements and find evidence of a mixed acidosis, where both the respiratory buffering and renal systems have become overwhelmed.

Each disturbance can be resolved by controlling or removing the cause; however, in many cases, prolonged disturbances prompt the body to attempt to return an abnormal pH to a normal pH. This process is known as *compensation* and

Table 2.7 Causes of respiratory acidosis.

Non-ventilated patient	Ventilated patient
Reduced surface area for gas exchange: • Primary disease of the lungs, e.g. pneumonia • Occlusion/limitation of airways, e.g. asthma, irritants, foreign objects • Depression of the respiratory centre, e.g. head injury, opiate induced • Mechanical difficulties, e.g. chest trauma, pneumothorax. Reduced blood flow to the lungs Persistent pulmonary hypertension	As with non-ventilated patient plus: • Inadequate inspiratory pressure (underinflation) • Excessive inspiratory pressure (overinflation) • Excessive PEEP (preventing adequate venous return)

Table 2.8 Causes of respiratory alkalosis.

Non-ventilated patient	Ventilated patient
Anxiety attacks, severe pain, irritant inhalation, asthma → deep and/or rapid breathing (blow off CO_2) Vigorous artificial ventilation → increased CO_2 excretion	As with non-ventilated patient plus: Excessively high rate or high minute volume ventilation (blows off CO_2)

Table 2.9 Causes of metabolic acidosis.

Non-ventilated patient	Ventilated patient
Metabolic acid load increased due to: • Lactic acid production in anaerobic respiration from any cause, reduced blood volume, reduced cardiac output, reduced perfusion in shock situations • Ketoacid, acetoacetic acid in untreated or poorly controlled insulin-dependent diabetes Bicarbonate losses due to: • Increased buffering in ketoacidosis • Poor re-absorption from the GI tract due to diarrhoea • Fluid shifts following burns	As with non-ventilated patient plus: • Insufficient oxygen. • Prolonged inadequate ventilation. • Hypotension and reduced organ perfusion.

Table 2.10 Causes of metabolic alkalosis.

Non-ventilated patient	Ventilated patient
Loss of acid due to: • Severe/excessive vomiting • Pyloric stenosis Bicarbonate gains due to: • Excess administration of bicarbonate via antacid • Potassium depletion from diuretics	As with non-ventilated patient plus: Loss of acids • Excessive aspiration of stomach acid Bicarbonate gains due to: • Excess administration of bicarbonate infusion

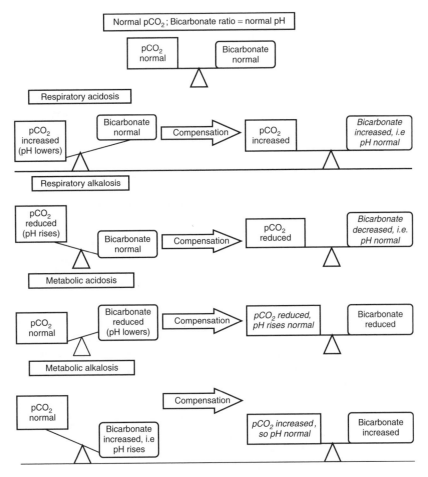

Figure 2.6 The compensation process in blood gases. Adapted from Higgins (2000).

involves restoring the ratio of carbon dioxide ions (in the form of carbonic acid) and bicarbonate ions to the correct level of 1:20 (Higgins 2000). Figure 2.6 demonstrates what occurs during this process. A guide to blood gas interpretation can be found in Chapter 3.

Blood gas sampling

As a general rule, arterial blood gas sampling is a medical responsibility and the technique will not be considered here. Although blood gas analysis should be obtained from an arterial site, often the initial blood gas result will come from other sources – particularly capillary sampling, which may be a nursing role.

Capillary blood sampling

Indications

Capillary blood sampling is carried out when urgent blood gas assessment is required by the medical team and to assist in assessment and management of a child receiving long-term oxygen therapy.

Equipment
- Pre-heparinised capillary tubes:
  - Plastic tubes reduce risks (US FDA, CDC, NIOSH 1999)
  - Generally 150-μl size but will depend on the local blood gas analyser
  - End caps ×2

- Alcohol wipe
- Lancet or similar device appropriate to age and site to be used
- Sterile gauze swab
- Plastic bag with ice for transportation
- Patient ID label

Method

- Discuss the need for the evaluation with the parents and child to gain consent.
- Preparing equipment away from the child and keeping it out of sight until necessary is suggested by Hockenberry *et al.* (2003) to minimise anxiety and trauma.
- Pain management should be considered; however, timing may limit this to non-pharmacological measures. Infants will respond well with non-nutritive sucking during heel pricks or the use of oral sucrose 2 minutes prior to the procedure. Older children can hold their breath during the puncture, then 'blow the pain away'. Parent participation will encourage positive results here.
- Good blood flow results from a well perfused site. A child could wash his or her hands under warm water; however, research has found that the application of a warm compress to the heel made little difference to the flow in infants (Barker *et al.* 1996). Yet Gray *et al.* (2000) suggest that 15 minutes of skin to skin contact has a positive impact in healthy infants, which may also occur in the sick infant.
- Identify the site to be used and put on gloves. For an infant, the fleshy lateral aspects of the heel provide good flow; however, to avoid problems of osteochondritis, infection and calcaneal damage, keep within the areas shown in Figure 2.7. Finger sites are on the fleshy finger pad. If ear lobes are large, this area can be used instead. All sites must be cleaned with an alcohol wipe prior to puncture and then allowed to completely dry – sampling when damp will alter the results obtained.

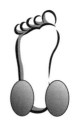

Figure 2.7 Sites on the infant heel for capillary sampling.

Stop and think

Petroleum jelly should not be applied to the skin as it can contaminate the capillary tube and subsequently the blood gas analyser, resulting in expensive repair bills (GOSH 2006).

- Pierce the skin using the lancet device. Choice must be influenced by the size/age of the child, and if in doubt check manufacturer's instructions. If the lancet is designed for use with a supporting device to prevent excessively deep piercing, this must be used. All designs should be pressed lightly against the clean, dry skin surface to achieve appropriate depth and flow.
- As the blood flows, the capillary tube should be placed at a 45-degree angle with one end in to the bead – capillary action will draw the blood steadily into a pre-heparinised capillary tube as a continuous column. When three-quarters full, the capillary tube should be removed and end caps applied. Local blood flow should be staunched with a sterile gauze swab – often held by the child or parent. If appropriate, a small plaster can be applied.
- Label the sample, place inside a plastic bag (surrounded by ice to prevent sample deterioration during transfer), and arrange urgent transportation to the local blood gas analyser (BGA). If this is located within another department, telephoning ahead ensures a smooth and efficient process.
- The patient ID and results should be recorded in the BGA log and entered onto the case notes – clearly indicating it as a capillary sample.

Table 2.11 Guidance for decision making with blood gas samples.

Source	Parameters to inform decision	Caution
Arterial sample	All parameters can inform decision	Must be free flowing with no air bubbles in sample
Capillary sample	Good indicator of pH and capillary pCO_2	Sample must be obtained without squeezing No air bubbles present
Venous sample	Indicates elevated venous pCO_2	Rarely useful

Caution

Different sites for blood gas analysis alter the usefulness of the parameters measured, so Table 2.11 should be used as a guide to impact decision making.

Arterial blood gas analysis

Collecting blood for arterial blood gas analysis can be performed by:

- Direct arterial stab to the femoral or radial artery.
- Aspiration from an indwelling arterial line (Hockenberry *et al.* 2003).

Direct arterial stabs can be used for intermittent or immediate assessment purposes, but they are more painful than venepuncture so topical analgesia should be applied if time allows (Higgins 2000). The sample will be collected in a pre-heparinised syringe by the physician, and the nurse will need to apply a pressure dressing to the stab area for 3–5 minutes after the event to prevent excess blood loss and encourage local clotting. To ensure the sample reflects the patient's status, the syringe should be sealed, labelled and packed in ice for transfer to the analyser.

When regular blood gases are required, an indwelling arterial line is the preferable source, since this line will also allow access for IABPM. Refer to the section on 'Invasive arterial blood pressure monitoring' to review the set-up procedure required.

Sampling from the arterial line

Generally this is a medical procedure in non-intensive areas. However, experience would suggest that the nurse should always be with the patient when samples are to be obtained since this will:

- Allow observation of the surrounding tissue, digits and limb for signs of cyanosis, swelling or arterial spasm that may be transient or newly occurring.
- Enhance the safety of the procedure as the nurse can confirm that the correct porthole is being used for sampling, that sufficient blood is withdrawn to prevent contamination of the sample (1.5–2 mL is sufficient), and that the aspirate is replaced, so preventing anaemia.
- Increase the survival of the IA line by ensuring that the line is adequately flushed to remove blood which can impact on pressure readings and cause blockage in the arterial catheter.

> **Top tip**
>
> Following sampling, it is good practice to re-establish zero (refer to section on 'Setting up invasive arterial blood pressure monitoring') to ensure trace accuracy prior to recommencing BP monitoring if in place.

Capnography

Theory

The measurement of carbon dioxide in the gas mix at the end of expiration is known generally as capnography when presented as a wave form, or capnometry when presented as numerical data alone. This indication of end tidal CO_2 is becoming an increasingly useful tool for decision making from a number of different perspectives. Similar to the historical spread of pulse oximetry, capnography was originally an anaesthetic tool and has now moved into the wider environment (Kodali 2007). Although currently not common in HD care, experience and research are already identifying situations where capnography offers potential insight to aid diagnosis in the sick child (Fearon and Steele 2002; Nagler and Krauss 2006). Significantly capnography provides indirect monitoring of ventilatory status which allows expeditious action to prevent significant hypoxia. Often this may be before hypoxia is recognised by pulse oximetry.

Traditionally respiratory status has been monitored using arterial/capillary blood gas sampling. Frequent blood gas sampling increases the potential for infection. More importantly this depletes the circulatory volume, reducing the oxygen carrying capacity of the patient as the blood cells and plasma cannot be returned after analysis. As capnography is a non-invasive method of determining carbon dioxide levels, these risks are reduced. It can be used in self-ventilating and intubated patients and works by sampling the exhaled air during respiration. Originally the technology was only useful in older children and adults due to the large sampling volumes and mode of action which potentially increased the dead space in the ventilation circuit. A change in design now means that different sampling/measurement techniques can be employed, so its usage can be extended.

Practice

Indications for use

In secondary care/general hospitals with HD areas, Kodali (2001) suggests that capnography should be used as a non-invasive predictor of CO_2 as follows:

As part of the triage/assessment process for the sick child:

- This can include those presenting with primary respiratory disorders

As part of the assessment of treatment/ interventions:

- As part of the assessment of the effectiveness of bronchodilators in severe asthma
- As part of the assessment of the effectiveness of adrenaline nebuliser in stridor

As part of pre-hospital stabilisation prior to transfer:

- To monitor ventilatory status whilst waiting for the transport team
- To confirm correct placement of ET if the child's condition deteriorates
- During transportation from secondary to tertiary care to confirm ET placement en route with minimal disturbance to the child

In addition there is emerging evidence that diagnosis of other conditions that result in acid balance disturbances can be facilitated by this monitoring, e.g. diabetic ketoacidosis (Fearon and Steele 2002) and gastroenteritis (Nagler et al. 2006).

Equipment

- Disposable colorimetric device – generally for confirming correct ETT placement; or
- A portable electronic capnograph. This will use infrared, photo-acoustic or mass spectrometry technology to sample exhaled air, providing a 'snapshot' of the end tidal CO_2 (etCO$_2$) which correlates well with the blood CO_2 levels (McArthur 2003). Sampling and analysis

use either a mainstream analyser (sampler/analyser inserted into the ventilator circuit) or a side stream analyser (micro-bore tube attached to circuit aspirates expiratory air sample, analysed externally). Devices are generally portable and have an internal filter, which needs to be changed between patients.

For non-ventilated children undergoing electronic capnography:

- Size-specific specialised nasal cannula compatible with capnograph to be used

For children about to be or already ventilated:

- Filtered circuit adapter – Flexlife® liquorice stick connector (with filter)
- etCO$_2$ sensor T-piece
- etCO$_2$ sensor tubing (clear plastic)
- Airway adapter (suction safe swivel Y connection)

Method for monitoring a non-ventilated child
- Discuss the need for monitoring with the parent and child to gain consent.
- Demonstrate how the prongs fit with a toy dolly or animal to reassure the child.
- Monitoring may be required continuously or intermittently to assess treatment effectiveness.
- Turn the monitor on – wait until self check and calibration are complete, silence alarms temporarily.
- Place the nasal cannula in position and alter the slide behind the head to draw the tubing taut but not tight on the child's face. Where the skin is excoriated, fragile or thin, place a small oblong of hydroactive dressing (e.g. Duoderm®) on the skin under the route of the cannula arms and secure with tape directly onto the dressing.
- Attach the cannula to the monitor, set alarms and commence monitoring.

- Record all events so comparisons can be accurately made.

Method for assessing ETT placement using disposable colorimetric device
Immediately following intubation, attach the colorimetric device so it is sandwiched in the circuit between the ends of the ETT immediately prior to the ventilation circuit (e.g. Ambubag®). Some devices show a change in the colorimetric wheel to indicate correct position.

Deliver five positive pressure breaths. The indicator colour will distinctly change during the different respiratory phases, e.g. purple → yellow → purple, indicating correct placement. Recent studies suggest that re-intubation times are shortened and that this approach can successfully be used in neonates even in delivery room resuscitation (Aziz et al. 1999; Molley and Deakins 2006).

Method for use with ventilated patients
- Turn monitor on to establish self check, calibration and correct function.
- Using the photograph in Figure 2.8 as a guide, attach one end of the et-sensor tubing to the monitor and the other to the et-sensor T piece.
- To the et-sensor T piece, add the airway adapter (suction safe swivel Y connector) to the front end and the filter circuit adapter (e.g. Flexlife® liquorice stick) to the back end. This end can then be attached to the ventilation circuit, whilst the Y connector is attached to the ETT in situ on the sick child.
- Keeping the sample port as close as possible to the patient enhances the correlation between etCO$_2$ and pCO$_2$ (McArther 2003).
- The additional equipment in the circuit adds to the weight so extubation risks are increased. Positioning and supporting the tubing will avoid this problem.
- Monitoring can then commence, etCO$_2$ should correlate well with arterial pCO$_2$ but

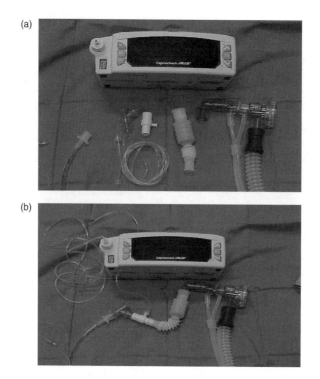

Figure 2.8 (a,b) Capnography equipment. Photographs by Leann Lancaster. Reproduced with permission.

Table 2.12 Troubleshooting etCO$_2$.

Problem	Action
Measurements become erratic with no other obvious changes in the child's state	Check for secretions/condensation – remove Reduce sampling tube length or remove kinks Sampling chamber obstructed – remove
The presence of antacids or carbonated liquids in the sick child's stomach can produce false positive results when the ETT is located in the pharynx	Prior to intubation, stomach contents should be aspirated to avoid this Record drug and drink inputs to allow correlation etCO$_2$ is not definitive – always auscultate chest to establish correct characteristics
Tidal volumes can be reduced if the sampling rate is too high specifically in volume control, volume-pressure control rate ventilation	Sampling frequency should be reduced
Large leaks around the ETT (especially uncuffed ETTs) and leaks from the ventilator circuit and around the nasal cannula ends reduce etCO$_2$ readings	Alter child's, ET or cannula position as this can reduce leaks; document, report and monitor If appropriate replace nasal cannula with larger size or re-intubate with larger bore ETT to reduce leak
The efficiency of the infrared technology can be affected by very high levels of oxygen/nitric oxide or both in the gas mix	Calibration can be adjusted by hospital support team or use alternative technology
Mass spectrometer efficiency is reduced by helium or freon in the gas mix (McArthur 2003)	Use alternative monitoring technology

intermittent ABGs will be required to confirm correlation. Additionally if $etCO_2$ trends identify constant rise/fall, then ABG should be performed. When calibrated and operated in line with the manufacturer's guidelines capnography is reliable and efficient; however, see Table 2.12 for troubleshooting.

- Normal record keeping protocols apply.

Stop and think

Raised $etCO_2$ due to increased resistance in the airways due to secretions can be resolved by suction. However, if $etCO_2$ trends show a continued rise or fall then alert the medical team so that ABG can be performed.

Chapter 3
RESPIRATORY

Caroline Haines

Introduction

Respiratory distress is the most common cause of illness in infants and children and although most will have self-limiting conditions, others will be severely affected, requiring ventilatory support for varying lengths of time. Recognition, assessment and treatment of the child's respiratory signs and symptoms is critical to prevent the respiratory distress progressing to respiratory failure.

Development of the respiratory system

The development of the respiratory system can be divided into five periods, which are shown in Table 3.1. Failure of these key stages may lead to the development of certain congenital malformations such as tracheo-oesophageal fistula (TOF) and congenital diaphragmatic hernia (CDH).

Overview of respiratory anatomy and physiology

The anatomical structures and physiological process of respiration are fundamentally the same in infants, children and adults. However, there are key differences linked to the developmental stage of infants and children that must be considered when discussing the respiratory system as they have a significant impact on the management principles for these age groups.

Anatomical differences in infants and children

- The head size – the large occiput of infants causes neck flexion.
- The mouth and nostril size are small and while infants have no teeth, older children have small loose teeth to be considered.
- The infant's tongue is relatively large in proportion to the rest of the oral cavity; hence it has the potential to more easily obstruct the airway.
- The larynx is higher in the neck (C3–4) than in an adult (C4–5).
- The infant's epiglottis enters the anterior pharyngeal wall at a 45° angle and therefore projects more posteriorly than in the older child.
- The cricoid ring is a complete ring of cartilage and the narrowest point of the upper airway (compared to the vocal cords in the adult). If tracheal intubation is required the tracheal tube will pass through the cords and be tightly fitted against the tracheal wall at the level of the cricoid. This can cause damage to the tracheal mucosa and potential sub-glottic stenosis or post-extubation stridor.
- The trachea is short in the infant, approximately 4–5 cm from cricoid to carina. It is narrow and soft.
- The airways are smaller and less developed than in the adults; hence a relatively small obstruction can compromise the airway radius, causing a significant increase in respiratory effort, e.g. a small amount of mucus or oedema.

Table 3.1 Embryological and fetal development of the respiratory system.

Gestational age	Development
Embryonic period: 26–52 days	The lung begins to appear as a ventral pouce from the foregut. The foregut divides into the dorsal portion, developing into the oesophagus, and the ventral portion develops into the trachea and lung buds. Development continues, giving shape to the left and right bronchial tree
Pseudoglandular period Day 52–16 weeks' gestation	Formation of all the major conducting airways and terminal bronchioles The diaphragm is formed between 8 and 10 weeks' gestation
Canalicular period Weeks 17–24 gestation	Development of the respiratory bronchioles. Each bronchiole ends with two or three terminal sacs or primitive alveoli
Saccular period Weeks 28–36 gestation	Increased vascularisation of the lung occurs. Elastic fibres develop and true alveoli are present at 34 weeks
Alveolar period Weeks 36 to term	Further development of the terminal sacs and formation of the walls of true alveoli. Columnar cells develop and differentiate within the alveoli into type I and II. Type I cells provide the alveolar surface area for gas exchange and type II cells secrete surfactant, necessary to lower the alveolar surface tension and sustain lung inflation

From Chamley (2003) and Moore and Persaud (2003).

- The number and size of the alveoli continue to increase until approximately 8 years of age, thus increasing the respiratory surface area available for gas exchange.
- Collateral ventilatory channels (Channel of Martin = interbronchiolar, Canals of Lambert = bronchiole-alveolar, and Pores of Kohn = interalveolar), which allow ventilation distal to an obstruction, are thought to develop after infancy and up to 6 years of age. Without these pathways infants and young children are at increased risk of atelectasis and hyperinflation associated with infection.
- In infants the ribs lie horizontally and the thorax is circular, with the anteroposterior diameter equal to the transverse diameter. This changes so that, by approximately 6 years of age, the thorax reaches the adult diameter and the rib cage is ellipsoid. In infancy the chest wall is thin with little muscle development and is very compliant. To compensate, infants use their abdominal muscles to assist with ventilation.
- The child's diaphragm is more horizontal in its position, resulting in a decreased efficiency of contraction.

Physiological differences in infants and children

- The lungs are less compliant in the infant, but this improves with age. The preterm infant (<37 weeks' gestation) is at particular risk of poor lung compliance and may also have reduced production of surfactant (a lipoprotein that coats the inner surface of the alveoli and reduces surface tension, thus facilitating alveolar expansion during inspiration).
- Infants, particularly those born prematurely, have irregular breathing patterns that make them prone to having apnoeas. Although short periods of apnoea are not uncommon, longer periods that require stimulation should be investigated.
- When infants suffer from respiratory distress they are unable to increase their lung volumes to the same extent as adults due to their rib cage structure. Instead they increase their respiratory rate to maintain minute volume.
- Because of the pattern of infant sleep, they have long periods of rapid eye movement (REM) sleep. During this time there is a decrease in

postural tone which can cause a drop in their functional residual capacity and so increase their effort in breathing.

- Despite similar perfusion patterns, children preferentially ventilate the upper lung regions, rather than the dependent sections as in adults (Pryor and Prasad 2002). For acutely ill children, with unilateral lung disease, placing the non-affected lung uppermost can optimise oxygenation.
- Children have a higher resting metabolic rate with an increase in oxygen demand. This increase in demand can lead to hypoxia more rapidly than in adults and the hypoxia may result in bradycardia.
- The diaphragm in infants is composed of 25% fatigue-resistant type-1 muscle fibres, in comparison to 50% in adults. This results in an increased susceptibility to fatigue of the diaphragm.
- In infants, the closing lung volume exceeds the functional residual capacity. In dependent regions, airway closure may occur during normal tidal breathing (Pryor and Prasad 2002).

Although there must be consideration of the above factors, the process of respiration remains the same in all ages and can be divided into four sections:

- Movement of gases into and out of the lungs. Factors influencing this include atmospheric air/lung pressure gradient, airway resistance, muscular function, lung compliance, intrapleural pressures and neural control
- Exchange of gases across a membrane by diffusion
- Carriage of gases to and from the tissues
- Metabolic processes of the cell to produce energy (Tortora and Derrickson 2005)

Respiratory assessment

Careful assessment of the respiratory system is essential in identifying any problems that require intervention (see below). Information should be obtained from the medical, nursing and allied health professionals' notes, from the children's parents/carers and, if appropriate, from the children themselves regarding their past and present history. Accurate documentation of findings must be made.

Key components

- Knowledge of paediatric anatomy and physiology
- Anatomical landmarks

Process

Structures involved in the respiratory system
- Sternum
- Manubrium
- Xiphoid process
- Costal cartilages
- Laterally – 12 pairs of ribs
- Posteriorly – 12 thoracic vertebrae
- Lungs
- Diaphragm
- Intercostals – external and internal
- Sternomastoid/scalenus muscles

Anatomical landmarks
- Manubriosternal junction (angle of Louis)
- Suprasternal notch
- Costal angle
- Vertebra prominens
- Clavicles
- Nipples/nipple line

Inspection
Inspect the general appearance of the child:

- Size and shape – anteroposterior diameter compared with transverse diameter
- Symmetry of thorax
- Rate and nature of breathing pattern, use of accessory muscles
- Colour, peripheral oedema, clubbing of fingers, anaemia

- Superficial venous patterns
- Rib prominence
- Marks/scars from previous interventions

Palpation
Palpate the thoracic muscles and skeleton:

- Bilateral symmetry
- Degree of elasticity of the rib cage
- Relative sternal/xiphoid inflexibility
- Thoracic spine rigidity
- Abnormal palpation
- Crepitus
- Pleural friction rub
- Tracheal position
- For presence of cardiac impulse on palpation of chest

Percussion
- Anterior, lateral and posterior chest wall
- Make comparisons from side to side to identify differences or similarities

Auscultation
Auscultate the four anterior and four posterior quadrants of the thorax, as well as the mid-axillae area.
   Normal breath sounds:

- Bronchial
- Bronchovesicular
- Vesicular

Abnormal breath sounds:

- Crackles
- Wheezes
- Stridor
- Pleural rub

Consider the above findings and possible effects on other systems
- Cardiac
- Renal
- Neurology
Adapted from Mosby 2001.

When undertaking a respiratory assessment it is important to also identify the presence of any signs of respiratory distress, such as those shown in the section on 'Additional considerations for respiratory assessment'. Frequent reassessment of the child for signs of increasing distress or tiring is paramount to providing effective and timely interventions.

Signs of respiratory distress

- Stridor

- Tachypnoea
- Recession – intercostal, subcostal, sternal, subcostal
- Head bobbing
- Abdominal breathing sounds
- Irritability/restlessness

- Tachycardia/bradycardia

- Colour – pallor/mottled/cyanosed
- Nasal flaring
- Expiratory grunting

- Neck extension
- Reluctance to feed

- Altered level of consciousness
- Hypertension/hypotension

Additional considerations

A number of features in the neonatal population could be recognised when carrying out a respiratory assessment:

- Cyanosis of hands and feet (acrocyanosis) is common in the newborn and may persist for several days in a cool environment.
- Respiratory pattern – infants are obligatory nose breathers and nasal flaring is common without clinical significance.
- Coughing in newborns is rare and is normally pathological in origin.
- Sneezing in newborns is frequent and expected.
- Hiccoughs in newborns are common, usually silent and associated with feeds. Frequent non-feed-associated hiccoughs may be suggestive of seizures, drug withdrawal or encephalopathy.

Table 3.2 Normal vital sign parameters in children.

Normal respiratory rates in children (breaths per minute)		Normal heart rates in children (beats per minute)	
Newborn	<60	<1 year	110–160
<1 year	30–40	1–2 years	100–150
1–2 years	25–35	2–5 years	95–140
2–5 years	25–30	5–12 years	80–120
5–12 years	20–25	>12 years	60–100
>12 years	15–20		

Non-invasive monitoring

Observations

The importance of regular and accurate documentation of the child's cardio/respiratory observations should not be underestimated. The broad parameters are replicated in Table 3.2. They are essential to inform the multi-disciplinary team of the child's condition and ensure complete, appropriate and timely care for the child. The regularity of documentation should relate to the individual child's condition. However, if receiving supplemental oxygen, a minimum of hourly recordings is required.

Recommended observations include:

- Temperature
- Respiratory rate
- Pulse rate
- Blood pressure
- Capillary refill time
- SpO_2

The observation chart should facilitate completion of the above parameters and allow for the recording of blood glucose levels and mode/percentage of oxygen delivery. Provision should also be available on the chart to document a brief respiratory assessment and chest drain observations.

Pulse oximetry

Pulse oximetry is widely available for use in various healthcare environments. It provides an estimate of arterial oxygen saturation (SaO_2) by utilising selected wavelengths of light to non-invasively determine the saturation of peripheral oxygen (SpO_2). A saturation recording of 95% means that 95% of the total amount of haemoglobin (Hb) in the blood is saturated with oxygen molecules. Pulse oximetry is considered a safe procedure, but, because of device limitations, underestimation and overestimation of SpO_2 may lead to inappropriate treatment of the patient. Remember to assess and treat the child, not the SpO_2 (For further information refer to Chapter 2, section on 'Pulse oximetry monitoring').

Within the hospital setting a multi-purpose observation document which includes a paediatric early warning (PEW) assessment tool (see below) is valuable in contributing to the care of the acutely ill child (see Table 3.3).

Peak expiratory flow rate (PEFR)

A PEFR provides information on the function of the large airways and can be obtained in a child over 4–5 years through the use of a peak flow meter. There will be a decreased PEFR in children who develop respiratory failure and those who have asthma or chronic airway conditions. Obtaining regular recordings during a child's acute illness can demonstrate a trend indicating improvement or deterioration in the child's respiratory status.

Oxygen therapy – methods of administration and humidification

Oxygen (O_2) administration

O_2 is required for cellular respiration and adequate oxygenation and is therefore vital to prevent tissue damage. Persistent hypoxia can

Table 3.3 Bristol paediatric early warning tool.

A	**Acute airway obstruction**
1	Child has required nebulised adrenaline
2	Clinically tiring or impending complete airway obstruction
B	**Breathing**
1	SaO_2 ≤92% in any amount of oxygen
2	SaO_2 ≤75% in any amount of oxygen (cyanotic heart disease)
3	Persistent tachypnoea (RR ≥70 under 6 months; ≥60 6–12 months; ≥40 1–5 years; ≥25 over 5 years)
4	Apnoea +/− bradycardia (HR ≤95 in children under 5 years)
C	**Circulation**
1	Persistent tachycardia following one bolus of 10 mL/kg fluid (HR ≥150 under 5 years; ≥120 5–12 years; ≥100 over 12 years)
2	Signs of shock: e.g. prolonged capillary refill (≥3 seconds); poor perfusion; +/− low BP
D	**Disability**
1	GCS ≤11 or unresponsive or responding only to pain
2	Convulsions unresponsive to anticonvulsant therapy (lasting ≥30 minutes)
E	**Other**
1	Hyperkalaemia K^+ ≥6.0 mmol/L
2	Any child with suspected meningococcus
3	Any child with diabetic ketoacidosis (DKA)
4	Any child whose condition is worrying

Haines *et al.* (2006).

lead to cell damage and death (Tortora and Derrickson 2005). The age of the child and amount of O_2 required will determine the mode of delivery and technique used.

The child

A normal healthy child's saturations (SpO_2) should be 98–100% (Campbell and McIntosh 1998). Children with a cardiac condition may have a lower SpO_2 even when healthy; similarly, some children with chronic conditions may also have SpO_2 levels below 'normal parameters'. These low SpO_2 levels are 'normal' for the individual. However, to optimise care delivery and prevent confusion, the expected or acceptable SpO_2 levels for every child should be clearly documented. The aim of O_2 delivery is to maintain a child's SpO_2 above 92–95%.

The neonate

The aetiology of retinopathy of prematurity, especially the role of O_2, is controversial. Care should be taken when supplemental O_2 is provided to preterm infants of less than 37 weeks' gestation (Myers 2002). The normal PaO_2 in utero is 30 mmHg, while a normal infant breathing room air will have a PaO_2 of 60–100 mmHg. It is suggested that the PaO_2 of a premature infant in an oxygen-enriched environment should not result in an arterial O_2 tension (PaO_2) of more than 80 mmHg and should be maintained at between 50 and 70 mmHg. An arterial oxygen tension of 40–50 mmHg may be adequate, providing cardiac output and peripheral perfusion are normal. A term infant may require a PaO_2 of 55–70 mmHg to be adequately oxygenated (Bell and Klein 2005).

Stop and think

Local guidelines should be consulted when providing supplementary oxygen therapy to the neonate.
Practitioners should discuss and confirm the prescribed oxygen therapy with the medical staff involved in the neonate's care.

O_2 and the child with a chronic condition

In children with chronic lung problems, administering a high concentration of O_2 can lead to respiratory failure. Normally the respiratory centres stimulate breathing in response to a rising concentration of CO_2. In chronic lung disease, the respiratory centres become used to the raised level of CO_2 and adapt. The increased level of CO_2 is no longer sufficient to stimulate breathing. Instead the centres respond to low levels of O_2 concentration in the blood. Giving high levels of O_2 to these children may remove the stimulus to which their respiratory centres respond to stimulate breathing. These children must only receive low-concentration O_2 therapy. However, giving high levels of O_2 may be judged necessary in the acute situation. In practice it is rare for children to have apnoea when given high concentrations of O_2.

The child with a cardiac condition

The administration of supplemental O_2 to patients with certain congenital heart lesions (e.g. hypoplastic left-heart, single ventricle or duct-dependent lesions) may cause an increase in alveolar O_2 tension and compromise the balance between pulmonary and systemic blood flow. Delivering high levels of O_2 may be judged necessary in the acute situation. However, it should be given with caution and with early and regular medical review.

The child with an oncological condition

The administration of O_2 to patients receiving certain chemotherapeutic agents (e.g. Bleomycin) may result in pulmonary complications such as O_2 toxicity and pulmonary fibrosis (Myers 2002). Delivering high levels of O_2 may be judged necessary in the acute situation. However, it should be given with caution and with early and regular medical review.

O_2 delivery

Delivery of supplemental O_2 to a child can be problematic. It can often be a challenge to encourage a child to tolerate the O_2 delivery equipment, and this can be especially difficult when a child is unwell or hypoxic. It is important to consider the nature of the illness, the therapeutic goals, the child's age and size, his or her wishes, and the amount of O_2 to be delivered (Table 3.4).

There are many different methods of administration, the most common being:

- Head box/incubator O_2
- Nasal cannula
- Simple face masks
- Non-rebreathing face mask
- Bucket mask/face mask
- 'Wafting' O_2

Other methods include:

- Resuscitation bags
- Nebulisers
- Continuous positive airway pressure (CPAP)
- Other ventilatory methods
- Partial-rebreathing masks
- Nasopharyngeal catheters
- Transtracheal catheters

Humidification

Normally the nose and upper respiratory tract warms, humidifies and filters inspired air. However, if a child is receiving high flow O_2 or where the upper airway is bypassed, as in a child with a tracheostomy, humidification should be administered. Dry gases have been associated with cilial dysfunction, drying, inflammation

Table 3.4 Key facts regarding common O_2 delivery devices.

Device	Approximate maximum FiO_2	Can be humidified?	Approximate age range
Nasal cannula	30% (variable)	X	Any
Simple face mask	40–50%	X	Any
Non re-breathe face mask	98–100%	X	12 months +
'Wafting'	21–30%	✓	Any
Head box	50–60%	✓	<8 months
Bucket mask	30–60%	✓	3 years +
Vapotherm®	21–100%	✓	Any
Incubator	21–70%	✓	Pre-term to newborn infant (NB: Consider size and weight of infant)

and ulceration of mucous membranes and an increase in the viscosity of secretions (Trigg and Mohammed 2006). Humidification may be administered via:

- Heated water bath humidifiers
- Heat and moisture exchangers (HMEs)
- Bubble-through humidifiers
- Nebulisers

Top tip

The decision on the device to be used will depend on the age of the child, the oxygen delivery system being used and the degree to which warming of the gases is required.

Low flow/ultra low flow O_2

Children on low flow O_2 will require a low flow meter that is capable of delivering small amounts of O_2. If a low flow meter is used a normal flow meter should be available and kept by the bed in case high flow O_2 is required. A cylinder of O_2 should also be readily available should an emergency situation arise. A nasal cannula is the most commonly used delivery method for a child who requires low flow O_2.

Nursing care and supportive interventions

Appropriate interventions for children with respiratory problems can often improve their condition and reduce their O_2 requirement. Effective and appropriate treatment of the underlying cause of respiratory distress is a priority.

- Positioning of the acutely unwell child is often a compromise between therapeutic aims. For the child in respiratory distress, particular positioning may be of benefit, e.g. to aid drainage of secretions, improve gaseous exchange and reduce the work of breathing. Children often benefit from being nursed upright, well supported with pillows. If the child is too ill to sit up, consider tilting the cot or bed to maintain a head-up position.
- Monitored babies can benefit from being nursed in the prone position, again with the head of the cot elevated to maintain a head-up position.
- Regular suctioning may also be beneficial.
- Referral for physiotherapy will be helpful in certain conditions.
- Supplemental humidity or saline nebulisers can often aid in the breakdown of secretions and clearing secretions.
- Feeding and fluid requirements should be given special consideration as the acutely unwell child may be tiring and not feeding well. Feeding may

also cause splinting of the diaphragm due to an increase in gastric contents. Consideration should be given therefore to using either nasogastric (NG) feeds or an intravenous infusion (IVI) to maintain adequate hydration and blood glucose levels. There is debate about the adverse effects of NG tubes blocking half of the upper airway of infants; therefore it may be more appropriate to use a well-secured orogastric tube. Accurate fluid balance, capillary refill time (CRT) and blood pressure (BP) will also need to be documented regularly in the dehydrated child.

- Children who present with lung pathology (i.e. asthma, bronchiolitis or pneumonia) may be at risk of developing inappropriate anti-diuretic hormone (ADH) secretion, which may contribute to the development of pulmonary oedema if fluid management is inappropriate. In view of this, maintenance fluids may be restricted to 80% of normal requirements.
- If oral feeding is reduced, extra mouth care should be given as mucous membranes may get dry.

Top tips

Children receiving O_2 therapy from a cylinder supply should not use Vaseline, oil-based lip balms or moisturisers as there is a risk of possible fire/explosion due to contamination of the regulator with grease (see http://www.dhsspsni.gov.uk/mdea(ni)2006-42.pdf for further information).

Saline nasal drops may be of benefit to help loosen thick secretions; however, there is very little supporting clinical evidence.

Monitoring and observations

- Children requiring O_2 therapy should receive at least hourly observations.
- All patients receiving O_2 should have continuous SpO_2 monitoring.

As a minimum, SpO_2, respiratory rate, heart rate and FiO_2 should be documented hourly and BP

daily. The frequency should be adjusted as the child's clinical condition dictates.

Regular clinical assessment, including neurological status and apparent respiratory effort, should be clearly documented, as should fluid balance. Any changes in the child's O_2 requirement should be reported promptly. If the child's oxygen requirement is increasing in order to maintain the desired saturations then a thorough respiratory assessment should be undertaken and findings reported in a timely and appropriate manner. If a child is on long-term O_2 therapy, the frequency of observations can be adjusted in line with his/her clinical condition after assessment and evaluation.

Discussion point

The evidence base for the use of respiratory monitors to detect apnoeas in the infant population is at best limited and is also controversial.

Practitioners should evaluate their use and utilise other monitoring devices where they are available in preference to reliance on the 'apnoea monitor'.

Physiotherapy techniques

Differing physiotherapy techniques can be a useful adjunct to managing the respiratory status of a child. Treatment should never be performed routinely as it can have detrimental effects (Krause and Hoehn 2000; Stiller 2000). However, following individual assessment of the child, treatment options that may be considered include the following.

Positioning

This can be one of the most fundamental, essential and effective elements of care that may optimise respiratory function.

- The supine position has been identified as the least beneficial (Pryor and Prasad 2002), with prone positioning being shown to improve respiratory function (Pryor and Prasad 2002), decrease oesophageal reflux and assist in reduced energy expenditure (Pryor and Prasad 2002). The prone position should only be used in monitored children within a hospital setting. Parents must be advised against using this position at home due to its association with sudden infant death (see http://www.fsid.org.uk/reduce-risk.html).

- Lateral positioning of a child is also beneficial; however, acknowledgement of the specifics of regional lung ventilation in children must be considered. Ventilation is preferentially distributed to the upper lung regions in infants and small children. Due to their altered rib cage dynamics, lung mechanics and ventilation/perfusion matching, children with unilateral lung disease have been shown to have a higher arterial oxygen tension when positioned with the affected lung down. This is a key issue to consider and is the opposite to care provision in adolescents and adults.

Chest percussion

- Chest percussion uses a hand, fingers or a face mask to percuss the chest wall and mobilise secretions.
- It is usually tolerated well by children.

Vibrations and shaking

- These can be undertaken when the respiratory rate is within normal or near normal limits.
- If an infant is breathing too rapidly the expiratory phase is too short to perform effective vibrations.

Postural drainage (gravity-assisted positioning)

- Postural drainage can be used in children to help assist the clearance of bronchial secretions, particularly those in the upper lobes

that tend to be more affected by respiratory problems.

- A head down position should, however, be avoided in children with raised intracranial pressure, those with abdominal distension where increased pressure on the diaphragm could further inhibit their respiratory performance, and those with a history of reflux.

Coughing

- Children over 18 months will mimic a cough if asked to do so; however, compliance in an acutely ill child may not be readily achieved.
- Altered positioning and play activity may assist in moving secretions and stimulating a cough reflex. Children <4 years will tend to swallow rather than expectorate secretions.
- Tracheal compression can be used to help stimulate a cough in those children who are unable to cough on request. A gentle pressure should be applied to the trachea just below the thyroid cartilage; however, care needs to be taken in small infants due to the possibility of vagal stimulation and bradycardia.
- Airway suctioning can be used to remove secretions.
- With appropriate education and training for staff, a cough assist device may be of use.

Mobilisation

- Ambulation and mobilisation should be encouraged as soon as possible according to the child's clinical condition.
- It stimulates deeper respiratory effort, increases perfusion, promotes secretion clearance and improves oxygenation.

Stop and think

Consider the child's clotting status before physiotherapy is administered.

Airway suctioning

Airway suctioning in the high-dependency child is likely to be naso- or oropharyngeal or via a tracheostomy tube (see the section on 'Nursing management of a child with a tracheostomy'). It assists in the removal of secretions from the upper airway.

- Care must be taken when suctioning a child as adverse effects such as hypoxaemia, pneumothorax, atelectasis and/or cardiac arrhythmias can occur.
- Oxygen and resuscitation equipment should always be available during any suction procedure and the child observed for any signs of hypoxia. Infants and children should be positioned on their side to avoid potential aspiration of stomach contents. They should be held firmly to avoid any trauma during the procedure and need to be constantly reassured.

Top tips

The child should be assessed and suction given prior to feeds where possible to reduce the risk of vomiting.

If the child has an NGT/OGT *in situ* and time allows, then aspirate the tube before suctioning; otherwise the tube should be opened to air.

- High vacuum pressure can cause trauma to mucous membranes; hence suction pressure should be as low as possible but should not compromise the efficiency of secretion removal.
- A flexible catheter of suitable size must be selected.
- Suction should not be applied as the catheter is passed through the nasal passage or into the side of the mouth. It should be curved down into the pharynx and suction applied when the child coughs or when the catheter is at the back of the pharynx. It may be necessary to pass the catheter further down into the trachea to stimulate a cough or remove the secretions.

Stop and think

Caution should be taken with nasopharyngeal suction in a child with stridor or who has been recently extubated, as the procedure may precipitate laryngospasm.

Continuous positive airway pressure (CPAP)

CPAP is a closed circuit system that delivers a raised airway pressure throughout the respiratory cycle. The child will breathe spontaneously while the system provides a constant positive end expiratory pressure (PEEP) in the airways.

Key features

- CPAP increases functional residual capacity (FRC) and pulmonary compliance and decreases airway resistance, allowing for a reduction in the work of breathing.
- It increases mean airway pressure in combination with increased FRC. This improves ventilation and perfusion relationships and potentially reduces oxygen requirements.
- It can help prevent further alveolar collapse and aides alveolar recruitment.
- Effective CPAP can complement and enhance the function of surfactant without interfering with spontaneous breathing.

Disadvantages

- CPAP increases mean airway pressure which can lead to reduced venous return.
- It can increase 'dead space' by impairing perfusion to hyperinflated areas.
- It can increase pulmonary vascular resistance and right heart dysfunction.

- It can alter renal blood flow with an increase in ADH release.
- It can cause barotraumas by increased airway pressure.

Care management

- CPAP is usually delivered non-invasively via a face mask or nasal cannulae or invasively via long nasal prongs or endotracheal tube (ETT).
- It is usually commenced at 4–6 cm H_2O, but this may increase depending on the child's condition and requirements.
- Check skin integrity around the nose and/or mouth and wash and dry 4–6 hourly, as pressure from equipment can cause reddening, excoriation and/or ulceration.

Top tips

For infants receiving CPAP the use of a dummy may be advantageous in helping to maintain the pressures generated by the circuit (by encouraging the infant to keep the lips together, thus forming a seal).

This must only be done after careful assessment of the infant's respiratory status and discussion with the infant's parents if the infant does not have a dummy when well.

Non-invasive ventilation (NIV)

Although NIV is increasing in popularity in paediatric settings, it is still not as commonly used as in the adult population. Differing manufacturers offer different options on bi-level non-invasive positive pressure ventilation and users should familiarise themselves with their specific equipment.

Bi-level non-invasive positive pressure ventilation alternates between two pressures, a higher one on inspiration (inspired positive airway pressure – IPAP) and a lower one on expiration (expired positive airway pressure – EPAP). This concept provides increased support during inspiration and creates less resistance on expiration, allowing larger volumes to enter and leave the lungs, thus improving carbon dioxide clearance.

In CPAP the level is often set at 5 cm H_2O, whereas in BIPAP commencement might be at IPAP 10 cm H_2O and EPAP 4 cm H_2O. By increasing the difference between IPAP and EPAP the 'pressure support' for each breath is increased, as well as the breath volume and carbon dioxide clearance. A back-up rate of 10–20 bpm is set; however, the infant's own respiratory pattern determines the ultimate rate.

Indications

The use of NIV may be indicated in any child with an acute or acute on chronic respiratory failure and no identified contraindications (see below). NIV is particularly worth considering in children with the following problems:

- Failure to wean/extubated from invasive ventilation
- Neuromuscular weakness/chest wall deformity
- Chronic lung disease, e.g. cystic fibrosis, broncho-pulmonary dysplasia
- Immunocompromised children, e.g. oncology or bone marrow transplant
- Cardiogenic pulmonary oedema
- Obstructive sleep apnoea

Contraindications

- Impaired consciousness
- Severe hypoxia
- Copious secretions
- Insecure airway, e.g. burns or epiglottitis
- Haemodynamic instability
- Respiratory arrest
- Vomiting
- Recent upper gastro-intestinal surgery
- Pneumothorax

Side effects

- Pressure sores on face, particularly the bridge of the nose
- Unprotected airway
- Gastric distension
- Intolerance of the system
- Volutrauma, e.g. pneumothorax
- Impaired venous return to the right ventricle
- Positive intrathoracic pressure can reduce ventricular filling pressure, causing hypotension

Care management

- Correct mask selection is crucial to the success of the therapy.
- Select the smallest mask that fits the child – use the sizing gauge that accompanies the machine. It may be necessary in a small child or infant to use an adult mask as a full face mask.
- Choose the correct size headgear and do not overtighten it – a leak is well compensated for by the machine.
- Release the mask every 2 hours. Wash the mask and the child's face regularly.
- Gastric distension is likely, so place the naso-/orogastric tube on free drainage and aspirate 2-hourly or as required.
- The child should have cardiovascular monitoring in place and observations recorded hourly (see Chapter 2), be cared for in an easily observed area, and have regular blood gas analysis.
- Carry out continual assessment of the child for improvement.

Intubation and principles of mechanical ventilation

If a child's condition deteriorates he/she may require intubation and ventilation for a period of time (see below). This should, wherever possible, be a planned and controlled procedure where all appropriate personnel, equipment and drugs are assembled.

Indications for intubation

- To maintain patency of the airway when actual or anticipated concern is present, e.g. airway trauma, oedema or infection
- To protect the airway from aspiration when the child has an altered level of consciousness or where airway-protective mechanisms are lost or impaired by injury or medication
- To facilitate pulmonary hygiene and avoid airway obstruction when atelectasis or pulmonary infection exists
- When positive pressure ventilation is necessary due to inadequate spontaneous ventilation
- To administer artificial surfactant therapy in the neonate diagnosed with surfactant deficiency

Adapted from Pryor and Prasad 2002.

Equipment required for intubation

- Face mask appropriate to child's size
- Oxygen and oxygen delivery system
- Stethoscope
- Oropharyngeal airway – correctly sized from the angle of jaw to centre of lips
- Yankeur suction catheter/fine bore suction catheters – to suction down ETT
- Working suction source (preferably main source)
- Laryngoscope with appropriate size and shaped blade:
  - Neonate – small straight blade
  - Small child – small curved blade
  - Older child – large curved blade

Note: Always check brightness of bulb prior to use.

- Paediatric Magill's forceps (for nasal intubation)
- Nasogastric tube
- Tape/ties/Duoderm® or Comfeel® to protect the skin
- End tidal CO_2 measurement (where possible – see Chapter 2)
- Endotracheal tubes (ETT) – see Table 3.5

Table 3.5 Considerations relating to endotracheal tubes.

Infants and children	Neonates
To estimate the size of ETT = age in years/4 + 4 = ETT size in mm (this refers to the internal diameter of the tube and only works when a child is 1 year old and above) To estimate the length of an oral ETT = age in years/2 + 12 cm To estimate the length of a nasal ETT = age in years/2 + 15 cm	~2 kg neonate Size 3.0 Fg tube, 7–8 cm at lips ~3 kg neonate Size 3.5 Fg tube, 8–9 cm at lips >3 kg neonate Size 3.5–4.0 Fg tube, 9–10 cm at lips An introducer may be inserted into the lumen to assist placement; however, this must not protrude beyond the end of the ETT as it can cause significant trauma to the neonate's airway

Adapted from International Guidelines for Neonatal Resuscitation (2000) and APLS (2005).

Note: Ensure one size above and one size below are available. Uncuffed ETTs are preferred up until approximately 8 years of age so as not to cause pressure and oedema at the cricoid ring, which may lead to stenosis.

Table 3.6 Common intubation drugs used in children.

Sedatives and narcotics	Morphine: 0.1–0.2 mg/kg IV Fentanyl: 1–5 μg/kg IV Midazolam: 0.1–0.2 mg/kg/dose IV
Anaesthetic agent	Ketamine: 0.5–2 mg/kg IV Thiopentone: 2–4 mg/kg IV
Neuromuscular blocking agent	Atracurium besylate: 0.5 mg/kg IV Vecuronium bromide: 0.1–0.15 mg/kg/dose IV Pancuronium bromide: 0.1–0.15 mg/kg/dose IV Suxamethonium: 1–2 mg/kg IV
Antimuscarinic	Atropine 20 μg/kg IV

Drugs for intubation will depend on practitioner preference and should be prescribed prior to the event. Examples of some commonly used drugs and doses are shown in Table 3.6. However, practitioners should refer to their local policies/guidelines and appropriate drug formularies such as the most recent British National Formulary (BNF) for Children. The administration of these drugs are incorporated into the intubation procedure as reviewed in Table 3.7.

Stop and think

Suxamethonium must not be used for children with renal failure or burns – it triggers the release of potassium which may cause a sudden rise in serum potassium levels and cardiac arrest.

In children with upper airway conditions such as croup and epiglottitis, inhalation anaesthetic agents are preferred to IV medications.

Stop and think

Intubation attempts should not last longer than 30 seconds. If unsuccessful remove the ETT and recommence bag-valve-mask ventilation/oxygenation.

If intubation attempts are unsuccessful and the child is clinically deteriorating, immediately seek senior help or put out an emergency call (if this has not already been done in response to the initial event necessitating intubation).

Tracheal suction

The recommended pressure that should be used for tracheal suction is 100–120 mmHg in children

Table 3.7 Guide to intubation – key steps in the procedure.

Intervention/action	Rationale
Prepare all equipment prior to commencing Ensure oxygen and suction equipment are available where the intubation is to occur, and that both are working	Thorough preparation of equipment can reduce the risks to the child during the procedure
Ensure appropriate monitoring is in place recording the child's heart rate, SpO_2 and blood pressure	Bradycardia and hypoxia are common side effects of intubation
Position the child appropriately and pre-oxygenate with 100% oxygen	The initial step of providing supplemental oxygen and basic airway manoeuvres must never be overlooked Good positioning will ensure the child's airway is patent Pre-oxygenation reduces the effects of possible hypoxia induced through the intubation
Give the prescribed drugs for intubation	The purpose of these drugs is for the child to experience no pain, to be unaware of the procedure and to be fully muscle relaxed. This reduces the risk of laryngospasm
The laryngoscope will be used to visualise the cords and when there is a clear view the ETT will then be passed into the trachea	Safe intubation practice
Observe the chest for equal, bilateral chest movement and if available attach end-tidal CO_2 monitor to confirm correct position of ETT	To ensure correct placement – it is possible that the tube may have been inserted into the oesophagus rather than the trachea
Resume hand ventilation and auscultate the chest for bilateral air entry	To ensure that the tube has not moved into either main stem bronchus
Cut tapes or assemble fixation device according to local policy as required and secure the tube in place	The tube will need to be secured to prevent accidental dislodgement when the child is moved or moves him-/herself
Apply skin protection, e.g. Duoderm®, to the child's face before any tape is applied	Skin of the infant and child is delicate and at risk of epidermal stripping after contact with strong adhesives (White and Denyer 2006)
Continue hand ventilation until child is placed on a mechanical ventilator	The child will be receiving sedative/analgesic agents and will therefore be unable to maintain effective ventilation him-/herself
Obtain a chest X-ray to confirm correct positioning of the ETT and nasogastric tube	Chest X-ray confirmation of tube placement is the gold standard in ensuring the safety of the child

Note: If not already in situ, pass a nasogastric tube which can be aspirated to deflate the stomach and reduce the risk of aspiration on intubation. In an emergency situation, however, this is normally done after the airway has been secured.

(Linton 2000). Table 3.8 gives a guide to the correct sized suction catheter to be used in relation to the ETT/tracheostomy tube size.

Principles of mechanical ventilation

The two key aims of mechanical ventilation are to maintain mean lung volumes and alveolar ventilation. Differing types of ventilators are available for use in paediatric care. These are described according to the ventilation variable in control during the inspiratory phase of each cycle (see section below).

Ventilator control settings

• Pressure controlled/limited – most infant ventilators are pressure controlled. Peak pressure

Table 3.8 Guide to suction catheter size. With French gauge (Fg) suction catheter, the size of catheter to use is double that of the tracheal tube size.

Endotracheal/ tracheostomy tube size (mm)	French gauge (Fg) suction catheter size
3.0	6
3.5	Ideally 7. Can use 6 or 8 depending on secretions
4.0	8
4.5	Can use 8 or 10 depending on secretions
5.0	10
5.5	Can use 10 or 12 depending on secretions
6.0	12
6.5	12
7.0	14

Note: If caring for a child over 50 kg or older than 15 years of age then adult guidelines may be used.

Table 3.9 Complications of mechanical ventilation.

Complication	Example
Air leak	Pneumothorax Pneumomediastinum Pneumoperitoneum Subcutaneous emphysema
Infection	Pneumonia
Airway	Dislodgement Occlusion Accidental extubation
Hyperinflation	Air trapping
Cardiovascular	Decreased venous return Decreased cardiac output Increased pulmonary vascular resistance
Mechanical	Ventilator malfunction Disconnection

remains constant, but tidal volumes change as lung compliance and resistance varies. There is a continuous gas flow that provides a gas source for spontaneous breaths.
- Volume controlled/limited – where the ventilator delivers a preset tidal volume. Airway pressure varies as compliance and resistance change.
- Pressure controlled and volume controlled – where either volume or pressure or a combination of both can be used to ventilate the child.

The mode of ventilation used or available will vary depending on the type of ventilator being used. The specific mode chosen to ventilate the child will depend on practitioner choice, experience and the condition of the child. Commonly used ventilator modes include:

- Intermittent mandatory ventilation (IMV)
- Synchronised intermittent mandatory ventilation (SIMV) – volume or pressure controlled
- Pressure controlled ventilation (PCV)
- Pressure support ventilation (PSV)
- Volume controlled ventilation

A number of short-term care management considerations and observations are required once mechanical ventilation is commenced. The complications associated with mechanical ventilation are detailed in Table 3.9.

- Respiratory assessment using visual assessment and auscultation
- Chest X-ray for ETT position, lung volumes and pathology, and position of nasogastric tube
- Arterial blood gas analysis – to assess pH, oxygenation and carbon dioxide levels
- Undertake and document cardio/respiratory monitoring
- Commence analgesia, sedation and muscle relaxants
- Undertake pulmonary hygiene as required. Consider diameter of the ETT and the secretions of the child. The smaller the tube and more tenacious the secretions the more regularly suctioning will be required
- Do not apply suction pressure as you introduce the catheter, only apply the suction pressure as you withdraw the catheter
- The process should take no more than 10 seconds

Table 3.10 Normal blood gas values.

Parameter	Arterial blood	Mixed venous blood	Capillary blood
pH	7.35–7.45	7.31–7.41	7.35–7.45
PO_2	80–100 mmHg (10.6–13.3 kPa)	35–40 mmHg (4.6–5.3 kPa)	Less than arterial
PCO_2	35–45 mmHg (4.6–6.0 kPa)	40–50 mmHg (5.3–6.6 kPa)	35–45 mmHg (4.6–6.0 kPa)
O_2 saturation	95–97%	70–75%	Less than arterial
HCO_3	22–27 mEq/L	20–27 mEq/L	20–27 mEq/L
Base excess	+2 to –2	+2 to –2	+2 to –2

See Chapter 2.

Note: Some areas prefer to express acidity in terms of hydrogen ions rather than the standard pH measurement noted in Table 3.10 (and also see Figure 3.1). Therefore it is important that practitioners are familiar with the terms and values used within their own clinical areas.

Introduction to blood gas analysis

Measurement of blood gases is an essential tool in the assessment and management of the respiratory status of children and their response to treatment. Normal blood gas values are noted in Table 3.10.

- pH is the term used to describe the acidity or alkalinity of a solution and is dependent on the concentrations of hydrogen ions (H^+) within the solution.
- pH is measured on a scale from 0 to 14, where 7 is neutral. A neutral solution, i.e. water, is one where the concentration of hydrogen ions and hydroxyl (OH^-) ions are equal.
- A pH below 7 = an acid solution, with more H^+ ions and less OH^- ions.
- A pH above 7 = an alkalotic solution, with less H^+ ions and more OH^- ions.

Blood gas result interpretation

A sequential approach to blood gas analysis can be helpful when reviewing results. This can be broken down into a number of easy steps, as shown in Figure 3.1.

A blood gas measurement outside the normal indices can indicate the nature of a problem. In the acutely unwell infant or child it is more likely that the primary imbalance will be an acidosis, which may be either respiratory in origin, metabolic in origin or a mixed picture (see Table 3.11).

Additional values

Oxygenation
Consideration will need to be given to the child's oxygenation status indicated by the PaO_2 (for arterial blood gases). If the child (in the absence of a cyanotic cardiac lesion or known chronic oxygen demand) has a PaO_2 of less than 80 mmHg (10.6 kPa) then hypoxia is present.

Lactate
An increased lactate value above 2 can be indicative of poor tissue perfusion and the presence of anaerobic (in the absence of oxygen) metabolism which may be related to poor cardiac performance or intravascular volume depletion. As with any single tool for clinical assessment the results should not be considered in isolation but

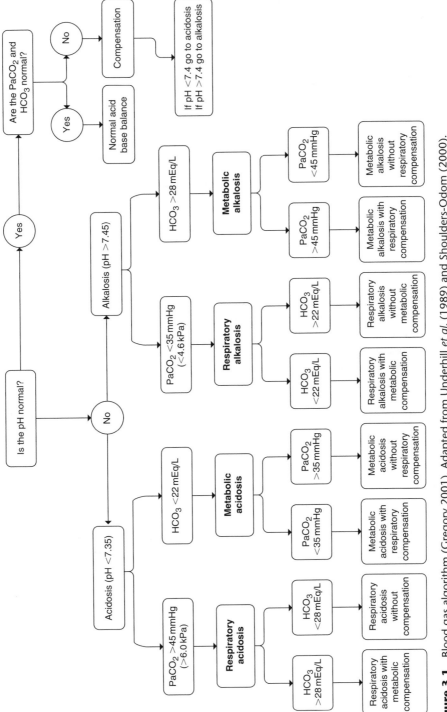

Figure 3.1 Blood gas algorithm (Gregory 2001). Adapted from Underhill *et al.* (1989) and Shoulders-Odom (2000).

Table 3.11 Summary of the alteration in blood gas indices.

Indices	pH	pCO$_2$	HCO$_3^-$	BE
Respiratory acidosis	Low (<7.35)	High	Normal	Normal
Respiratory alkalosis	High (>7.45)	Low	Normal	Normal
Metabolic acidosis	Low	Normal	Low	Low (–ve)
Metabolic alkalosis	High	Normal	High	High (+ve)
Mixed acidosis	Low	High	Low	Low

in conjunction with a thorough evaluation of the child's condition.

Nursing management of a child with a tracheostomy

A number of children who have specific clinical conditions and the need for long-term ventilatory support will have a tracheostomy (artificial airway) (Table 3.12). A tracheostomy tube is usually inserted through a surgical incision made in the trachea just below the vocal cords.

Many children who may be admitted to the HDU with a tracheostomy will have an established stoma. However, you may encounter children who have only just undergone tracheostomy formation. In either case the bed space must contain the following emergency equipment:

- Tracheal dilators
- Spare tracheostomy tubes – one same size/one a size smaller
- Stitch cutters (if new tracheostomy)
- 10-mL syringe for cuff deflation (if child has cuffed tube *in situ*)
- Collar and/or tape
- One Lyofoam® dressing (or the dressings being used by the child)
- Water-based lubricant

In addition there must be all the equipment necessary to provide suction:

- Suction unit – (suction pressure <120 mmHg)

Table 3.12 Examples of conditions in which children may require a tracheostomy.

Classifications	Example
Congenital malformations	Subglottic stenosis Tracheal stenosis Micrognathia (underdeveloped mandible) associated with Pierre–Robin syndrome/Treacher–Collins syndrome Laryngeal web Haemangioma/cystic hygroma
Acquired airway problems	Subglottic stenosis (after long-term intubation) Airway obstruction secondary to acute infection, e.g. epiglottitis Airway obstruction secondary to foreign body inhalation Tumours affecting head and/or neck
Other	Post-traumatic brain injury – poor or absent protective reflexes Guillain–Barré syndrome Degenerative neuromuscular disorders

- Suction catheters (appropriate catheter size; see Table 3.8 for further information)
- Oxygen supply tracheal mask and/or bagging circuit/Ambubag
- Syringes – 5 mL or 10 mL
- 0.9% Saline for irrigation
- Gloves
- Aprons and eye protection
- Pulse oximeter (if the child is receiving oxygen therapy)
- Yankeur sucker

- Clinical waste bin for disposal of used catheters
- Tap water in clean container
- Tracheostomy care record sheet

A technique for performing suction via a tracheostomy is suggested below. However, local policies and/or guidelines should be used wherever they are available.

- Be alert for signs of the need to perform suction.
- Wear gloves, apron and eye protection.
- Use a clean, non-touch technique.
- Ask patient to take a couple of deep breaths (if appropriate age) or pre-oxygenate if required.
- Insert catheter without suction up to 0.5 cm from the end of the tube.
- Apply suction gently, withdraw the catheter but do not rotate. This process should take no longer than 5–10 seconds.
- Once the catheter is withdrawn allow the patient to breathe and recover before suctioning again.

Top tip

If secretions are very thick and sticky the catheter may be inserted to the end of the tube or up to 0.5 cm beyond the end of the tube.

This should not be undertaken routinely.

- Dispose of catheter and glove in an appropriate bag as per local guidelines.
- Repeat suctioning if required using clean gloves and suction catheter.
- Record outcome and observe for changes in mucus, colour and smell. Report findings and prepare to send specimen.
- Rinse suction connection tubing with water after suctioning and connect new catheter.

The major complications associated with a tracheostomy tube normally relate to mechanical problems relating to the actual tube, i.e. it is blocked, dislodged or displaced.

In each of these scenarios the priority is to establish a patent airway for the child, and therefore prompt action is required. Flow charts for the management of the child with a tracheostomy are shown in Figures 3.2–3.4.

Care of a child with an intra-pleural chest drain

A chest drain is used to drain any abnormal collection of fluid or air from the thoracic cavity. Indications for insertion include the presence of conditions outlined in Table 3.13.

Children may require drain insertion post thoracic or cardiac surgical procedure. This section will focus on the care of intrapleural drains rather than those inserted into the mediastinum post cardiac surgery. A chest drain will be inserted into the pleural space either in an apical position to remove air or in a basal position to remove fluid. The chest drain will be attached to tubing that feeds into a drainage bottle, the end of which is under water. This creates a siphon effect that will draw air or fluid to a lower level. It is essential therefore that the chest drain bottle remains lower than the child's chest, to prevent the content of the bottle being siphoned back into the pleura. The water in the bottle creates an 'underwater seal' which prevents air entering the pleural space. A second tube will lead out from the collection chamber of the drainage bottle and will either remain open to air or be attached to low flow suction.

Nursing care and assessment of a child with a chest drain

Fluid level and type of fluid in the chest drain bottle

Hourly measurements of fluid drainage must be recorded, together with documentation of the type of fluid draining. If the fluid becomes blood stained or changes dramatically it must be reported immediately. If it becomes cloudy, it

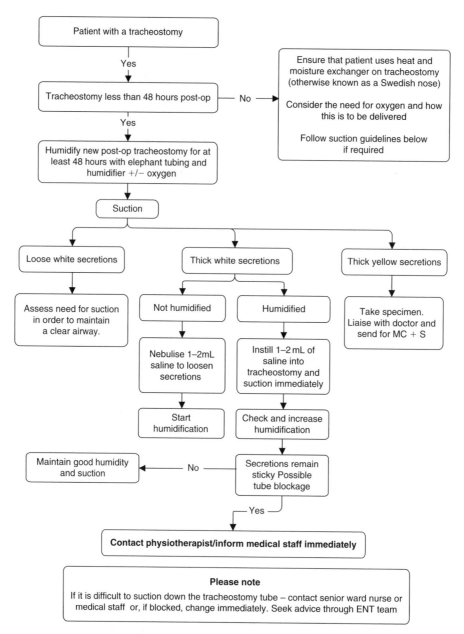

Figure 3.2 Flow chart for tracheostomy care.

may be infected and a specimen should be sent for culture and sensitivity.

Fluid swing
A 'fluid swing' should be present in the chest tubing during inspiration and expiration. This

should be documented and if not present could indicate a blockage of the tube.

Bubble or air leak
'Bubbling' of the water in the chest drain bottle will be present if the drain has been inserted to

Changing of tracheostomy tubes must always be a two person procedure with each individual having a clear understanding of their role

Rationale
- To prevent a buildup of secretions within the tube
- To prevent infections of the trachea and stoma
- To maintain patient safety throughout procedure

When
- First post-operative tube change is usually performed by the ENT surgeon
- Tubes changed weekly or more frequently as necessary

Equipment required	
- Material roll (blanket or towel)	- New dressing
- New tracheostomy tube of the same size	- Sterile saline
- New tracheostomy tube 1 size smaller in case of difficulty during insertion	- New tracheostomy tapes/Velcro holder
- Sterile lubricant – optional (water based gel or saline)	- Gloves
Tracheal dilators (for emergency use)	- Working oxygen delivery system
	- Working oxygen delivery system
	Round-ended scissors

Changing tracheostomy tubes
Step by step guide

1   Prepare the new tube with clean tapes or Velcro ties. (The use of twill (strong cotton) tapes or Velcro ties to secure the child's tracheostomy tube will depend upon individual hospital/unit policies and the preference of the child (where appropriate) and their parents/caregivers. This information should be documented in the child's nursing notes to ensure there is continuity in care.)
2   Perform suction if required.
3   Place roll under the shoulders to expose neck.
4   Remove soiled dressing and clean around stoma site (see Figure 3.4).
5   With a colleague holding the tube securely in position, cut tapes with round-ended scissors.
6   With a colleague holding the child still, remove the tube.
7   Insert newly prepared tube (anatomical insertion i.e. tube in line with direction of trachea). NB: Occasionally the stoma may require dilation using the tracheal dilators; in this event call for senior assistance.
8   Remove introducer.
9   Secure the tie furthest away first, then repeat this procedure with tie closest to you, leaving sufficient room to insert the dressing.
10 Insert new dressing, then check overall fit – the gentle insertion of a single finger between the tapes and the child's neck indicates an appropriate fit.

Figure 3.3 Changing tracheostomy tubes.

resolve a pneumothorax and will continue until it has resolved.

Respiratory status
Continual assessment of the child's respiratory status whilst the drain is *in situ* is essential to identify and prevent complications.

Infection
A chest drain is a source of infection for the child and the longer the drain remains *in situ* the greater the risk. Observation of the fluid drainage, as indicated above, is essential, as well as monitoring the child's cardiovascular status for signs of infection, noting any complaint of pain

As when changing a tracheotomy tube, changing of tapes must always be a two person procedure with each person having a clear understanding of their role	
Rationale	
• To keep the neck clean and dry, reducing the risk of skin irritation and infection • To maintain patient safety throughout the procedure	
When	
• Daily or if wet or soiled	
Equipment required	
• Roll to go under the neck e.g. towel or blanket • Tapes (twill) cut to size or Velcro holders • Gloves • Round ended scissors • Gauze swabs	• Sterile saline • Sterile dressing • Tracheal dilators for emergency use • Spare tubes for emergency use • Working suction equipment

Changing tracheostomy tapes/Velcro holders and fasteners
Step by step guide

1	Wash hands.
2	Perform suction if required.
3	Carefully remove soiled dressing and dispose as per local guidelines.
4	Clean area – use saline soaked swabs, starting at stoma site and sweeping outwards. Gently dry.
5	Place clean holders behind neck.
6	Place roll under child's shoulders to expose neck.
7	With your colleague holding the tube securely in position, undo the tie furthest away; immediately attach new tie and secure.
8	Repeat this procedure with the tie closest to you leaving sufficient room to insert the dressing.
9	Insert new dressing then check overall fit – the gentle insertion of a single finger between the tapes and the child's neck indicates an appropriate fit.

Figure 3.4 Changing tracheostomy tapes/Velcro holders and fasteners.

Table 3.13 Indications for chest drain insertion.

Condition	Definition
Simple pneumothorax	The presence of air or gas in the pleural cavity between the visceral and parietal pleura. There is a variable amount of lung collapse dependent on the size of the pneumothorax
Tension pneumothorax	Tension pneumothorax is a life-threatening emergency. It is caused when air enters the pleural space during inspiration but cannot exit during exhalation. There is significant cardiovascular impairment associated with a tension pneumothorax, which can if untreated lead to cardiac arrest
Haemothorax	Haemothorax is a collection of blood in the pleural space and may be caused by blunt or penetrating trauma
Pleural effusion	Pleural effusion is defined as an abnormal accumulation of fluid in the pleural space
Empyema	A collection of pus in the cavity between the lung and the membrane that surrounds it
Chylothorax	A chylothorax will occur due to the presence of lymphatic fluid in the pleural space secondary to leakage from the thoracic duct or one of its main tributaries

or discomfort, and observing for any inflammation or signs of infection around the entry site.

Dressings

This depends upon individual hospital guidelines; some advocate airtight dressings, others gauze keyhole dressings or transparent bio-occlusive dressings. Irrespective of the dressing, the tubing should be securely fixed to the child, to prevent accidental dislodgement, and the entry site should be easily visualised.

Pain management

Chest drains can be uncomfortable and restricting and can prevent the child breathing deeply and coughing. Regular pain assessment and treatment should be an integral part of chest drain management.

Mobilisation

Encouragement to mobilise, move and take deep breaths is recommended, based upon the clinical condition of the individual child. It is important that the drain is kept below thoracic level at all times.

Continuous low-grade suction

This may be required if the pneumothorax is large and to ensure the drainage exceeds the air leak. Suction pressures applied to pleural drains must be delivered via a low flow suction device. The drain must never be attached to the suction unit used for airway suctioning.

Milking/stripping the tubing

The chest drain *should never* be milked or stripped unless it is blocked and the decision specifically made to do so. Milking a drain will increase the intrathoracic pressure and may cause further pneumothoraces or a tension pneumothorax.

Clamping

A chest drain should only be clamped when the bottle is being changed or a specimen being taken.

It *should never* be clamped when moving a patient as this may cause a tension pneumothorax.

Changing a chest drain bottle

This should only be undertaken when the bottle is full. Regular and unnecessary breaking of the underwater seal increases the risk of introducing infection.

Top tips

As noted above it is important that the chest drain is kept below thoracic level at all times.

Heimlich or sealed valves can be used in place of underwater sealed chest drain bottles, however only where there is no active fluid drainage. They can be particularly useful when transporting the child.

Complications of pleural drains

- Infection
- Blocked drain
- Air leak from insertion site
- Tension pneumothorax
- Displaced drain
- Surgical emphysema
- Pain

Drain removal

- The chest drain will be removed when the lung has re-expanded, the air leak resolved or the drainage ceased.
- After an appropriate explanation has been given to the child and family and analgesia administered as prescribed, the stay sutures should be removed.
- The chest drain should be removed during expiration. Pleural pressure is +1 cm in expiration and −4 cm in inspiration. Pressure within the intrapleural space will be higher than atmospheric air and therefore there will be a reduced risk of air entrapment. This will

therefore reduce the risk of a pneumothorax developing. While this is the optimum method of chest drain removal it is acknowledged that it is dependent on the age and co-operation of the child.

- The purse string suture should be gently tied to prevent skin puckering, which could then lead to scarring.
- Steristrips should be applied if skin closure around the entry site has not occurred with the purse string suture and a dry gauze dressing applied.

Appendix

The treatment and management of acute respiratory conditions is explained in Table A1. Table A2 tabulates common drugs and their mode of delivery.

Table A1 Acute respiratory conditions – treatment and management.

Condition	Definition and Cause	Clinical manifestations	Diagnostic tests	Treatment and Management
Asthma	A chronic inflammatory disorder of the airway with acute exacerbations and increased airway responsiveness to stimuli Inflammation during acute episodes causes bronchial constriction, airway swelling and mucus production Mucus clogs the small airways, trapping air below the plugs Decreased perfusion of the alveolar capillaries leads to hypoxaemia Repeated episodes of bronchospasm, mucosal oedema and mucous plugging cause chronic inflammation	Productive cough Expiratory wheeze Shortness of breath Rapid and laboured respirations Respiratory fatigue Nasal flaring Intercostal recession Decreased air movement Chest tightness Head bobbing when using accessory muscles Agitation and irritability due to hypoxia and side effects of medication Inability to converse Pallor, mottled or cyanosed	History, signs and symptoms Chest X-ray Peak flow expiratory flow rate (PEFR) or spirometer test	Assess airway/breathing/circulation Administer humidification and supplemental oxygen Nebulised bronchodilators and oral steroids – if severe use IV mediations Continue respiratory assessment Continue SpO_2 and cardio-respiratory monitoring Assess PEFR Carry out blood gas analysis Manage hydration fluids and balance Offer supportive care
Bronchiolitis	Inflammation and obstruction of the bronchioles Causes: respiratory syncytial virus (RSV), bacteria, Mycoplasma RSV is commonest cause in infants and most severe in those <6 months, born prematurely, with chronic lung disease, congenital heart disease or immunodeficiency	Sharp, dry cough Tachypnoea Inspiratory and expiratory wheeze Nasal flaring Marked intercostal and subcostal recession Fine end-inspiratory crackles Fever and tachycardia Mottling progressing to cyanosis Irregular breathing pattern/recurrent apnoeas Decreased breath sounds	Nasopharyngeal aspiration – direct fluorescent assay Chest X-ray shows hyperinflation, air trapping and patchy atelectasis Blood gas analysis will show lowered arterial oxygenation and raised carbon dioxide levels	Humidified oxygen Cardio/respiratory monitoring SpO_2 monitoring Positioning with head up. Minimal handling Intubation and mechanical ventilation if in severe respiratory distress Hydration with IV or oral fluids Nebulised epinephrine (adrenaline) and steroids are used, but their value is inconclusive Nebulised bronchodilators have not been shown to reduce severity or duration of illness The antiviral drug Ribavirin marginally shortens viral excretion and clinical symptoms

(Continued)

Table A1 Continued.

Condition	Definition and Cause	Clinical manifestations	Diagnostic tests	Treatment and Management
Pneumonia	Inflammation or infection of the bronchioles and alveolar sacs of the lungs Causes: viral, bacterial, Mycoplasma or fungal infections	History and signs and symptoms Fever Cough Tachypnoea Grunting on expiration Pleuritic chest pain, neck stiffness and abdominal pain if pleural inflammation is present Lethargy Consolidation on chest X-ray Dullness on percussion Decreased breath sounds and bronchial breathing often absent	Blood culture Nasopharyngeal aspirate for viral isolation	Assess airway/respiratory status Administer humidification and supplemental oxygen as required Administer IV or oral antibiotics – depending on disease severity Pain management Physiotherapy Hydration
Pertussis (whooping cough)	A specific and infectious form of bronchitis Cause: Bordetella pertussis Transmitted by respiratory droplet and direct contact with discharge from the respiratory mucous membranes Incubation is 7–21 days Most contagious before the paroxysmal cough stage	Paroxysmal or spasmodic cough followed by a characteristic inspiratory whoop Cough spasms are often worse at night and may culminate in vomiting During a paroxysm the child goes red and/or blue in the face and mucus flows from the nose and mouth. Epistaxis and subconjunctival haemorrhages can occur with vigorous coughing	The organism can be identified on a per-nasal swab	Assess airway/respiratory status Administer humidification and supplemental oxygen Sit the child up and forward and give additional oxygen during a paroxysm Administer IV antibiotics as prescribed Offer supportive care

	Laryngotracheobronchitis (Croup)	Epiglottitis
	Viral illness affecting larynx trachea and bronchi Common in children between 3 months and 4 years old Causes: parainfluenza type I, II and III; influenzae A and B; adenovirus; RSV Inflammation and oedema narrow the subglottic area of the airway	An acute and life-threatening condition Cause: *Haemophilus influenzae* type b (the introduction of the HIB vaccination has significantly reduced the incidence of this infection) Intense swelling of the epiglottis and surrounding tissue, with associated septicaemia Most common in 1–6 year olds but can affect any age
	Cough and hoarseness Low-grade fever Tachypnoea Inspiratory stridor Seal-like barking cough Progression of symptoms include: Expiratory stridor Severe tachypnoea Recession Exhaustion	Can present with similar signs and symptoms to viral croup, but treatment is very different Very acute onset High temperature Toxic-looking child Intensely painful throat that prevents the child from talking or swallowing; saliva drools down chin Soft inspiratory stridor Tachypnoea Child will sit in an upright position with an open mouth, to optimise airway
	History and clinical signs No throat cultures or visual inspection of the mouth should be undertaken due to the possible initiation of laryngospasm	History, signs and symptoms No attempt to lie the child down, examine the throat or perform a lateral neck X-ray should be made as they can precipitate total airway obstruction and death Once the airway has been secured and the child is in a safe environment, blood cultures can be taken
	Assess airway/respiratory status Administer humidification and supplemental oxygen Monitor for airway obstruction and respiratory distress Beta-agonists and beta-adrenergics, e.g. salbutamol and epinephrine (adrenaline) If airway compromise or obstruction is severe, intubation and ventilation may be required Monitor conscious level Administer medications as prescribed Allow child to find the most comfortable position to maintain airway patency	Keep the child calm Administer oxygen only if the child allows Monitor respiratory status Once diagnosis has been made, immediate intubation in a controlled and safe environment, by a senior, experienced anaesthetist is required Intubation and mechanical ventilation (usually only required for 24 hours) Administer IV antibiotic and fluid therapy Prophylaxis with Rifampicin should be offered to close family members

(Continued)

Table A1 Continued.

Condition	Definition and Cause	Clinical manifestations	Diagnostic tests	Treatment and Management
Bacterial tracheitis	A secondary infection of the upper trachea flowing viral laryngotracheitis Causes: *Staphylococcus aureus*, *Haemophilus influenzae* Subglottic area is oedematous and ulcerated Thick muco-purulent exudates may obstruct the trachea/bronchi and are evident at tracheal intubation	High temperature Tachypnoea Tachycardia Respiratory distress Toxic in appearance	Blood culture	Administer humidified oxygen Allow child to find the most comfortable position to maintain airway patency Intubation and mechanical ventilation is usually required Administer IV antibiotic and fluid therapy
Bronchopulmonary dysplasia (BPD) (chronic lung disease)	A chronic lung disease caused by the need for positive pressure ventilation and oxygen therapy for respiratory distress syndrome, which causes inflammatory changes in the airways and persistent hypoxia in the neonatal period	Signs of respiratory distress: tachypnoea, wheezing, crackles, nasal flaring, grunting, recession, irritability, pulmonary oedema and failure to thrive Intermittent bronchospasm and mucous plugging leads to persistent air trapping Episodes of sudden respiratory deterioration with dusky or cyanotic colour, agitation and limited expiratory air flow	Chest X-ray shows hyperexpansion, atelectasis and interstitial thickening	Assess airway/respiratory status Administer humidification and supplemental oxygen Monitor for airway obstruction and increased respiratory distress Physiotherapy may help to clear the airways A tracheostomy for long-term airway management may be required Increase caloric intake to promote growth and development Administer prescribed medication, e.g. diuretics, bronchodilators, anti-inflammatory drugs and corticosteroids

Table A2 Common drug therapy.

	Drug	Method of delivery and dosage	Points of note
Bronchodilators	Aminophylline[a]	Oral or IV	If receiving IV aminophylline, the child must be on a cardiac monitor, observing for tachycardia and/or ectopic beats Monitor blood levels of K^+ – this can be low Check blood levels to ensure they are within the therapeutic range
	Theophylline[a]	Oral	Helps relax airway muscles by stopping mast cells in the lining of the air passages from releasing chemicals that cause muscle spasm and bronchoconstriction
	Salbutamol[a]	Nebuliser or IV	If receiving IV salbutamol, the child must be on a cardiac monitor, observing for tachycardia and/or ectopic beats
	Ipratropium bromide (Atrovent)[a]	Nebuliser	Monitor peak expiratory flow rate (PEFR)
Corticosteroid therapy	Budesonide[a]	Nebuliser	Corticosteroids act within the body's cells to decrease the release of chemicals involved in the immune system, which initiate an inflammatory reaction. By decreasing the release of these chemicals, corticosteroids help to reduce inflammation
	Dexamethasone[a]	Oral or IV	Use in children with croup to help reduce airway inflammation
	Prednisolone[a]	Oral	Check blood glucose levels if doses are increasing
	Hydrocortisone[a]	IV	Check blood glucose levels if doses are increasing
Respiratory stimulant	Caffeine citrate[a]	Oral or IV	Helps increase central respiratory drive
Mucolytic agents	Dornase Alfa (rhDNAse)[a]	Nebuliser	Used primarily in children with cystic fibrosis or those with thick respiratory secretions For use in children >5 years old
Other	Epinephrine (adrenaline)[a]	Nebuliser	Use 1–5 mL 1:1000 strength epinephrine (adrenaline) Produces a transient improvement in airway patency and can have a dramatic rebound effect. Observe closely with cardio-respiratory monitoring and SpO_2

[a] For clarification on delivery and dosage see British National Formulary for Children (2007) BMJ Books. London

Note: Nebuliser therapy – in an acutely ill child, nebuliser therapy should *always* use oxygen (unless specifically stated) to produce an aerosol of a drug in solution, which can then be inhaled either by a mask or mouthpiece into the airway.

Chapter 4

CARDIAC

Sandra Batcheler and Michaela Dixon

Introduction

Primary disease of the cardiovascular system in children may be attributed to the presence of a structural lesion such as those seen in congenital heart disease (CHD), as a component of a syndrome, e.g. Barth's syndrome, which is a combination of cardiomyopathy, neutropenia, general weakness and faltering growth, or as a consequence of an infective process. It is rare that primary cardiovascular disease in children can be linked to lifestyle such as those disorders that affect the adult population.

Cardiovascular performance in the acutely unwell child is often decreased secondary to hypoxia, acidosis or the presence of both. Effective assessment, recognition of the factors affecting cardiovascular performance and timely management are all essential in preventing further deterioration in the child's condition.

Development of the cardiovascular system

The embryological development of the whole cardiovascular system is a topic that is beyond the remit of this chapter, given the complexity of the structures involved. This section identifies the key stages in the development of the heart (Table 4.1) and its associated structures but will not look at the development of the vascular (veins and arteries) system. Failure of any of these key stages may lead to the development of certain congenital heart lesions; however, the exact mechanism for the lack of completion of one or more of these stages is not always clear (see section on 'Congenital Heart Disease').

Overview of cardiac anatomy and physiology

The basic anatomical structures of the heart are essentially the same across the age range from infant to adult. There are a number of important limitations based on size and immaturity of the contractile fibres (myofibrils) which influence the ability of the heart to modify its performance to meet the increased demands placed upon it when the child is unwell.

- At birth the two cardiac ventricles are of a similar weight.
- By 2 months of age the RV/LV weight ratio is 0.5:1 and by the age of 1 year the relative sizes of the ventricles are approximate to that of the adult heart ratio 1:2 (RV:LV).
- The infant's ECG reflects these changes:
  - 0–3 months: RV dominance is apparent;
  - 4–6 months: LV dominance is evident.
- As the heart develops during childhood, the size of the P wave and QRS complexes increases and the P–R interval and QRS duration become longer.

Table 4.1 Embryological and fetal development of the heart and its associated structures.

Gestational age	Development
Up to 21 days	The origin of cardiac tissue is the mesoderm of the embryo. Around day 18, during the third gestational week, a crescent or arch of mesoderm is formed from a pair of endothelial tubes The endothelial tubes fuse and grow, establishing a single straight primitive heart tube at around day 20 A rhythmic ebb and flow of blood (which precedes heart beats) is a chief characteristic of the primitive heart
Days 21–28	The heart twists, loops to the right and develops from two lateral endothelial tubes into the beginnings of four chambers with blood flow through them and a truncus arteriosus. Looping to the right known as dextro or D looping results in the right ventricle (RV) lying to the right of the primitive left ventricle (LV) (anatomically correct) Looping to the left (levo or L looping) results in ventricular inversion
Weeks 4–5 gestation	Two truncal swellings combine and the aorticopulmonary (or truncal) septum will complete the division of the common ventricular outflow tract into the pulmonary artery and the aorta Atrial septation also occurs at week 4. The ostium primum and the ostium secundum divide the atria into left and right, with just the flap-like structure of the foramen ovale allowing blood to flow through the septum from right to left atrium *Endocardial cushions* are areas of the fibrous skeleton which form between the atrium and ventricle. They serve two important functions: (1) They form a partition in the heart tube between the atrium and ventricle known as the AV canal. The resulting two channels represent sites for the future tricuspid and bicuspid valves (2) They provide a 'scaffold' to which the interatrial septae and the interventricular septum will grow towards and fuse with
Weeks 4–8 gestation	The ventricles fuse, forming the muscular portion of the ventricular septum. This then grows towards the endocardial cushion whilst the endocardial cushion itself and conal swellings from the base of the truncus also develop towards the muscular septum to complete septation Over the next 3 weeks a number of key stages occur which complete individual atrial and ventricular development, septation and the establishment of separate outflow tracts (aorta and PA)
Weeks 8–12 gestation	By the end of week 8 the structural development of the heart is complete Refinement and continued development of the atrioventricular valves (mainly tricuspid valve) continues to about 12 weeks' gestation

Sources: Curley and Moloney-Harmon (2001); Moore and Persaud (2003); Abdulla *et al.* (2004).

- Infants have a small stroke volume – 1.5 mL/kg at birth.
- Stroke volume increases as the heart grows.
- As stroke volume is relatively fixed in infants and small children, cardiac output is determined by heart rate. Heart rate is inversely proportional to age (see Table 4.2).
- By the age of 2, myocardial function is similar to that of an adult.

Table 4.2 Range of normal heart rate values.

Age range	Awake heart rate	Sleeping heart rate
Neonate	100–180	80–160
<2 years	100–160	75–160
2–5 years	80–110	60–90
5–12 years	65–110	60–90
>12 years	60–90	50–90

Stop and think

Prolonged tachycardia in infants and small children will reduce cardiac output as the time for coronary artery perfusion and ventricular filling will be decreased.

Both of these occur during the diastolic component of the cardiac cycle which is reduced in the presence of a tachycardia.

- Systemic vascular resistance: this rises after birth and continues to rise until adulthood is reached – this is reflected in blood pressure values seen in infants and children (see Table 4.3).
- Circulating blood volume is higher per kilogramme of body weight (70–80 mL/kg) than that of adults but involves much smaller actual volumes; therefore neonates and infants are at greater risk with fluid loss.
- Myocardial cells in infants are smaller and have an increased number of non-contractile elements.
- Degree/velocity of fibre shortening is less in the newborn heart and therefore less force is generated.
- Increased afterload decreases functional capacity far quicker in neonates than in the mature heart.
- Newborn myocardium lacks complete development of sympathetic innervation, but parasympathetic innervation is complete at birth.
- Cardiac stores of noradrenaline in the ventricular myocardium are less; therefore there is a limited response in the neonate to alter contractility.
- Neonatal hearts function at near capacity with minimal reserves.

Cardiac assessment

Apart from blood pressure, heart rate, pulse character and rhythm there are several other means by which the nurse can assess the condition of the child's cardiac system. How alert, responsive and well developed the child is may seem to be crude indicators, but they are indicative of a child's wellbeing and physiological stability. Significant heart disease restricts growth and development. Children may be mottled, cyanosed, pale or plethoric depending on how well perfused they are, how much haemoglobin they have in circulation and how well this is saturated with oxygen. The skin should be dry to touch and not sweaty. The child may have oedema, and this swelling may be centrally generalised, gravitationally dependent or restricted to the peripheral parts. It may be worse at certain times of the day, may indent and leave the imprint of fingers if touched.

Experienced nurses may choose to auscultate and listen for any deviation from the normal heart sounds heard as a result of the closure of the cardiac valves. Murmurs are caused by turbulence in the flow of blood in the heart. Some are innocent; they are graded 1–6 according to how loud they are and if there is a thrill present. A thrill is a palpable murmur and is always abnormal.

Sluggish capillary refill is an indication of poor peripheral circulation or if central a late sign of shock. Finger and toe clubbing is indicative of a long-standing condition in which there is ongoing cyanosis.

Table 4.3 Range of systolic blood pressure values based on age.

Age (years)	Systolic blood pressure (mmHg)
<1	70–90
1–2	80–95
2–5	80–110
5–12	90–110
>12	100–120

Blood pressure quick calculation: 80 + (2 × age in years) = systolic value.

The shocked child

In the HDU, the recognition and prompt management of the shocked child are paramount to effecting a good recovery. An understanding of the underlying physiological processes involved provides practitioners with the rationale for their interventions. It is important therefore to consider the following issues:

- Definition of shock – types of and common causes in children
- The shock process
- Recognition of a shocked child
- Management of a child in shock

Definition of shock

A wide range of shock definitions are available; however, they all acknowledge the following process as being key to the development of shock: an inability or failure of the cardiovascular system to deliver adequate amounts of essential nutrients, especially oxygen, to meet the metabolic needs of the cells, or impaired use of essential cellular substrates by the cells themselves. In addition to this there is impaired clearance of the by-products of cellular metabolism.

Shock is a complex progressive syndrome which, without appropriate management, will lead to continued deterioration in the child's condition. There are a number of different types of shock, which are summarised in Table 4.4 along with some of the common causes seen in the child.

The shock process

The shock process can be divided into three distinct phases each with their own specific clinical signs as a consequence of physiological processes occurring within the body. The three phases are:

- Compensated
- Uncompensated
- Irreversible

Table 4.4 Types and common causes of shock in children.

Type of shock	Common causes
Hypovolaemic	Diarrhoea and vomiting Peritonitis Burns Haemorrhage
Septic	Bacterial infection Meningococcal disease *Varicella* infection Pneumococcal disease
Anaphylactic	Exposure to triggering allergen Peanuts Eggs Milk products
Cardiogenic	Cardiomyopathy Dysrhythmias Heart failure Myocardial infarction/contusion Congenital heart disease
Obstructive (flow restrictive)	Tension pneumothorax Haemopneumothorax Cardiac tamponade Flail chest
Dissociative (tissue perfusion is adequate but oxygen release is abnormal)	Carbon monoxide poisoning
Neurogenic (changes in systemic vascular resistance and a loss of arterial and venous tone)	Head injury Spinal cord injury (rare in children)

Compensated shock

As a response to the causative mechanism the body triggers a series of compensatory pathways involving the sympathetic nervous system (SNS). The responses seen are present irrespective of the cause of shock.

This is known as the 'fight or flight' mechanism and its aim is to preserve vital brain and cardiac function, thereby ensuring survival. The key hormone responsible for the majority of the changes seen is *adrenaline* along with *noradrenaline*, adrenocorticotrophic hormone (ACTH), cortisol and many others.

Key physiological events/changes of the 'fight or flight' mechanism

- Heart rate and blood pressure increase.
- Pupils dilate (to take in as much light as possible).
- Veins in skin constrict to send more blood to major muscle groups (responsible for the 'chill' sometimes associated with fear – less blood in the skin to keep it warm).
- Blood-glucose level increases.
- Smooth muscle relaxes in order to allow more oxygen into the lungs.
- Muscles tense up, energised by adrenaline and glucose (responsible for goose bumps – when tiny muscles attached to each hair on the surface of skin tense up, the hairs are forced upright, pulling skin with them).
- Non-essential systems (like digestion and the immune system) shut down to allow more energy for emergency functions.
- Trouble focusing on small tasks (brain is directed to focus only on the big picture in order to determine where the threat is coming from).

Clinical presentation – key signs to note

- Tachycardia
- Decreased urine output
- Increased respiratory rate and increased depth of each breath
- Relative hyperglycaemia
- Cool peripheries
- Normal-for-age blood pressure values on sequential readings. (*Note*: A single blood pressure reading is of little help except in establishing a baseline value. Frequent reassessment is important in the management of the shocked child)

Stop and think

Hypotension is a late and worrying sign in the unwell child. Always seek advice from more senior staff if you are concerned and/or uncertain.

Uncompensated shock

The compensatory pathways of the 'flight or fight' mechanism fail to maintain adequate perfusion to the tissues and as a consequence some significant changes occur at a cellular level.

Normal cellular metabolism takes place in the presence of oxygen. This is known as aerobic metabolism. As cellular energy demands now have to be met in a state of reduced oxygen delivery or in the complete absence of oxygen, metabolism switches from aerobic to anaerobic and there is a buildup of lactic acid.

There is an overall energy deficit at the cellular level because anaerobic metabolism is a very inefficient mechanism which does not adequately meet the energy needs of the cell. Consequences of this changed state of metabolism are shown in Figure 4.1.

Clinical presentation

- Tachycardia leading to progressive bradycardia
- Tachypnoea leading to slowing of respiratory rate and development of shallow ineffective breathing
- Altered level of consciousness – agitation leading to progressive drowsiness
- Hypotension (particularly low diastolic values)
- Prolonged capillary refill time >3 seconds (note: must be tested centrally)
- Hypoglycaemia
- Pallor/mottled skin
- Weak peripheral pulses
- Reduced/no urine output
- Metabolic acidosis evident on a blood gas

Other clinical signs will be evident depending upon the underlying cause of the shock, e.g. the child may well be febrile (septic shock) and there may be a rash/the presence of petechia (meningococcal/pneumococcal septicaemia).

Irreversible shock

As the name suggests this phase of the shock process is a retrospective diagnosis only.

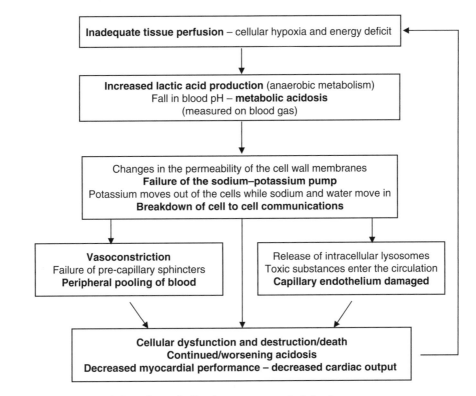

Figure 4.1 Consequences of altered metabolism in uncompensated shock.

Table 4.5 Summary of recognition of the shocked child.

Heart rate	Tachycardia progressing to bradycardia
Blood pressure	Phase 1: normal values for age (increased diastolic) Phase 2: hypotension (decreased diastolic)
Peripheral pulses	Phase 1 – bounding Phase 2 – weak
Capillary refill (central)	Prolonged >3 seconds
Respiration	Increased rate and depth progressing to slow shallow breathing

Continued dysfunction of the myocardium causes decreased cardiac output to the point at which cardiac standstill/arrest occurs.

Thorough assessment is the key to effective management of the shocked child; therefore recognition of the clinical signs is important (Table 4.5).

While practitioners working within the Emergency Department may have encountered all the types of shock identified previously, most staff working in the HDU will probably encounter predominantly either hypovolaemic, septic or cardiogenic shock as the child's primary presentation. A summary of the clinical presentation of these three types of shock is shown in Table 4.6. While there are a number of identical signs associated with the general presentation of the shocked child, there are a number of important differences in each clinical presentation as well. It is important that practitioners are familiar with these differences as it may well have an influence on the management of the individual child.

It is also important to elicit a thorough history from parents relating firstly to the child's current

Table 4.6 Specific clinical presentation of three types of shock.

Septic shock	Hypovolaemic shock	Cardiogenic shock
Early		
Hyperdynamic cardiovascular function	Tachycardia	Tachycardia
Increased cardiac output	Decreased perfusion	Decreased skin perfusion
Warm extremities	Prolonged capillary refill	Diminished peripheral pulses
Hyperpyrexia	Decreased urine output	Mottled, pale appearance
Hyperventilation	Decreased mean blood pressure	Hepatomegaly
Tachycardia	Increased oxygen demands	Pulmonary oedema/increasing
Altered level of consciousness	Decreased level of consciousness	O_2 demands
	No cardiomegaly on chest X-ray	Altered level of consciousness
		Cardiomegaly on chest X-ray
Late		
Poor cardiovascular function		
Decreased cardiac output		
Cold extremities		
Hyperpyrexia		
Slowing respiratory rate		
Slowing heart rate		
Obtunded		

presentation and secondly any previous/ongoing medical conditions which may be significant in the child's illness course.

Management of the shocked child

The priorities of management for the shocked child may be divided into two, the primary assessment and initial emergency treatment, followed by reassessment and the institution of further therapies as determined by the child's clinical condition. These interventions will overlap and while for ease of presentation they are divided into two, the assessment and management of the shocked child is a continuous process.

Primary assessment

Any assessment of the acutely unwell child must be logical and incorporate respiratory and circulatory components. It is sensible therefore to identify the Advanced Paediatric Life Support Group's (APLS 2005) structured approach as the most appropriate assessment of the shocked child as it is recognised throughout the United Kingdom (UK) both in

nursing and medical education (Table 4.7). In addition it is the approach advocated for the assessment of the acutely unwell adult, so there is minimal chance of confusion arising amongst practitioners working in adult environments who may only occasionally encounter the acutely unwell child.

Once initial assessment has been undertaken, secondary and ongoing management can be instituted. It is possible that the child will require admission to an Intensive Care Unit, but this will depend on the child's response to initial interventions and his or her need for more invasive monitoring and/or therapies (Table 4.8). Consideration must be given at all times to also supporting the parents/child's care givers.

Management of cardiac arrest

Primary cardiac arrest is not as common in children as it is in adults, and more often than not the event is preceded by a period of hypoxia. Common arrest rhythms in children are asystole (Figure 4.2) and pulseless electrical

Table 4.7 Primary assessment and management of the shocked child.

Primary assessment	Immediate management
Airway Assess patency and presence of protective reflexes (cough and gag)	It not patent/reflexes absent, consider use of Guedel airway and/or possible intubation
Breathing Assess rate, depth, effort and efficiency of respirations	Give high flow O_2 via face mask with reservoir bag
Circulation Assess HR, BP, CRT, colour	Apply monitoring – ECG, NIBP and SPO_2 as a minimum Assist with gaining IV/IO access Volume resuscitation – 20 mL/kg of prescribed fluids (0.9% saline/4.5% HAS)
Disability Assess AVPU, pupils, posture	Inadequate perfusion to the brain causes altered levels of consciousness in the child and also poor handling in the infant
Exposure Assess – look for an identifiable cause, e.g. bleeding/rash	Assess temperature Petechial rash or areas of purpura may be indicative of meningococcal or pneumococcal sepsis

Adapted from APLS (2005).

Table 4.8 Ongoing management priorities.

Intervention	Rationale
Increase oxygen supply and delivery Administer warmed and humidified oxygen using age-appropriate delivery method and sufficient concentration of O_2 to maintain saturations above 95% If airway is compromised contact anaesthetist/ICU for intubation and ventilation	Prevent drying of upper airway mucosa, which may increase tenacity of secretions and impede the function of the mucocillary escalator Avoid desiccation and damage of the lower respiratory tract, which may impede oxygen diffusion Prevent secondary cell damage and cell death from hypoxia Maintain patent airway and effective means of pulmonary ventilation
Administer IV fluids Maintain patent IV access Administer fluid boluses 20 mL/kg PRN (prescription required as needed) and evaluate effect Use blood products Ensure maintenance fluids are prescribed and administered Maintain fluid balance chart	Maintain circulating volume, blood pressure and tissue perfusion Correct anaemia, replace blood loss, and maintain osmotic and oncotic homeostasis Prevent potential overload
Administer drugs and electrolytes as prescribed Give inotropic support Monitor electrolytes Administer prescribed electrolyte replacements	Optimise cardiac function, support cardiac action, maintain blood pressure, and maximise circulation and perfusion Prevent complications such as arrhythmia as a result of deviations in normal ions
Take samples for investigation Send bloods Take blood cultures Administer IV antibiotics	Isolate causative organism and treat

(Continued)

Table 4.8 Continued.

Intervention	Rationale
Monitor temperature Administer paracetamol as prescribed/appropriate Apply cooling measures Apply active warming	Correct hypo-/hyperthermia to prevent secondary cellular insult and make child feel more comfortable
Monitor blood glucose Maintain serum glucose levels within normal limits Give dextrose as required if child is hypoglycaemic (5 mL/kg of 10%)	Maintaining serum glucose levels promotes cellular metabolism and helps prevent secondary cell death
Administer analgesic and sedative agents as prescribed	Prevent/reduce distress for the child and reassure the family Relieve pain to reduce risk of continued activation of the stress cycle, which may exacerbate circulatory instability

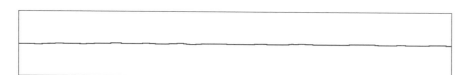

Figure 4.2   Monitor waveform of asystole.

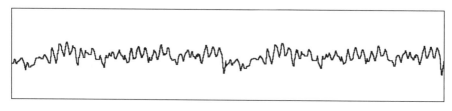

Figure 4.3   Monitor waveform of ventricular fibrillation.

activity (PEA), but ventricular fibrillation (VF) (Figure 4.3) is also seen in children and may be as a consequence of CHD or accidental ingestion of certain drugs such as tricyclic anti-depressants.

The guidelines for the management of paediatric cardiac arrest have been changed in the last 2 years and are now simplified into two pathways (Figure 4.4).

Congenital heart disease (CHD)

CHD is the most frequently diagnosed congenital condition in the newborn baby (www.patient.co.uk). The number of babies in the UK born with CHD each year is approximately 4600. This equates to 6.9/1000 births or one baby in every 450 (www.bhf.org. uk). Of these, the majority (3479) are diagnosed within the first year of life. Survival rates have improved dramatically, from a 20% survival rate at 1 year in 1940–1960 to a 90% survival rate at 1 year in 1980–1990 (www.heartstats. org). As children with CHD are now surviving to have families of their own it can be seen that children of mothers with CHD have an increased risk of 25–180/1000 births and

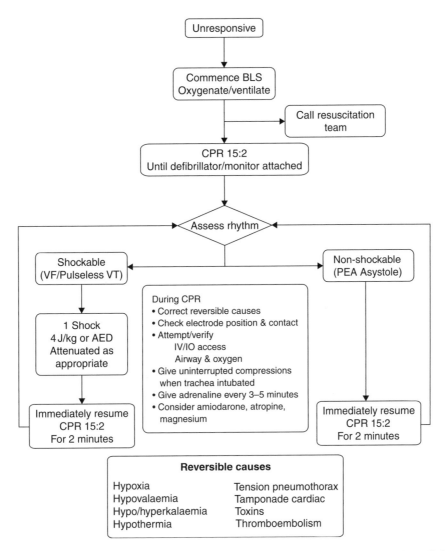

Figure 4.4 Paediatric cardiac arrest algorithm. Adapted from the European Resuscitation Council Guidelines for Resuscitation (2005), Section 6 – Paediatric life support.

children of fathers with CHD have an increased risk of 15–30/1000 births (www.patient.co.uk).

Causes

In the majority of cases the cause of CHD is unknown. However, there is a higher incidence associated with maternal rubella, diabetes and phenylketonuria (www.patient.co.uk). In addition, some anti-epileptic medications, smoking, alcohol and illegal drugs are also known to adversely affect cardiac development in the fetus. A higher incidence of CHD is also associated with chromosomal disorders of the fetus such as Down's syndrome or Turner's syndrome.

Congenital heart lesions are difficult to classify due to the many complicated variations that are seen, but it is common for them to be described according to:

- Area of the heart affected
- Direction of shunt caused

Accordingly classification can be as follows (Table 4.9):

- Affecting the heart generally
- Left to right shunt lesions

- Obstructive lesions
- Cyanotic lesions with increased pulmonary blood flow
- Cyanotic lesions with decreased pulmonary blood flow
- Cyanotic lesions with variable pulmonary blood flow

Antenatal diagnosis:

- Ultra-sound scan (USS).

Table 4.9 Classification and examples of types of lesions/conditions.

Classification	Examples of lesions/conditions	Key features
Affecting the heart generally	Cardiomyopathy Congenital arrhythmias	Conditions that produce an overall reduction in the performance of the myocardium
Acyanotic lesions	Patent ductus arteriosus (PDA) Atrial septal defect (ASD) Ventricular septal defect (VSD) Atrio-ventricular septal defect (AVSD)	Lesions that produce a left to right shunt (blood is pushed from the left side of the heart to the right side of the heart) at varying points in the circulation lead to increased blood flow to the lungs As the shunt is left to right, there is no evidence of cyanosis because the mixing that occurs is the addition of oxygenated blood to deoxygenated blood
Obstructive lesions	Coarctation of the aorta Aortic stenosis (AS) Pulmonary stenosis (PS) Interrupted aortic arch	Lesions in this group will increase the work of the heart, especially the left ventricle, leading to either left or right ventricular hypertrophy As there are no abnormal connections between the systemic and pulmonary circulations, there is no shunting, no cyanosis and essentially normal pulmonary blood flow.
Cyanotic lesions with increased pulmonary blood flow (PBF)	Total anomalous pulmonary venous drainage (TAPVD) Truncus arteriosus Hypoplastic left heart syndrome	Lesions in this group arise from the failure of the heart and blood vessels to differentiate into pulmonary and systemic circulations. Blood shunts from right to left, meaning that deoxygenated blood enters the systemic circulation, resulting in cyanosis. The reasons for increased pulmonary blood flow are related to specific lesions
Cyanotic lesions with decreased pulmonary blood flow	Tricuspid atresia Fallot's tetralogy Pulmonary atresia with intact ventricular septum	Decreased pulmonary blood flow is usually caused by an obstruction at some point in the right side of the heart These lesions have an abnormal opening between the pulmonary and systemic circulations or the persistence of fetal shunts, which result in right to left shunting and cyanosis
Cyanotic lesions with variable pulmonary blood flow	Transposition of great arteries with intact septum Transposition of great arteries with a VSD Transposition of great arteries with a VSD and sub-pulmonary stenosis	Lesions in this group have mixing of blood, resulting in cyanosis but variable pulmonary blood flow dependent on the degree of right-sided obstruction and/or the presence of an intact septum

Postnatal diagnosis:

- Clinical presentation
- ECHO
- CXR
- Hyperoxia test

Hyperoxia test – key facts

The nitrogen washout test is helpful in trying to distinguish between cardiac and respiratory causes of cyanosis. It works on the assumption that if there is right to left shunting in cyanotic heart disease then no amount of oxygenation in the pulmonary circulation will alter the desaturating effect of the shunt. However, if there is a pulmonary defect causing cyanosis this may be corrected by increasing the inspired oxygen.

The test is carried out by placing the infant in 100% oxygen normally given via a head box or close-fitting face mask for 10 minutes. If the infant remains cyanotic after this period the cyanosis is said to be secondary to cyanotic heart disease. This can be defined in blood gases as follows:

- PaO_2 <20 kPa (148 mmHg) – cyanotic heart disease likely
- PaO_2 <27 kPa (199 mmHg) but >20 kPa (148 mmHg) – result equivocal
- PaO_2 >27 kPa (199 mmHg) – primary respiratory disease

Clearly there are exceptions to this rule and severe respiratory disease may result in persistent cyanosis, even in 100% inspired oxygen. It remains a helpful test in the absence of imaging and may avoid an inappropriate referral and transfer of a neonate and family.

Care of an infant receiving a prostaglandin infusion

If there is suspicion that an infant may have a duct-dependent lesion then a continuous infusion of prostaglandin will be necessary to maintain the patency of the duct. Duct-dependent lesions cover a wide range of different anatomical anomalies but can be broadly defined as follows:

Duct-dependent systemic flow lesions: obstructive left-sided lesions which affect the circulation of blood to the body (systemic flow) such as coarctation of the aorta/critical aortic stenosis or hypoplastic left heart syndrome.

Duct-dependent cyanotic lesions: cyanotic lesions which require a degree of mixing between pulmonary (lungs) and systemic (body) blood flows to maintain adequate oxygenation/tissue perfusion such as transposition of the great arteries (TGA) or lesions with restricted/obstructed pulmonary blood flow such as pulmonary stenosis/pulmonary atresia.

Prostaglandin is a potent vasodilator of all arterioles within the body and has an effect on the walls of the ductus arteriosus which causes relaxation and opening of the pathway required by the infant, regardless of the underlying pathology.

There are two types of prostaglandin currently used in the UK, prostaglandin E1 (Alprostadil) and prostaglandin E2 (Dinoprostone). Both are detailed in the British National Formulary for Children (2007) and use is determined by local policy and practice. It is important that individual practitioners are familiar with the brand used in their locality, while remembering that they both achieve the same result – the maintenance of duct patency.

Stop and think

Prostaglandin must never be given as an intravenous bolus dose; therefore the infant should have a second working intravenous cannula for the administration of bolus medications.

Table 4.10 Side effects of prostaglandin infusions and care priorities.

Side effect	Notes/considerations
Apnoeas	Very common in low-birth-weight infants (2 kg or less)/preterm infants • Monitor infant's respiratory rate and pattern • Monitor infant' saturations (SpO_2) • Ensure there is a documented acceptable SpO_2 in the infant's notes • Inform medical staff if the infant's saturations fall below the prescribed limits
Bradycardia/hypotension	More common at higher doses, but awareness important to avoid deleterious changes in the infant's condition • Monitor infant's heart rate and blood pressure • Ensure there are documented acceptable cardiovascular parameters in the infant's notes • Inform medical staff if the infant's cardiovascular signs fall outside of prescribed limits
Fever	Normally resolves when infusion is discontinued – it is important to observe for additional signs of sepsis • Monitor infant's temperature • Maintain thermoneutral environment to avoid possible overheating of infant
Irritability/poor handling	Infants are often jittery and irritable – important to rule out other causes of irritability such as low blood glucose levels, although hypoglycaemia can be a side effect of prostaglandin infusions • Monitor infant's blood glucose level regularly • Assess infant's neuro status regularly – observe for signs of seizures (lip smacking, eye rolling, hypertonia)
Poor feeding/diarrhoea	Pre-term infants at increased risk of developing necrotising enterocolitis (NEC), although it is thought all infants may be at risk due to altered/reduced blood supply to the gut • If infant is receiving oral feeds, maintain feed chart in addition to intravenous infusion chart • Observe infant for abdominal distension, blood in stools, bilious vomiting • Inform medical staff if the infant develops any of the above signs

Note: The administration of oxygen to an infant receiving a prostaglandin infusion should only be commenced after careful consultation with the medical staff involved in the infant's care. A persistently high PaO_2 can stimulate the closure of the duct over a period of time; therefore oxygen should only be given to the infant in the presence of marked hypoxia.

The specific priorities of care for the infant receiving a prostaglandin infusion relate to detection and management of the side effects associated with the drug therapy. There are a number associated with each of the different preparations available, the most frequent of which are detailed in Table 4.10.

The complex nature of congenital heart disease makes it impractical to discuss the specific management of each individual lesion within this chapter; however, care of the infant with two of the more common lesions presenting in the neonatal period is detailed within the next two sections. The general principles identified apply to the care of most infants with CHD, but advice can and should always be sought from the specialist centre involved in the child's treatment.

Useful resources

www.ccad.org.uk/congenital – provides information and statistics about UK centres offering cardiac services.

www.lhm.org.uk – provides information and support for parents and children with single ventricle heart conditions (e.g. hypoplastic left heart syndrome).

Coarctation of the aorta

Definition
- A narrowing of the aorta distal to the left subclavian artery
- It accounts for 8–10% of congenital heart lesions and affects more boys than girls

Depending upon the site of the narrowing, a coarctation may be described as:

- Pre-ductal: proximal to PDA
- Juxtaductal: opposite the PDA
- Post-ductal: distal to the PDA

Clinical presentation
Clinical presentation is dependent upon the degree of aortic narrowing and the timing of ductal closure. Severe coarctation and early duct closure will mean presentation in the neonatal period; therefore infants with small and/or narrow ducts and severe coarctation may commonly present to the Emergency Department at between 3 and 10 days of age. Conversely, a mild coarctation may not present until later in childhood, although duct closure will have occurred in the neonatal period as normal.

Increased left ventricular pressure occurs as a consequence of the ventricle attempting to pump blood past the obstruction. Again the severity of the obstruction will determine the degree of strain placed on the ventricle but can lead to left ventricular failure and poor cardiac output.

Clinical signs evident in the neonate with a coarctation may be those generally associated with the generally unwell neonate, such as a history of poor feeding, minimal weight gain and poor handling. Additionally, parents often report breathlessness or fast breathing patterns in the infant. More specific clinical signs following duct closure include:

- Tachycardia
- Tachypnoea
- Mottled look
- Poor peripheral perfusion
- Prolonged capillary refill
- Decreased urine output
- Diminished/absent femoral pulses
- Significant gradient between upper and lower extremity blood pressure measurements

Management
The infant will require surgery to repair the aorta which is normally undertaken once the infant's condition has been stabilised and ventricular function has been assessed. Transfer to a specialist centre will be required for these infants. Initial assessment of the infant on presentation should follow the usual logical approach and concerns relating to airway, breathing and circulation must be addressed appropriately. More specific management priorities relating to the presence of the coarctation are highlighted in Table 4.11.

Transposition of great arteries (TGA) with intact septum

Definition
The aorta arises from the right ventricle and the pulmonary artery from the left ventricle, but the ventricles are in the correct position and have normal structure. The aorta is in front of and to the right of the pulmonary artery instead of in its usual position behind. It accounts for between 4 and 5% of congenital heart lesions. Within this broad definition there are a number of complex

Table 4.11 Initial management of the infant with coarctation.

Aim of management	Actions
Restore perfusion to the lower body	Commence prostaglandin infusion to improve and maintain duct patency
Improve tissue oxygenation	If required administer humidified and warmed oxygen therapy as required to maintain saturations at prescribed levels Assess effectiveness of therapy Reduce FiO_2 as able according to the infant's clinical condition (discuss with medical staff)
Correct metabolic acidosis	Administer small aliquots of volume as prescribed Monitor effect
Support left ventricular function	Commence inotropic infusion to support ventricular function (see section on 'Vasoactive medications') Intubation, mechanical ventilation and appropriate use of analgesia and sedative agents can reduce the demands placed on the cardiovascular system

anatomical variations such as transposition of great arteries with a ventricular septal defect (VSD) or transposition of great arteries with a VSD and sub-pulmonary stenosis, the management of which will not be discussed here.

The mechanics of a TGA with an intact septum means that there are two separate circulations. The systemic circulation is de-oxygenated as it feeds off the right side of the heart; however, no blood within this circuit passes through the lungs while pulmonary circulation which feeds off the left side of the heart is completely oxygenated as the blood circulates through the lungs. The systemic circuit is therefore reliant upon the presence of either a patent ductus arteriosus or a patent foramen ovale which allow some mixing of the blood and a small amount of oxygenated blood to be available to the body.

The condition is incompatible with life unless there is a communication between the two circulations.

In an infant with TGA and intact septum, clinical presentation almost always occurs within the first 6–8 hours of life. Clinical signs

- Tachycardia
- Tachypnoea
- Central cyanosis – unresolved by the administration of oxygen
- Saturations likely to be in the mid-30s (on SpO_2 monitor)
- Grunting
- Cardiomegaly on chest X-ray
- Plethoric lung fields on chest X-ray
- Marked metabolic acidosis

As with any acutely unwell infant the initial assessment on presentation should follow the usual logical approach, and concerns relating to airway, breathing and circulation must be addressed appropriately while confirming the diagnosis. With these infants the immediate specific priority is to create a communication between the two circulations to improve the flow of oxygenated blood to the body (Table 4.12). Transfer to a specialist centre will be necessary for the ongoing management of these infants.

Once infants have undergone balloon septostomy, there is usually a marked improvement in their systemic oxygenation (indicated by saturations in the low to mid-70s and improving blood gas results). Infants do not normally require prolonged intensive care at this stage, although a small number will. Surgical repair is normally undertaken at between 10 and 14 days of life, which allows time for the elevated pulmonary vascular pressures associated with fetal circulation to fall.

Table 4.12 Initial management of the infant with TGA and intact septum.

Aim of management	Actions
Create a communication between the two circulations	Commence prostaglandin infusion to improve and maintain duct patency
Improve tissue oxygenation	Once transferred to a specialist centre the infant will undergo a balloon septostomy which opens and enlarges the foramen ovale, making a permanent opening. (This will be closed when the infant undergoes surgical repair)
Correct metabolic acidosis	Administer small aliquots of volume as prescribed Monitor effect
Support left ventricular function	Commence inotropic infusion to support ventricular function (see section on 'Vasoactive medications') Intubation, mechanical ventilation and appropriate use of analgesia and sedative agents can reduce the demands placed on the cardiovascular system

Cardiomyopathy and myocarditis in infants and children

The disease processes of cardiomyopathy and myocarditis in children refer to a group of diseases that predominantly affect myocardial function. Although less common than CHD, cardiomyopathy and myocarditis can lead to significant myocardial dysfunction, morbidity and mortality.

Hypertrophic cardiomyopathy (HCM)

Hypertrophic cardiomyopathy is the most common cause of sudden death in people under 35 years of age (www.c-r-y.org.uk/hypertrophic_cardiomyopathy).

The myocardium of a healthy heart consists of an organised arrangement of muscle fibres which is usually less than 11 mm thick (www.c-r-y.org.uk/hypertrophic_cardiomyopathy). However, with HCM there is myocardial disarray: the arrangement of the myocardial cells, myofibrils and myofilaments is unsystematic and it is thought that it is this abnormality that predisposes the damaged heart to life-threatening dysrhythmias. In addition, the myocardium becomes thickened and this adversely affects both systolic and diastolic

function as the stiff muscle relaxes poorly, which impairs filling and also has poor compliance, which affects contractility and compromises cardiac output.

The most common area of myocardial thickening caused by HCM is the upper portion of the ventricular septum. This is known as asymmetric septal hypertrophy. Due to its location, the thickening intrudes into the left ventricular chamber and may cause outflow tract obstruction which subsequently affects cardiac output. The function of the mitral valve may also be affected by the thickened myocardium, resulting in mitral regurgitation. Alternative patterns of myocardial thickening can also be found: symmetric or concentric left ventricular hypertrophy is where the myocardial thickening is evenly distributed over the left ventricle, and atypical hypertrophy is where myocardial thickening is focused on the apex of the ventricle.

Occasionally there is no familial link to HCM, but with the vast majority of cases it is caused by inheriting an autosomal dominant defective gene from one parent. Children of an affected parent will have a 50% chance of inheriting the gene and developing the disease. This defective gene causes an abnormality of the sarcometric contractile proteins which affect myocardial contraction.

Although the disorder will be present in utero, signs and symptoms may only become evident in infancy or later life, depending on the severity of the disease process.

Clinical presentation
- Dysrhythmias
- Chest pain, due to thickened coronary arteries within the ventricular septum
- Dyspnoea, especially on exertion
- Syncope
- Heart murmur, due to mitral regurgitation and/or turbulent flow resulting from outflow tract obstruction

Diagnosis
An ECG will demonstrate hypertrophy and diagnosis is usually confirmed following a cardiac echo.

Management
Medical treatment, often with beta-blockers or calcium antagonists, aims to control symptoms and prevent complications by slowing the heart rate and producing a more effective contraction which improves cardiac output. Fluid restriction, electrolyte management and diuretics are also key therapies in controlling the degree of heart failure. Anti-arrhythmics should be used with care as the majority have a negative inotropic effect. ECG and invasive blood pressure monitoring will be required. Implantable pacemakers or defibrillators may be required to effectively manage dysrhythmias if anti-arrhythmics prove insufficient.

If there is concern about stasis and possible clot/thrombus formation due to the low cardiac output, anti-coagulation may also be required. On occasion, the surgical option of a myectomy may be advised. This involves resecting the left ventricular outflow tract in an attempt to relieve the obstruction and improve cardiac output. In severe HCM a cardiac transplant may be necessary.

Dilated cardiomyopathy (DCM)

With DCM the ventricles become enlarged and the myocardium becomes thin and weak, resulting in decreased contractility and reduced cardiac output. The resulting left ventricular failure produces increased left ventricular and left atrial pressures and increased end-systolic volumes, and the ensuing pulmonary congestion causes dyspnoea. Right-sided heart failure may also cause increased systemic venous congestion and result in ascites and peripheral oedema.

In the majority of cases the cause of DCM is idiopathic. However, dilated cardiomyopathy can also be caused by a viral illness per se or by an auto-immune process which may be triggered by a viral illness. In these situations the immune system is activated by the virus, but then aberrantly begins to attack itself. In DCM approximately 30% of patients are found to have this auto-immune form of the disease. Dilated cardiomyopathy also has some genetic links and has been shown to be familial in around 20% of cases.

Clinical presentation
- Dyspnoea due to pulmonary venous congestion
- Lethargy due to poor cardiac output
- Peripheral oedema due to systemic venous congestion
- Chest pain at rest or on exertion
- Dysrhythmias, either brady or tachycardias, which may result in reduced cardiac output
- Syncope – the sudden faint/temporary loss of consciousness owing to a sudden drop in blood pressure

Diagnosis
Diagnosis is based on physical examination of the child, history of the illness and results from ECG, cardiac echo and exercise tolerance tests.

Management
Treatment primarily aims to control the heart failure and any dysrhythmias with the use of diuretics and anti-arrhythmic agents. Beta-blockers and

angiotensin converting enzyme (ACE) inhibitors may also be used to reduce left ventricular afterload and optimise cardiac output. If medical treatment is unsuccessful, cardiac transplant may be required.

Arrhythmogenic right ventricular cardiomyopathy (ARVC)

ARVC is the second most common cause of unexpected sudden death in the young (www.c-r-y.org.uk) and often presents in the teenage years. The illness typically presents with the development of fibrous tissue and fat in place of the normal right ventricular myocardial cells. At the outset only localised regions of the right ventricular myocardium are involved, but the disease becomes more profuse as it progresses. Whilst ARVC predominantly affects the right ventricle, the left may also be involved. As the myocardium becomes more diseased it becomes progressively thinner and less contractile, which results in dilation and dysrhythmias.

The cause of ARVC is unknown, but it is familial and is most commonly passed on as an autosomal dominant trait. This means that children of an affected parent will have a 50% chance of inheriting the deviant gene. However, ARVC has 'incomplete penetrance', which means that those with the defective gene may still not develop any signs of the condition.

Clinical presentation

Dyspnoea is uncommon with this form of cardiomyopathy and many patients are asymptomatic until dysrhythmias occur. Signs and symptoms are then usually those associated with dysrhythmias, such as palpitations and syncope. However, peripheral oedema, ascites and dyspnoea may develop as a consequence of progressive heart failure and sudden death may also occur.

Diagnosis

ARVC can be quite difficult to diagnose as the signs and symptoms may be quite subtle in the early stages of the illness. Cardiac echo and ECG may be useful and MRI may detect the abnormalities of the right ventricle.

Management

Treatment aims to control any dysrhythmias with anti-arrhythmics such as Amiodarone or Sotalol. Ablation of aberrant pathways may be required if medical treatment fails and occasionally an implantable defibrillator is needed.

Restrictive cardiomyopathy

This is the least common form of cardiomyopathy and is defined by an increased rigidity of the myocardium, which restricts filling. Often the origin of the stiffness is unclear, but it may be a result of infection, drugs or infiltrative diseases such as sarcoidosis. There is also evidence to suggest that some cases may be caused by a defective gene which affects the protein responsible for normal myocardial contraction (www.cardiomyopathy.org). With restrictive cardiomyopathy, even though the myocardium is stiffer than normal, it is not usually thickened.

In advanced stages of the disease the stiff myocardium results in increased right- and left-sided heart pressures. These increased pressures within the heart result in increased pressures within both the pulmonary and venous system and can result in pulmonary oedema and ascites as a consequence.

Clinical presentation

The clinical signs are very much associated with the venous congestion which is caused by the increased filling pressures and will include:

- Dyspnoea due to pulmonary venous congestion
- Ascites and peripheral oedema due to systemic venous congestion
- Dysrhythmias may also occur and can result in sudden death
- Fatigue

Diagnosis

A combination of ECG, cardiac echo and cardiac catheterisation confirms the diagnosis.

Management

Treatment is aimed at controlling the heart failure and the dysrhythmias, diuretics and anti-arrhythmics being the drugs of choice. If the heart failure becomes unmanageable on drug therapy then cardiac transplantation may be required.

Myocarditis

Myocarditis refers to the myocardial inflammation associated with infection and may be caused by virtually any pathogen. However, it is usually viral in origin. The most common causative organisms are Coxsackie B and enteroviruses and it is most often seen in children less than 1 year old. The causative organism interferes with cell function, resulting in myocardial necrosis in the very early stages of the disease process. Subsequent inflammation and thickening of the ventricular wall causes impaired contractility, reduced cardiac output and rhythm disturbances. The majority of cases resolve with treatment; however, 10% will develop dilated cardiomyopathy and require additional or life-long treatment.

The incidence of myocarditis is difficult to estimate. It can be very mild and relatively asymptomatic and so remain undiagnosed, or severe and associated with sudden death.

Clinical presentation

- Dysrhythmias
- Fever
- Tachycardia
- Heart failure
- General malaise
- Dyspnoea
- Lethargy

Diagnosis

A cardiac echo will demonstrate hypertrophy and poor contractility and this associated with fever should suggest a diagnosis of myocarditis.

Management

Treatment of the infective cause and rest are the main priority. If signs of heart failure are evident then diuretics and fluid restriction may be required. Anti-arrhythmics may be used to control dysrhythmias. Steroids may also be beneficial in reducing inflammation and helping to relieve symptoms, although their effect should be balanced with the potential of steroid-induced immune suppression.

Useful resources

www.c-r-y.org.uk – provides information relating to cardiomyopathies and other heart disease (e.g. Kawasaki's disease) in children and adolescents.

www.cardiomyopathy.org – provides general information for children, families and adults affected by cardiomyopathy.

www.sads.org.uk – provides information and support about sudden arrhythmic death syndrome in adolescents.

www.bhf.org.uk – general information about heart disease, with a subsection relating to cardiomyopathy.

Rhythm recognition and pacing

Physiology of cardiac muscle contraction

Cardiac muscle is stimulated to contract when an electrical impulse is generated, and then spread throughout the network of specialised muscle fibres which infiltrate the myocardium. The impulse is generated intrinsically in the right atrium by the sino-atrial (SA) node and although the SA node is innervated by the autonomic nervous system, this merely affects the rate of the impulse generation. From the SA node the impulse spreads throughout both atria, causing simultaneous atrial contraction. The impulse then reaches the atrio-ventricular (AV) node, where it pauses for 0.1–0.2 ms before being conducted through both ventricles by the bundle of His, the right and left bundle branches and finally

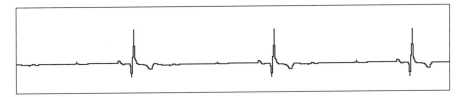

Figure 4.5 Monitor waveform of sinus bradycardia.

the Purkinje fibres. Once more, this spread of the electrical impulse along the network of specialised muscle fibres results in simultaneous ventricular contraction.

The spread of the electrical impulse along the specialised muscle fibres is known as depolarisation and results in myocardial contraction, or systole. During depolarisation there is a rapid influx of positively charged sodium ions into the cell. This influx then stops suddenly and calcium ions now move into the cell whilst potassium ions slowly leave, and it is this that generates the electrical impulse. The fibres then return to their pre-impulse state as potassium rapidly leaves the cell and sodium slowly leaks back in. This is known as repolarisation and results in myocardial relaxation, or diastole.

If this cycle is disturbed by hypoxia, acidosis, electrolyte imbalance, surgical trauma, drug toxicity or for idiopathic reasons, then an abnormal conduction pathway and an abnormal cardiac rhythm will result. In such situations temporary and/or permanent pacing may be required to effect sequential atrial and ventricular contraction and so maintain cardiac output.

Rhythms requiring pacing

Bradydysrhythmias which result in compromised cardiac output may require pacing. However, it is always essential to ascertain the cause of the dysrhythmia, e.g. hypoxia, and ensure that this is also comprehensively treated.

Sinus bradycardia

The electrical impulse is being generated and conducted in the appropriate manner, but the rate is slower than is normal for the child's age/condition. This can be caused by hypoxia, vagal stimulation or damage to the SA node, amongst other reasons. It will usually result in compromised cardiac output and require immediate treatment of the cause. Full resuscitation may be required until the heart rate and cardiac output improves or pacing can be established (Figure 4.5).

First-degree heart block

The SA node generates impulses as normal which spread across the atria, resulting in atrial contraction. However, the AV node delays the impulse slightly longer than normal, resulting in an abnormally long P–R interval. However, all impulses are conducted from the atria to the ventricles and the overall heart rate and cardiac output are usually unaffected. In many situations, no treatment is required (Figure 4.6).

Second-degree heart block

This can be further divided into Mobitz type I and Mobitz type II. Mobitz type II is also known as Wenckebach's phenomenon.

Mobitz type I occurs when the AV node blocks a regular number of impulses from the atria to the ventricles. It may block alternate impulses, allowing one P wave to result in ventricular contraction but not the next. On the ECG this would be visible as two P waves to every QRS, i.e. a 2:1 block. Alternatively, the AV node may block two atrial impulses but allow the third through to the ventricles. This would be visible as three P waves to every QRS, i.e. a 3:1 block. With Mobitz type I the block is regular, and the QRS rate will determine whether cardiac output

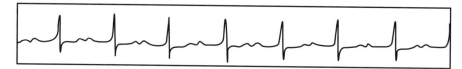

Figure 4.6 Monitor waveform of first-degree heart block.

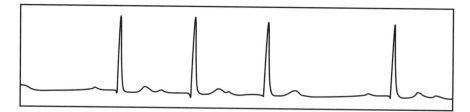

Figure 4.7 Monitor waveform of second-degree heart block.

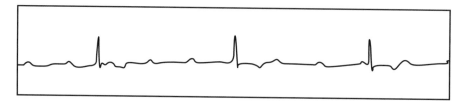

Figure 4.8 Monitor waveform of complete heart block.

is adequate or not. Pacing may be required to increase the ventricular rate.

Mobitz type II occurs when the conduction time of the AV node becomes progressively longer. The first P wave may be conducted to the ventricles in a relatively normal time. However, the next P wave takes slightly longer to be conducted through the AV node and so on, until eventually the P wave is blocked at the AV node and a QRS complex is dropped completely. This is visible on the ECG as an increasing P-R time with subsequent complexes until a QRS complex is omitted. The cycle then begins again. Overall heart rate is usually sufficient to maintain adequate cardiac output, but, if not, pacing may be used to increase the ventricular rate (Figure 4.7).

Third-degree heart block

This is also known as complete heart block. The AV node is unable to conduct any impulses from the SA node through to the bundle of His and the ventricular conduction network. The ventricular myocardium recognises that no impulse is being received and an area of myocardium takes over as the ventricular pacemaker, but with a slower intrinsic rate than that of the atria. Consequently, the atria and the ventricles are contracting independently and this impairs ventricular filling. The combination of poor ventricular filling and slow ventricular rate will usually result in a compromised cardiac output. This is visible on the ECG as P waves and QRS complexes which have no relationship to each other.

Complete heart block may be congenital, or due to hypoxic or surgical trauma to the AV node. Pacing is usually required to ensure sequential contraction of the atria and ventricles and improved cardiac output (Figure 4.8).

Some tachydysrhythmias may require overdrive pacing as cardiac output is compromised

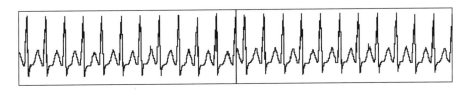

Figure 4.9 Monitor waveform of supraventricular tachycardia.

by the fast ventricular rate and subsequent decrease in both ventricular filling and coronary perfusion time. The associated increase in myocardial oxygen consumption also warrants quick and effective treatment even if output is not initially compromised as it renders the rhythm unsustainable for any prolonged period of time.

Supraventricular tachycardia (SVT)

The rhythm is usually regular but the rate will be greater than 220 beats/minutes in infants and greater than 180 beats/minutes in children. P waves are lost in the preceding QRS or T wave, making it difficult to determine whether the impulse originates from the atria or the AV node. QRS complexes are narrow. The fast rate results in a compromised output, and treatment with over-drive pacing, adenosine or cardioversion is required (Figure 4.9).

Pacing modes

Demand

Demand pacing complements the child's intrinsic rhythm by 'filling the gaps' between what is sensed and what is required. If the child's atrial or ventricular rate falls below that set, then the pacing box will stimulate an impulse. Demand pacing can stimulate an atrial impulse, a ventricular impulse or both in sequence, i.e. sequential pacing.

Fixed

Fixed pacing refers to when the pacing box is set to stimulate an atrial and/or ventricular impulse regardless of the child's intrinsic rhythm. Whilst fixed atrial pacing has value within the clinical setting, fixed ventricular pacing is rarely used as it can have potentially fatal results. If the pacing box delivers a ventricular impulse on the T wave of an intrinsic beat then this may induce ventricular fibrillation and the child will require immediate resuscitation.

Over-drive

This style of pacing can be used to gain control of tachydysrhythmias which originate above the AV node. The pacing box is initially set to deliver a rate that is faster than the child's intrinsic rate. Once the pacing box 'captures' the atrial rate, the rate can then be gradually turned down with the intention that the atria will then follow the pacing stimuli rather than continue to generate an aberrant rhythm. Other causes of the tachydysrhythmias, such as pyrexia, should also be treated to ensure maximum effectiveness.

Common pacing modes

Pacing modes are identified by a three-letter code, e.g. DDD. The first letter refers to which chambers are paced, the second letter refers to which chambers are sensed and the third letter will verify that if an intrinsic beat is sensed the pacing box will be 'inhibited' from pacing that chamber:

- D – Dual
- A – Atrial
- V – Ventricular
- I – Inhibited
- O – Off

The required rate and the AV delay time must also be set. The AV delay mimics the natural pause in conduction which occurs at the AV node. The strength of the impulse required to achieve myocardial contraction should be checked by the cardiologist and from this the stimulation settings can be determined. Similarly, the strength of any intrinsic impulses must be ascertained to ensure that the sensitivity thresholds are set appropriately.

DDD is one of the most frequently used pacing modes: in this mode the pacing box will sense for an atrial impulse, and if one is not detected within the time determined by the set rate, then the atria will be paced. The pacing box will then sense for a ventricular impulse, and if one is not detected within the time determined by the set AV delay, then the ventricles will be paced. If intrinsic atrial or ventricular impulses are sensed that are stronger than the set threshold, then the pacing box will be inhibited from pacing that chamber, i.e. this is demand, sequential pacing.

DVI is another pacing mode which is used reasonably frequently: in this mode, whilst both chambers are paced (the first letter is D), only the ventricles are being sensed (the second letter is V). Essentially this is fixed atrial pacing, as the atrial activity is not being sensed, but demand ventricular pacing – the ventricular activity – is being sensed. The third letter, I, reflects that as only one chamber is being sensed, only one chamber can be inhibited from pacing.

DOO is fixed atrial and ventricular pacing: in this mode both chambers are paced (the first letter D), but no chambers are being sensed (the second letter O), and as the pacing box is not sensing for any activity it cannot be inhibited from pacing (the third letter O). This pacing mode should never be used because of the risk of stimulating a ventricular contraction mid-repolarisation and inducing ventricular fibrillation.

Temporary pacing

Temporary pacing is used to maintain effective cardiac output until the cause of the dysrhythmia has been treated and a rhythm with adequate cardiac output established. Alternatively it can be used to maintain effective cardiac output until a permanent pacing system can be established. Temporary pacing can be epicardial, transvenous, oesophageal or external.

Summary of different temporary pacing modes

Epicardial pacing. During most open heart surgical procedures it is acknowledged that dysrhythmias are a potential post-operative complication, especially if surgery has been close to the SA or AV node, or any of the conduction pathways. Temporary pacing wires are therefore attached to both the atrial and ventricular epicardium prior to closing the child's chest to facilitate management of any such problems. Universally, atrial wires exit to the right of the child's sternum and ventricular wires exit to the left of the child's sternum. It is imperative that the exit site is kept clean and dry to minimise the risk of any infection. A 12-lead ECG and clotting profile are checked prior to removal of the wires as there is a risk of bleeding and cardiac tamponade after the wires have been removed. The child's haemodynamic observations must be monitored carefully during this time. Epicardial pacing is always a temporary measure.

Transvenous pacing. Transvenous pacing is generally used in children weighing over 10 kg, although it has also been used in the management of neonates (www.emedicine.com). Size of the wires tends to be the limiting factor. Insertion of the wires is performed by a cardiologist and takes 10–20 minutes. A large vein needs to be accessed and the subclavian or the femoral are common entry sites. The pacing wire is then threaded through to the right atrium and/or the right ventricle where it is fixed to the endocardium. Pacing can then be controlled by an external pacing box as with epicardial wires. Lower stimulation thresholds are required with transvenous pacing than epicardial pacing due to the fixation of the pacing wires to the endocardium rather than the epicardium, thus generating less tissue resistance. Once more it is imperative that the exit site is kept clean and dry to minimise the risk of infection.

Transvenous pacing can also be used as a permanent pacing system. Wires are inserted in a similar way to that described but are attached to a small, matchbox-sized implantable pacing box.

Trans-oesophageal pacing. Trans-oesophageal pacing can be commenced within a relatively short period of time and can prove a valuable method of pacing in children without epicardial wires, and can provide some stability until transvenous wires have been inserted. A flexible pacing catheter is inserted into the oesophagus and advanced until it is at atrial level. A specific trans-oesophageal pacing box is also required.

External pacing. External pacing is achieved through the use of large electrodes which are positioned anteriorly and posteriorly on the child's thorax. These are attached to the defibrillator which is set to 'pacing' mode with appropriate values entered for rate and stimulation threshold. Large stimulation thresholds are required as only a fraction of the set current will be delivered to the myocardium. Although this method of pacing causes discomfort to the child it can be instigated in seconds and can be used as a bridge to the insertion of transvenous wires.

Care of the child

Whichever technique is being employed to pace the child it is vital that the nurse ensures that the values set on the pacing box translate into the appropriate response on the child's heart rate and rhythm. The effect of pacing can be visualised on the child's ECG. Any stimulation from the pacing box is graphed as vertical line, or pacing spike, on the ECG and should be followed appropriately by a P wave or QRS complex. As the origin of the impulse is the tip of the pacing wire rather than the SA or AV node, the subsequent wave will be a different form to intrinsic activity. If the pacing spike is not followed by an appropriate response then the stimulation threshold may need to be increased. Conversely if the pacing spikes appear to be competing with intrinsic activity the sensing threshold may need to be decreased.

It is also important to ensure that all connections are secure and that a spare battery is available for the pacing box. As with any ECG interpretation it is also essential to ensure that the electrical activity visualised on the ECG converts into effective myocardial contraction and an adequate cardiac output.

Vasoactive medications

Throughout children's healthcare experience they may require the use of a variety of drug therapies to optimise their cardiac function and well-being. It is vital that the nurse ensures the child receives the correct dose of the prescribed drug and has knowledge of the drug's desired effect and potential side effects in order to effectively monitor the child's response to the therapy.

Within this broad grouping of vasoactive medications a number of different types of drug may be found, classified by the specific actions or effects they produce within the body; e.g. inotropes, beta blockers, cardiac glycosides and vasodilators.

Inotropes

Inotropes may be termed positive or negative and will also produce chronotropic effects. (Chronotropic effects influence the rate of the heart beat and may also be positive or negative.)

- Positive inotropes: enhance the contractility of the myocardium
- Negative inotropes: decrease the force of myocardial contractility and slow AV node conduction, thus decreasing the heart rate and blood pressure

These can be used to manipulate the child's preload, afterload and contractility in order to improve the cardiac output. They predominantly affect the autonomic nervous system (ANS). The ANS consists of the parasympathetic and the sympathetic system. The vagus nerve contains 75% of the parasympathetic nerve fibres and its main effect is to decrease heart rate and contractility. Acetylcholine is the neurotransmitter for the parasympathetic nervous system.

In contrast the sympathetic nervous system achieves its effect through the release of adrenaline and noradrenaline which are secreted by the adrenal medulla. These neurotransmitters act on adrenergic receptors which are found mainly in the heart, blood vessels and the airway. These adrenergic receptors can be further divided into alpha, beta and dopaminergic receptors. Alpha (α) receptors are found in the smooth muscle of the peripheral vasculature and the bronchi. Stimulation of these receptors produces vasoconstriction. Beta (β) receptors are categorised as $\beta 1$ or $\beta 2$, depending on the effect they have on the cardiovascular system. $\beta 1$ receptors are innervated and located within the myocardium. Stimulation of these receptors produces a positive chronotropic effect (i.e. an increased heart rate), an increase in atrio-ventricular conduction velocity and an increase in contractility. $\beta 2$ receptors are not innervated; they are found in smooth muscle and are affected by circulating catecholamines. Stimulation of these receptors produces vasodilation and bronchial dilation.

Dopaminergic receptors are situated in the myocardium and the renal, coronary and intestinal blood vessels. Stimulation of these receptors produces vasodilation.

It can be seen that by selecting drugs according to the receptors they affect allows us to quite specifically control the way in which cardiac function is altered. Stimulation of alpha receptors will increase blood pressure through vasoconstriction. This will also increase left ventricular afterload; afterload can be defined as the resistance against which the ventricle contracts and increasing afterload increases the workload and oxygen demands of the myocardium.

Stimulation of $\beta 1$ receptors will increase cardiac output and blood pressure by increasing both the rate and force of contraction of the myocardium. This increase in contractility will also increase the myocardium's oxygen requirement. Whilst stimulation of either alpha or $\beta 1$ receptors will produce an increase in blood pressure, it can be seen that the mode of increase varies depending on the receptor stimulated. $\beta 2$ receptors produce vascular and bronchial vasodilation and their main clinical use is to relieve the bronchospasm associated with asthma. Dopaminergic receptors also produce vasodilation but mainly of the coronary and renal vasculature. The benefit of this is improved coronary perfusion which aids oxygen delivery to the myocardium. The improved renal perfusion helps to maintain an acceptable glomerular filtration rate and a good diuresis. This is beneficial in managing the child's fluid status and maintaining optimal cardiac function.

It is evident that the drugs used in the clinical arena affect more than one adrenergic receptor: knowledge of their effects will influence the choice of drug used. A summary of the effects of stimulation of each of the receptors and the drugs that commonly produce the effects are detailed in Table 4.13.

Care of the child receiving specific vasoactive medications

A number of infants and children may require continuous infusions of vasoactive medications to support their cardiac function, e.g. the child with dilated cardiomyopathy. These children will not necessarily require an intensive care bed but may be managed within either a designated HDU or a specialist clinical area. The aim with the majority of these children is to gradually

Table 4.13 Summary of adrenergic receptors, effects of stimulation and medications involved.

Receptor	Effects	Agonist (drugs that enhance the effect)	Notes
$\alpha1$ (alpha 1)	Vasoconstriction of veins and arteries Increases myocardial contraction	Adrenaline Noradrenaline Dopamine	Increases blood pressure Decreases urine output Reduces skin and splanchnic blood flow
$\alpha2$ (alpha 2)	Vasodilation Negative chronotropic effect	Adrenaline Noradrenaline	
$\beta1$ (beta 1)	Tachycardia Improves contractility Speeds up conduction velocity	Isoprenaline Adrenaline Dopamine Noradrenaline Dobutamine	Increases heart rate Increases systemic perfusion
$\beta2$ (beta 2)	Vasodilatation Bronchodilation	Isoprenaline Adrenaline Dopamine Noradrenaline Dobutamine	Increases skin blood flow Reduces wheeze
Dopaminergic	Dilation of renal mesenteric coronary and cerebral vascular beds	Dopamine	Increases urine output

convert them to oral medications which will continue to support their cardiac function, allowing time for myocardial recovery.

The majority of vasoactive medications require central access for delivery due to their pharmacological properties. Care of the child with either a short-term central venous line (CVL) or a long-term tunnelled line such as a Hickman line should be carried out according to local policy and guidelines.

Dobutamine is the only vasoactive medication that can be safely administrated via a peripheral cannula over a long period of time and it is recommended that it is only run at doses of 10 µg/kg/min or less if being given via this route. If children are receiving peripheral Dobutamine they must have a second working cannula *in situ* through which bolus drugs may be given and which may be used should the infusion cannula fail.

- Full monitoring must be used for children receiving infusions until their clinical stability is established. As a minimum, ECG/NIBP/ SpO_2 monitoring should be in place and observations should be recorded hourly (or according to local policy).
- Invasive monitoring via an arterial line may be available; however, this will depend upon local policy and guidelines. The care and management of children with an arterial line *in situ* is discussed in more detail in Chapter 2 and in particular section on 'Blood pressure monitoring'.
- The infusions should be on a dedicated line which must be clearly identified. The

Table 4.14 Vasoactive medications and their effects.

Vasoactive drug	Effect	Side effects
Adrenaline (epinephrine)	α and β agonist, $\beta1$ effects Increased α effect at high dose	Tachycardias Increases myocardial work Increases O_2 consumption Splanchnic constriction
Calcium gluconate	Increases myocardial contractility Enhances ventricular automaticity	Bradycardia Hypotension Tissue necrosis with extravasations Digoxin and high calcium doses can cause arrhythmias
Dobutamine	Predominantly $\beta1$ effect with some $\beta2$ and α effects can be given peripherally	Tachyarrhythmias Hypotension Pulmonary constriction
Dopamine	Low dose: dilation of vascular beds and increased heart rate High dose α stimulation	Tachyarrhythmias increases PAP Inhibits thyroid stimulation hormone and aldosterone production
Enoximone	Phosphodiesterase inhibitor Increases intracellular cyclic AMP Increases cardiac contractility Vasodilatation	Arrhythmias Hypotension Liver and GI dysfunction Administration site pain Thrombocytopenia
Epoprostenol	Relaxation of vascular smooth muscle leading to a decrease in systemic vascular resistance Increases heart rate Lowers diastolic blood pressure Inhibits platelet aggregation Vasodilation	Cerebral vasodilation which increases cerebral blood flow Hypotension Bradycardia
Esmolol	Negative inotrope and chronotrope Blocks beta-adrenoreceptors – $\beta1$ Lowers blood pressure and (dose-dependent) lowers heart rate Slows atri-ventricular conduction	Severe bradycardia Hypotension Asystole Very short acting/half-life
Glyceryl trinitrate (GTN)	Low-dose venodilation High-dose venous and arterial vasodilation Blockade of alpha-receptors in pulmonary circulation Increases heart rate	Hypotension Tachycardia/bradycardia Headache
Hydralazine	Peripheral vasodilator Predominantly an arteriolar vasodilator → decreases systemic vascular resistance Increases heart rate Increases cardiac output	Tachycardia Palpitations Hypotension Headaches
Isoprenaline	Positive inotrope and chronotrope Potent bronchodilator Reduction in peripheral vascular resistance – $\beta2$ effects Increases automaticity and enhances atrioventricular nodal conduction	Palpitations Headaches Cardiac arrhythmias if other drugs, e.g. digoxin or beta-adrenoreceptors, are being given

Table 4.14 Continued

Vasoactive drug	Effect	Side effects
Labetolol	Anti-hypertensive Lowers systolic and diastolic blood pressure Decreases heart rate and cardiac output	Liver damage Hypotension
Lignocaine	Anti-arrhythmic Local anaesthetic	Seizures Heart block Hypotension
Milrinone	Phosphodiesterase inhibitor Increases intracellular cyclic AMP Increases cardiac contractility Vasodilatation	Arrhythmias Hypotension Liver and GI dysfunction Administration site pain Thrombocytopenia
Noradrenaline (norepinephrine)	Alpha and beta agonist Vasoconstriction Increases heart rate and blood pressure High doses may increase afterload and therefore worsen effect and reduce tissue perfusion	Tachyarrhythmias Increases myocardial work Increases O_2 consumption Hepatic and mesenteric ischaemia
Phenoxybenzamine	Vasodilator (predominantly arterial) Lowers peripheral vascular resistance Lowers diastolic blood pressure Increases heart rate Increases cardiac output	Idiosyncratic profound hypotension
Sodium nitroprusside(SNP)	Vasodilation and hypotension Lowers blood pressure Increases heart rate	SNP breaks down to cyanide Ensure levels of cyanide are measured if infusion continues for more than 72 hours

compatibilities of vasoactive infusions running together must also be ascertained before commencing new infusions.

- Volume boluses or bolus drugs must be given on a separate line to prevent children receiving an inadvertent bolus of their inotropes.
- Most vasoactive medications have very short half lives; therefore the effects of disruption to infusions are seen in seconds to minutes. It is essential that the nurse maintains continuity of these infusions at all times to avoid deleterious changes in cardiac output (see Table 4.14).

Appendix

A list of commonly used drugs and their action are explained in Table A1.

Table A1 Commonly used drugs.

Drug	Action	Administration	Notes
Diuretics			
Frusemide (loop diuretic)	Acts on the ascending limb of the loop of Henlé Increases potassium loss as well as sodium and water *Adverse effects:* Hyponatraemia, hypokalaemia	Oral/intravenous – may be bolus or infusion	Diuretics are drugs that improve urine production. They are useful in the management of heart failure in maintaining an optimum circulating volume and so reducing the workload of the heart Most diuretics work by increasing the excretion of sodium and thus water by the kidneys Careful assessment of the child's fluid balance as well as evaluation of the response to diuretics are important in maintaining stability Monitoring of potassium levels should be considered in children on diuretic therapy
Spironalactone (potassium-sparing diuretic)	Acts on the distal convoluted tubule by inhibiting the action of aldosterone *Adverse effects:* Gynaecomastia, hirsuitism, menstrual irregularities	Oral	
Angiotensin converting enzyme (ACE) inhibitors			
Captopril	Prevents conversion of Angiotensin I to angiotensin II *Adverse effects:* Dizziness, tachycardia, hypotension	Oral	ACE inhibitors are used to lower blood pressure, but they achieve their effect through disruption of the angiotensin cycle. They reduce the amount of angiotensin II production and so decrease sympathetic nervous stimulation. This prevents vasoconstriction and reduces systemic vascular resistance In addition, the reduction in angiotensin II decreases the amount of aldosterone produced by the adrenal cortex and so decreases the amount of water and sodium retained by the kidneys, resulting in a decrease in blood pressure The overall effect of these drugs is a reduction in both preload and afterload It is very important that a child receiving diuretics and ACE inhibitors as part of anti-failure management has doses timed to avoid simultaneous administration of frusemide and captopril.

Beta blockers (beta adrenergic receptor antagonists)

Propanolol (non-selective)	Oral/intravenous – bolus	Blocks the action of adrenaline on beta 1 and beta 2 receptors Depresses renin secretion Useful in treating tachyarrhythmias caused by excessive catecholamines	Act by blocking catecholamine-induced increases in heart rate and contractility and so induce a slower rate and a decrease in contractility An adverse effect can be bronchoconstriction which results from blockage of β2 receptors
Atenolol (cardio-selective)	Oral	Selectively blocks beta1 receptors, slowing heart rate and decreasing contractility Decreases renin secretion *Adverse effects:* Bradycardia, Hypotension	
Metoprolol (cardio-selective)	Oral	Selectively blocks beta 1 receptors, slowing heart rate and decreasing contractility Decreases renin secretion *Adverse effects:* Bradycardia, AV block	
Labetolol (non-selective)	Oral/intravenous – infusion	Blocks alpha and beta receptors, slowing heart rate, decreasing contractility and reducing vasoconstriction *Adverse effects:* Fatigue, headache, ventricular arrhythmias	

Cardiac glycosides

Digoxin	Oral intravenous – bolus	Increases AV conduction time, thus slowing the overall ventricular rate Useful in controlling the ventricular rate in children with atrial fibrillation/flutter, although it does not resolve the abnormal rhythm *Adverse effects:* Bradycardia, AV block, loss of appetite, drowsiness	Used less in clinical practice now than in the past Their main use is in the treatment of heart failure and rhythm disturbances They work by increasing intracellular calcium availability and so improving contractility and by slowing conduction through the AV node, i.e. they slow and strengthen the heart rate

(Continued)

Table A1 Continued.

Drug	Action	Administration	Notes
Anti-arrhythmics			
Nifedipine	Primarily act on the smooth muscle in arterial walls Dilate coronary and systemic arteries and so reduce blood pressure *Adverse effects:* Headache, oedema	Sublingual	Inhibit the influx of calcium ions across the cellular membrane in smooth and cardiac muscle The effect of this is to reduce contractility, slow conduction within the heart and cause arteriolar dilation This then reduces cardiac output and also blood pressure
Amiodarone	A class III anti-arrhythmic agent which prolongs phase three of the cardiac action potential and also slows the intrinsic rate of the SA and AV nodes Useful in treatment of SVT and atrial dysrhythmias *Adverse effects:* Hypokalaemia, bradycardia, pulmonary toxicity and hepato-cellular toxicity	Oral/intravenous – continuous infusion	Loading dose normally given over 20 minutes prior to starting intravenous infusion Monitoring of serum potassium levels required while infusion being administered Has a very long half-life; therefore adverse effects may still be present after discontinuing therapy
Adenosine	A class V anti-arrhythmic which causes a temporary block of the AV node Causes a transient ventricular asystole Useful in the treatment of SVT and re-entry tachycardias *Adverse effects:* Chest pain, dyspnoea, dizziness, nausea and severe bradycardia (requiring temporary pacing)	Intravenous – bolus dose	Must be given rapidly into a large peripheral or central vein and followed by a rapid 0.9% saline flush

Phosphodiesterase inhibitors

Milrinone	Intravenous – infusion	A group of drugs that increase stroke volume by enhancing diastolic relaxation, improving contractility and decreasing vascular resistance
		Their clinical value in afterload reduction is used to enhance both right and left ventricular function
		Milrinone has a long half life of up to 10 hours, which can make dose management difficult

Used to reduce systemic vascular resistance and optimise left ventricular function

May be administered via a peripheral line

Adverse effects:
Dysrhythmias, hypotension, thrombocytopenia

Sildenafil	Oral	Works by increasing the levels of c-GMP which results in pulmonary vascular relaxation
		(Cyclic-guanosine monophosphate acts at the cellular level as a regulator of various metabolic processes)

Primarily used for its pulmonary vasodilation and reduction in right ventricular afterload

Augments the effects of inhaled nitric oxide (iNO) therapy

Prevents the pulmonary vasoconstriction and rebound PHT associated with weaning of iNO

Has been shown to increase cardiac output by as much as 30%

Adverse effects:
Headache, dizziness, visual disturbances, flushing.

Note: It is the responsibility of the individual practitioner to check prescribed medications against recognised National Formularies such as the British National Formulary (BNF) for Children (2007).

Chapter 5

CARING FOR A HIGHLY DEPENDENT CHILD WITH FLUID, ELECTROLYTE AND NUTRITIONAL REQUIREMENTS

Jill Cochrane, Doreen Crawford, Michaela Dixon and Janet Murphy

Introduction

The gastro-intestinal tract (GIT) is an enormously complex system and this chapter is not an exhaustive review. It focuses on the core principles of the anatomy and physiology of the tract, considers the importance of fluids, electrolytes and nutrition to a child and reviews how these can be administered. All children, regardless of their primary pathology, need fluid and nutritional support. The chapter will consider alterations from the normal gastro-intestinal function related to some of the more common conditions seen by children's nurses in high dependency areas.

Adequate fluid, electrolyte and nutritional status are essential for growth, development and homeostasis of children. It is even more important that the highly dependent child is adequately hydrated and nourished in order to support bodily functions and systems at a time of potential stress and higher metabolic demand. The needs of one child may differ greatly from the needs of another depending upon age, stage of illness/disease and condition. Different situations require different strategies, ranging from natural breast feeding, 'normal' free diet and drinks, to complex dietary supplements and fluid restrictions. The number of interventions required, e.g.

blood sugar testing or blood sampling for urea and electrolytes (U&E), and the frequency in which they are carried out depend on the above variables.

Eating and drinking is so much a part of daily living and central to many cultural celebrations that, whenever possible, the oral and enteral route is chosen, but this might not always be possible.

Embryological development of the GIT

See Table 5.1 for details of this.

Overview of the postnatal anatomy and physiology of the GIT

Following is a brief review of the structure and function of the GIT. For a more detailed perspective readers are advised to refer to an anatomy and physiology book of their choice. The GIT is often referred to as the digestive tract, reflecting its function, or the alimentary canal. It is a continuous tubular structure commencing at the mouth and ending with the anus. The oral and pharyngeal structures are shared with the

Table 5.1 Embryology and fetal development of the GIT.

Gestational age	Development
Weeks 2/3	Gastrulation comes from the Greek word for stomach but is also used to define the trilaminar embryo (this is made up of three layers: the ectoderm, mesoderm and endoderm). A cavity (intraembryonic coelom) forms with a layer of endoderm and mesoderm. This is still in communication with the yolk sac but will extend and grow later to become a continuous tubular structure which will extend from the pharyngeal membrane to the cloacal (meaning sewer) membrane
Week 4	Three distinct portions can be identified: the foregut, midgut and hindgut. These extend the length of the embryo and outgrowths will contribute different components of the GIT (see Table 7.1 in the metabolic chapter). The large midgut is generated by lateral embryonic folding which 'pinches off' a pocket of the yolk sac. The two coelomic compartments continue to communicate through the vitelline duct. The blood vessels are derived from the vessels that supplied the yolk sac. The terminal expanded part of the hindgut is the embryonic cloaca and this develops a fork-like projection which grows downwards towards the tail
Weeks 5/6	Lateral folds have given the embryo a cylindrical appearance. The development of the umbilical cord and the regression of the yolk sac reduces the communication between the intraembryonic coelom and the extracoelomic coelom. The foregut, midgut and hindgut are suspended from the posterior abdominal wall by the dorsal mesentery. The portion of the foregut destined to become the stomach is already dilating and rotating. Growth of the stomach is not equal and this results in the curvatures. Migration of the neural crest cells into the colon begin to enervate the walls of the intestine
Weeks 7/9	Massive growth and differentiation of the liver and heart results in a limited amount of intraembryonic space for the developing midgut loop and this projects and herniates into the base of the umbilical cord where the intestines lengthen and rotate. The proliferations of the epithelial cells which line the gut actually occlude the lumen. The cloaca has now divided into the urogenital sinus and the structure which will become the rectum and anal canal. By the end of the seventh week the anal membrane ruptures to form the anal opening. By week eight there are gastric pits, rughae and smooth muscle in the walls of the stomach.
Week 10	With a relative increase in the size of the abdominal cavity the intestines migrate back into this cavity and the developing peritoneal cavity loses its connections with the extraembryonic coelom. A key step in development is the rotation of the midgut that occurs to place the intestines in the correct abdominal position with its associated mesentry. An increasingly rich blood supply is provided by branches of the superior mesenteric artery
Weeks 11–20	By week 11 the caecum is in the right iliac fossa and there are villi increasing the surface area of the small intestine. The liver produces bile which is secreted into the duodenum. Increasing cellular differentiation allows for the unique and specialist histology within the GIT. This is mainly endodermal in origin. Chief cells and parietal cells are present by week 16. The fetus can swallow amniotic fluid, stimulating a limited peristalsis. The framework of the GIT is established. All that is required is growth and maturity. The surface mucosa will not mature fully until after birth and exposure to milk

From Chamley (2003) and Moore and Persaud (2003).

respiratory tract and will not be considered here. The functions of the GIT are supported by a range of accessory glands and organs.

Basic functions of the GIT

- Ingestion
- Digestion
- Absorption
- Egestion and elimination

Ingestion

This is the physical process of taking in food and fluids for processing in the GIT. In sick children this process often has to be supported by the selected use of nasal or oral tubes. Nurses are skilled at and accustomed to passing these into the stomach, but if the stomach has to be bypassed for any reason the tubes can be passed through the pylorus and placed into the duodenum or the jejunum. If the requirement for support is likely to be long term then a gastrostomy or a jejunostomy could be performed. These are surgical openings into the stomach or jejunum.

Digestion and absorption

This process is divided into two complementary functions: mechanical digestion and chemical digestion. The result is to process food and fluid into small enough component parts to facilitate absorption across the gastro-intestinal membrane and transportation in the circulation. The ultimate stage in these digestive processes is assimilation into the cells to provide the raw materials for metabolism. The function of digestion is supported by peristalsis (a powerful rhythmic sequential unidirectional muscular contraction, propelling gut contents forward). In high dependency children there are many reasons why this might not happen normally:

- There could be altered anatomy with insufficient surface area to absorb required nutrients, e.g. short gut syndrome as a result of surgical resection for necrotising enterocolitis.

- The surface area may not be compromised, but the child's metabolic needs are increased because of illness.
- There could be sensitivity or inflammatory conditions impeding the absorption of nutrients or liquid from the gut, e.g. coeliac and Crohn's disease.
- There could be physical problems with the gut motility. This may be a result of sedation or related to the GIT itself, e.g. malrotation, volvulus, intussusceptions causing acute obstruction, or Hirschsprung's disease, which may present as a more chronic condition. Alternatively the process could be dramatically speeded up as a reaction to infection, toxins or irritation, causing diarrhoea.

Egestion and elimination

This is the process of excretion of waste and of non-absorbable bulk. Defecation is a painless process and the quantity and content of the stool passed reflects the quantity and content of the diet, the state of the GIT and the general wellbeing of the individual. Bowel patterns change with developmental maturity of the GIT and bowel habits can vary enormously between individuals. Many children in high dependency areas will be unable to evacuate their bowels normally and many of the children will have stoma of various types, such as a colostomy (a surgical opening into the colon). The higher up the intestinal tract the stoma is formed, the more liquid the stool and the greater the need for nutritional support.

Overview of the physiology of fluid and electrolyte balance

Body fluids are necessary for the transportation of gases, nutrients and waste, they help with the electrical activity needed for body functions and they are involved in the process of converting food into energy. The total volume of water and its distribution in the child changes with age and amount of fat present. Those with more body fat have a lower proportion of body water than children with less fat. The approximate water content and blood volume in the body related to age is shown in Table 5.2.

Distribution and movement of body fluids

The water content of the body is contained within various compartments. Intracellular fluid (ICF) is water contained within the cells. Extracellular fluid (ECF) is water outside of the cells. ECF fluid can be further divided into intravascular fluid (plasma), interstitial fluid (fluid surrounding tissue cells) and transcellular fluid (cerebral spinal fluid, synovial fluid, pleural fluid and peritoneal fluid). ECF contains large amounts of sodium and chloride, moderate amounts of bicarbonate and small amounts of potassium, magnesium, calcium and phosphate. This is very different from the content of ICF which has hardly any calcium, small amounts of sodium, chloride, bicarbonate and phosphate, moderate amounts of magnesium and large amounts of potassium.

Table 5.2 Body water content and blood volume.

Age group	Approximate water content in body (%)	Approximate blood volume (mL/kg)
Premature infant	90	85–90
Newborn infant	70–80	80–90
12–24 months	64	75–80
Adult	60	65–70

Top tip

When measuring levels of substances/electrolytes in a patient's blood it is the ECF levels that you are measuring.

Several factors influence the movement of fluid in and out of the vascular space; these are osmotic, oncotic and hydrostatic pressure, together with changes in capillary permeability (Table 5.3).

Table 5.3 The distribution and movement of body fluids.

Pressure or mechanism	Contributing factors
Osmotic pressure	Directly related to number of particles dissolved in a fluid. The number of dissolved particles per litre of fluid is known as osmolality. These particles are mainly electrolytes and proteins. Sodium is the main electrolyte determining intravascular osmotic pressure. The osmotic pressure of intravascular, interstitial and intracellular fluids will be equal; however, if there is an acute fall in osmotic pressure of the intravascular compartment then fluid will move out into the tissues
Oncotic pressure	Mainly determined by plasma proteins. A normal level of plasma proteins will keep fluid within the intravascular space. Significant loss of plasma proteins will result in water moving from the intravascular space to the tissues, causing tissue oedema and hypovolaemia
Hydrostatic pressure	This can be described as the pressure of water in the blood vessels or tissues. The force of the heart pumping the blood through the blood vessels causes a hydrostatic pressure that is slightly higher than that in the tissues. This is counteracted by the oncotic pressure so that there is no net loss of fluid into the tissue spaces
Capillary permeability	In health capillary pores are too small to allow the passage of plasma proteins. However, if capillary permeability increases, plasma proteins will leave the capillaries, taking water with them into the interstitial space, leading to hypovolaemia. The permeability of the capillary wall changes in inflammatory disease states

In addition to these mechanisms of body fluid distribution, fluid balance is influenced by changes in both the osmolality and volume of the plasma (Pearson 2002). Water is lost from the body by insensible loss (skin and respiration) and sensible mechanisms (kidneys and urine production).

Regulation of water balance

Total body water (TBW) varies with gender, weight and age. Infants and young children have a greater water concentration than adults, with TBW approximating 75–80% of body weight in the full-term infant and an even greater proportion in the premature infant. In older children and adolescents the range is from 40 to 60%. In addition to having more TBW, infants have more water in their ECF compartments than adults. The infant also has a greater water turnover due to its higher metabolic rate, larger surface area in relation to body mass and the infant's inability to concentrate urine due to immature kidneys.

Stop and think

Infants and children under 2 years of age are more vulnerable to fluid loss and dehydration due to the proportion of ECF than older children and adults and will become dehydrated much quicker.

Water is taken into the body by the oral intake of fluid and food. The water from fluids and solid foods is absorbed from the gastrointestinal tract. A small amount of water is gained from metabolic processes. Regardless of age, all healthy persons require approximately 100 mL of water per 100 calories metabolised for dissolving and eliminating metabolic wastes. It should be remembered that the metabolic rate will increase with fever. Water loss is mainly through the kidneys although it is also lost through the skin, lungs and gastrointestinal tract.

There are two main physiological mechanisms important in regulating body water: thirst and the antidiuretic hormone (ADH). Thirst is controlled by the thirst centre in the hypothalamus. This centre is stimulated by two stimuli: cellular dehydration, caused by an increase in extracellular osmolality and detected by osmoreceptors situated near the thirst centre, and a decrease in blood volume. Stretch receptors, known as baroreceptors, which are situated in the carotid sinus and aorta are sensitive to changes in arterial blood pressure together with low pressure baroreceptors which are located in the left atrium and major thoracic veins.

A third important stimulus for thirst is angiotensin 2. Its secretion increases in response to low blood volume and low blood pressure. ADH is responsible for the reabsorption of water by the kidneys. ADH is also known as vasopressin. If too little ADH is secreted then the kidneys' ability to reabsorb water diminishes, resulting in excessive urine output (polyuria). The levels of circulating ADH are controlled by extracellular volume and osmolality.

In the highly dependent and critically ill child there is a propensity for the child to retain fluid due to increased production of ADH and aldosterone. Factors that may cause this to occur include hypotension, pain, stress, positive pressure ventilation and severe pulmonary hypertension. Increased production of ADH results in an increase in intravascular volume and a reduction in intravascular osmolarity, while increased secretion of aldosterone results in increased sodium and water reabsorption. It is therefore essential that the nurse is able to accurately assess the fluid balance status of the child.

Daily fluid requirements

The daily fluid requirement of children varies with age and condition. Consideration must also be given to the route and efficiency of fluid administration when fluid is not always administered by the enteral route. Standard fluid allowance for neonates, infants and children is calculated in terms of volume of oral feed required to meet the calorific needs of the

Table 5.4 Fluid requirements.

Daily fluid requirements	Hourly fluid requirements
Preterm infants 200 mL/kg/day	1–10 kg: 4 mL/kg/h
Term infants 150 mL/kg/day	11–20 kg: 2 mL/kg/h
Children/adolescents 2–3 L/day	>20 kg: 1 mL/kg/h

Adapted from APLS guidelines (2005).

healthy growing child. Table 5.4 illustrates normal fluid requirements according to age.

Clinical considerations

Dehydration

Infants under the age of 2 years are more at risk of becoming dehydrated due to their physiology. However, dehydration can occur in any age of child and may occur more readily in a child with high dependency needs. Some causes of dehydration include vomiting, poor absorption, diarrhoea, diabetes, not replacing gastric or intestinal aspirate, thermal injury, fever and the use of diuretics. Dehydration can result from either inadequate fluid intake or excessive fluid loss. In addition to dehydration it is likely that the child will also have abnormal levels of electrolytes. Dehydration is usually classified according to its level of severity, i.e. mild, moderate or severe, but also according to the serum sodium and osmolarity levels, thus:

- Isotonic
- Hypotonic (hyponatraemic)
- Hypertonic (hypernatraemic)

Isotonic dehydration occurs when the loss of water and sodium are proportional. Serum sodium remains normal and as a result there is equal distribution of fluid loss between the interstitial and intravascular spaces.

Hypotonic dehydration results if a greater proportion of sodium is lost than that of water. Serum sodium falls, resulting in decreased serum osmolarity and shifting of fluid from intravascular to interstitial and cellular spaces. Children with hypotonic dehydration are likely to quickly show signs and symptoms of low intravascular volume.

Hypertonic dehydration occurs when water is lost in greater proportion to sodium. Serum sodium increases which shifts fluid from the cellular and interstitial spaces to the intravascular space. This will help maintain intravascular volume, so signs of dehydration may not be evident until fluid loss is substantial. Classification and signs and symptoms of dehydration are shown in Table 5.5. When assessing children for signs of dehydration it is always essential that a complete history is taken and that the child's age and type of dehydration are taken into account, as signs and symptoms may vary.

Treatment

Unless treated, moderate to severe dehydration will lead to a compromise of cardiac output and systemic perfusion. If this occurs, the body uses compensatory mechanisms to try to maintain systemic and essential organ perfusion, which in turn may lead to metabolic acidosis, multi-system failure and ultimately death. As the systems are so interdependent, readers should refer to Chapters 4 (Cardiac) and 8 (Renal) to augment their understanding.

Whether the dehydration is isotonic, hypotonic or hypertonic in origin the aims of treatment are restoration and maintenance of intravascular volume and systemic perfusion together with correction of any electrolyte imbalance. In mild dehydration and, depending on cause and the age of the child, rehydration may be achieved through oral therapy. However, in the child with high dependency needs the insertion of one or preferably two wide-bore intravenous catheters should be established. If access is difficult to obtain, an intraosseous needle should be considered while preparation is made for a cut down into a vein. When access to the circulation is established, the insertion of a central venous pressure monitor should be considered (see Chapter 2).

Stop and think

A central venous catheter (CVP) may be appropriate as this provides good access for the administration of fluids while also allowing measurement of central venous pressure as an indication of intravascular volume. However, CVPs are not without risk and should only be used in areas where the doctors and nurses are used to caring for them.

The dehydrated child must be assessed for signs of shock. This is ascertained by clinical (Table 5.5) and biochemical examination. The cause of the dehydration also needs to be established together with an effective treatment regime to allow for rehydration and correction of abnormalities in electrolyte balance over a 24 to 48 hours period (APLS 2005). The acid–base balance of the child also needs to be considered

and treated accordingly. For details on the maintenance of body pH refer to Chapter 3.

The fluid resuscitation of a child in hypovolaemic shock, secondary to fluid loss, involves the rapid administration of crystalloid. The starting volume is 20 mL/kg. This can be repeated if there is inadequate clinical response (with no evidence of intravascular overload). The type of fluid used should approximate in electrolyte concentration to that of serum. Commonly used fluids are 0.9% saline or Hartmann's® solution. The presence of hyper-/hyponatraemia does not affect the choice of fluids during this stage of resuscitation (APLS 2005).

Stop and think

If the primary cause of shock is cardiac dysrhythmia caused by electrolyte imbalance, specifically potassium, then correction of the electrolyte abnormality is required.

Over-hydration and fluid overload

The highly dependent child may be more susceptible to fluid overload and oedema. There should be hourly calculation of fluid input and output

Table 5.5 Classification and signs and symptoms of dehydration.

Clinical presentation	Mild dehydration	Moderate dehydration	Severe dehydration
Body weight loss	Infant: 5% (50 mL/kg) Child: 3% (30 mL/kg)	10% (100 mL/kg) 6% (60 mL/kg)	15% (150 mL/kg) 9% (90 mL/kg)
Heart rate	Mild tachycardia	Moderate tachycardia	Extreme tachycardia
Blood pressure	Normal	Normal	Hypotensive
Peripheral pulses	Normal	Weakened	Absent
Skin perfusion	Normal/warm	Pale/cool	Mottled/grey/cold
Skin turgor	Slightly reduced	Moderately reduced	Severely reduced
Mucous membrane	Dry	Very dry	Extremely dry
Capillary refill time	Normal to slightly prolonged	Slightly/moderately prolonged	Severely prolonged
Urine output	Slightly reduced	Mild oliguria	Severe oliguria or anuria
Neurological	Normal/irritable	Irritable/lethargic	Unresponsive
Anterior fontanels	Flat or depressed	Moderately depressed	Significantly depressed

Adapted from Hazinski (1992).

and continuous monitoring supplemented by frequent clinical reassessment.

Four main factors can cause oedema and they are listed in Table 5.6.

Signs and symptoms of fluid overload include:

- Oedema
- Tachycardia
- Hypertension
- Breathlessness
- Decrease in saturations
- Enlarged liver
- Raised central venous pressure
- Weight gain
- Signs of a 'wet' chest on X-ray
- Frothy pink secretions if intubated

Treatment of fluid overload will be determined by the cause, e.g. if the primary cause of fluid overload is due to cardiac failure then the use of inotropic and/or diuretic therapy may be indicated in order to increase cardiac output. However, if the fluid overload is due to over-hydration and intravascular overload then the patient is likely to need fluid restriction and the administration of diuretics.

Electrolytes

Electrolytes are ions with the ability to conduct a charge and they account for approximately 95% of the solute molecules in body water (see Table 5.7). The other 5% of solutes are

Table 5.6 Factors contributing to oedema.

Circulatory disturbance	Reason
Increased capillary pressure	A result of increased vascular volume caused by heart failure, kidney disease or thermal injury A result of venous obstruction caused by acute pulmonary oedema or liver disease with portal vein congestion A result of decreased arteriolar resistance caused by drugs blocking the calcium channels
Decreased colloidal osmotic pressure	A loss of plasma proteins caused by kidney disease, such as nephrotic syndrome, or extensive burns A decrease in the production of plasma proteins as a result of liver disease, starvation or malnutrition
Increased capillary permeability	A result of extensive tissue injury or thermal injury, allergic reactions or inflammation
Obstruction of lymphatic flow	A result of malignant obstruction or obliteration of lymphatic structures

Adapted from Matfin and Porth (2004).

Table 5.7 Normal values of electrolytes.

Electrolyte	Premature infant (mmol/L)	Term infant (mmol/L)	Child (mmol/L)	Daily requirements (mmol/kg/day)
Potassium	4.5–7.2	3.6–6.4	3.5–5.0	1–2
Sodium	135–145	135–145	135–145	2–4
Calcium	2.1–2.7	2.1–2.7	2.1–2.7	0.3
Magnesium	0.6–1.0	0.6–1.0	0.6–1.0	0.07–0.2
Phosphate	1.0–2.6	1.0–1.8	1.0–1.8	0.04–1.5

Adapted from Pearson (2002).

non-electrolytes such as glucose, urea and creatinine (McCance and Huether 2002). The main electrolytes are sodium, potassium, calcium, magnesium, chloride, bicarbonate and phosphate. The main intracellular electrolyte is potassium while the main extracellular electrolyte is sodium.

Stop and think

Normal values and daily requirements differ according to age of the child and the different techniques used by different laboratories. Refer to local policy and seek advice if you are unsure about a value for a particular child.

Electrolyte action

Having an excess or deficiency of electrolytes can potentially be dangerous for any child and even more so for the child with high dependency needs.

Sodium (Na+)

As the main electrolyte in the ECF compartment, sodium (Na+) has a major effect on osmosis and osmolality. Hyponatraemia is classified as a sodium level less than 135 mmol/L. Deficits of sodium alter the ability of cells to depolarise and repolarise normally .

Signs and symptoms of hyponatraemia may include lethargy, headaches, seizures and coma. If hyponatraemia is accompanied by a loss of ECF then signs of hypovolaemia may be displayed, including tachycardia hypotension and diminished urine output. In other situations hyponatraemia may be due to water retention, detected by weight gain and oedema (McCance and Huether 2002). Treatment will depend on the cause, biochemical results and clinical manifestation. Rapid falls in sodium can be corrected quickly, but these situations are unusual. Sodium levels usually fall gradually and correction should also be so. Natural correction with fluid restriction is possible.

Stop and think

Hypertonic saline should be given with care as this can result in fluid shifts.

Hypernatraemia is a sodium level in excess of 145 mmol/L. It can be caused by excessive water loss, decreased water intake or excessive sodium intake. Signs and symptoms may include thirst, oliguria/anuria, high specific gravity of urine and increased serum osmolality. If decreased intravascular volume occurs then tachycardia, hypotension and peripheral shutdown may also present. Neurological symptoms resulting from the movement of water out of brain cells may include headache, seizures and coma. Identification of the cause by history, clinical examination and biochemical investigations will define treatment. The cause needs to be treated but will also include rehydration.

Potassium (K+)

Potassium is the most common intracellular ion, with a normal intracellular concentration of 140–150 mmol/L. The extra cellular levels are much lower (please refer to Table 5.7). Potassium is regulated by two main mechanisms: through the kidneys, which either conserve or eliminate potassium, and through the transcellular shifts between the intracellular and extracellular compartments, which allows potassium to enter body cells when plasma levels are high and move out when plasma levels are low (Matfin and Porth 2004). The control of potassium within the normal range is essential as only a slight derangement from normal levels can result in life-threatening cardiac dysrhythmias.

Potassium is essential for many body functions including growth, conduction of nerve impulses, acid–base balance and the use of carbohydrates for energy. Hypokalaemia is a plasma potassium level below 3.5 mmol/L. Causes of hypokalaemia include inadequate intake, excessive loss, usually through gastrointestinal, skin and renal losses, and redistribution of potassium between the ICF and ECF compartments.

Signs and symptoms can include polyuria, vomiting, muscle cramps, confusion, metabolic alkalosis and cardiac arrhythmias. Treatment consists of treating the cause and if necessary administering potassium supplements either by the oral route or if necessary intravenously.

Top tip

Potassium is a powerful electrolyte. Children with abnormal potassium levels ought to be electro-cardiographically monitored. Hypokalaemia can cause (ECG) changes including prolonged PR interval, depression of ST segment and the flattening of the T wave.

Stop and think

IV potassium *must* be administered by a nurse or doctor who is appropriately trained and skilled in its administration. It needs to be given slowly. potassium should only be administered through a good central vascular access and infusion rate should not exceed 0.4 mmol/kg/h. The child should be ECG monitored.

Hyperkalaemia is an increase in plasma potassium level above 5.0 mmol/L. It is a condition that is very rarely seen in the well child but can occur in the highly dependent patient. The main causes are excessive rapid administration of potassium, decreased renal excretion, as in acute renal failure, and movement of potassium between the ICF and ECF compartments. The signs and symptoms include nausea and diarrhoea, dizziness and muscle cramps. The main risk of hyperkalaemia is cardiac dysrhythmia which could lead to cardiac arrest. The child should be ECG monitored. Treatment options include decreasing or stopping intake, increasing renal excretion and increasing cellular uptake (Matfin and Porth 2004).

Calcium (Ca^+), phosphate (PO_4^-) and magnesium (Mg)

Calcium and magnesium are closely linked to phosphate levels (Pearson 2002). They are obtained from the diet and absorbed from the intestines, with any excess being eliminated in the urine. Most of the body's calcium and phosphate and 50% of magnesium are found in the bones. Most of the remaining amounts of each electrolyte are found intracellularly. Only very small amounts of calcium, magnesium and phosphate are present within the extracellular fluid and are regulated by vitamin D, parathyroid hormone and calcitonin production.

Calcium: The major source of calcium is milk and milk products. The calcium content of the bone provides strength and stability to the skeletal system. It is also used to maintain extracellular levels. The small amount of extracellular calcium is either a protein-bound complex or ionised. It is only the ionised form that is free to leave the vascular compartment and participate in cellular function. Functions of ionised calcium include participation in enzyme reactions, an effect on membrane potential, neuronal excitability, which is necessary for contraction in skeletal, cardiac and smooth muscle, and influencing cardiac contractility and automaticity. It is also essential for blood clotting (Matfin and Porth 2004).

Children with critical illness or high dependency needs are at risk of suffering from hypocalcaemia as they may have impaired ability to gain calcium from bone stores, high losses from the kidneys or more may bind with protein and then be unavailable. Hypocalcaemia may be acute or chronic. In the acute stage it can cause jittery symptoms, convulsions, ECG abnormalities, arrhythmias and heart failure. Treatment will be to identify and treat the cause and administer calcium infusion according to local treatment regime and policy. Hypercalcaemia is rare but may occur because of excessive bone resorption as a result of cancer, with bone metastases, leukaemia, lymphoma and multiple myeloma. It may occur as a result of prolonged and extensive immobilisation and in paraplegics and quadriplegics. Other causes include endocrine diseases, the recovery phase of acute renal failure and Williams syndrome. Signs and symptoms include seizures, muscle flaccidity and tachyarrhythmias. Many patients with hypercalcaemia will be volume depleted and will respond to fluid resuscitation followed by diuretic therapy. Other forms of treatment include renal replacement therapy (Pearson 2002).

Hypocalcaemia

Clinical manifestations of hypocalcaemia are due to disturbances in cellular membrane potential, resulting in neuromuscular irritability. Muscle cramps involving the back and legs are common. Insidious hypocalcaemia may produce symptoms of encephalopathy. Papilloedema occasionally occurs, and cataracts may develop after prolonged hypocalcaemia. Severe hypocalcaemia with plasma Ca <1.75 mmol/L may cause tetany, laryngospasm and generalised seizures.

Stop and think

Measurement of calcium can be done as total calcium or ionised calcium. The value range differs so it is important you know which one has been measured and requested.
Total: 2.0–2.7 mmol/L
Ionised: 1.20–1.3 mmol/L

Phosphate (HPO₄): Negative electrolyte

Phosphate is essential for many bodily functions. It helps bone formation, is essential for certain metabolic processes, including the formation of ATP and the enzymes necessary for metabolism of glucose, fat and protein, and serves as an acid–base buffer in ECF and in the renal excretion of hydrogen ions (Matfin and Porth 2004). Like calcium, only a small amount of phosphate is located in the ECF compartment. Causes of hypophosphataemia include decreased intestinal absorption, e.g. by severe and prolonged diarrhoea, lack of vitamin D, increased renal losses and malnutrition. The treatment is by replacement therapy and treatment of the cause. The most common causes of hyperphosphataemia is impaired renal function and tumor lysis syndrome. If hyperphosphataemia is present then symptoms similar to hypocalcaemia will be seen.

Hyperphosphataemia

Skeletal fractures or disease, kidney failure, hypoparathyroidism, haemodialysis, diabetic ketoacidosis (DKA), acromegaly, systemic infection and intestinal obstruction can all cause phosphate retention and buildup in the blood, known as hyperphosphataemia. The disorder occurs concurrently with hypocalcaemia. Individuals with mild hyperphosphataemia are typically asymptomatic, but signs of severe hyperphosphataemia include parathesia, tingling in the hands and fingers, muscle spasms and cramps, convulsions and cardiac arrest.

Hypophosphataemia

Low serum phosphate levels may be caused by hypomagnesaemia and hypokalaemia. Severe burns, DKA, kidney disease, hyperparathyroidism, hypothyroidism, Cushing's syndrome, malnutrition, haemodialysis, vitamin D deficiency, and prolonged diuretic therapy can also diminish blood phosphate levels and cause hypophosphataemia. There are typically few physical signs of mild phosphate depletion. Symptoms of severe hypophosphataemia include muscle weakness, weight loss and bone deformities (osteomalacia).

Magnesium

Magnesium is a very important electrolyte. It is essential for all reactions that require ATP, for replication and transcription of DNA and for the translocation of messenger RNA. It is required for cellular energy metabolism, functioning of the sodium potassium membrane pump, nerve conduction and calcium channel activity (Matfin and Porth 2004). Magnesium is found in green vegetables, meats, nuts and seafood and body levels are mainly regulated by the kidney.

Hypomagnesaemia can be caused by impaired intake or absorption as in starvation and malabsorption. It can also be caused by increased losses due to diuretic therapy and DKA. Signs and symptoms include tetany, cardiac arrhythmias and nystagmus. Treatment is by magnesium replacement, but caution is required if the intravenous route is used.

Hypermagnesaemia is rare and is mainly caused by renal failure. Signs and symptoms include lethargy, confusion, hypotension and cardiac arrhythmias. Treatment should include stopping any administration and the administration of calcium which is an antagonist of magnesium.

Nutritional needs of the child

About 11–12 million children die each year before the age of 5. Malnutrition is considered to be the sole contributing cause in about 60% of these deaths. Nutritional needs for the high dependency infant and child must equate or meet the total metabolic needs of the body allowing for tissue repair and/or catch-up with growth. Energy input is obtained from three main classifications of food groups – carbohydrates, fats and proteins. Energy is derived from the oxidation of carbon and hydrogen in dietary molecules. Terms that are associated with metabolism are shown in Table 5.8.

Carbohydrate

Carbohydrates are absorbed from the digestive tract. During digestion large carbohydrate molecules such as starch and lactose are broken down to simple sugars such as glucose, fructose and galactose. These are then absorbed into the bloodstream and transported to the liver by the hepatic portal vein. From the liver they are then transported systemically. Any excess of these substances is stored as glycogen in the liver and skeletal muscle. This storage of glycogen can be readily broken down into glucose when required. The importance of this mechanism is that some cells, e.g. brain cells, rely almost exclusively on glucose as their source of energy for ATP production.

Fat

Fat molecules are absorbed from the digestive system in small clusters known as chylomicrons. These chylomicrons tend not to enter the bloodstream directly but are absorbed by the lymphatic system. This means they are transported directly to the heart and the rest of the body. Fat consists of glycerol and fatty acids and both of these can be used to produce energy. Glycerol is a carbohydrate and the liver uses it to synthesise glucose. Fatty acids are fed into the Krebs cycle in the mitochondria, leading to further production of ATP. Fat contains more energy per gram than carbohydrate.

Protein

Proteins consist of chains of amino acids. These chains are broken down by enzymes in the digestive system, releasing amino acids which are then absorbed into the bloodstream. Amino acids are

Table 5.8 Terms associated with metabolism.

Term	Definition
Homeostasis	The maintenance of a stable environment
Anabolism	The building of large molecules from smaller ones, requiring energy; e.g. making fat from fatty acids and glycerol
Catabolism	The breakdown of large complex molecules into smaller ones, releasing energy; e.g. releasing amino acids from a peptide chain
Adenosine tri-phosphate (ATP)	Energy generated and used by the cells
Glycolysis	A stage in glucose metabolism where glucose is broken down, resulting in the production of ATP

first transported to the liver and then to the rest of the body. Amino acids are not usually used as a source of fuel, their primary function being for growth and development. However, if other sources of energy are not available then they are utilised as a source of energy. The breakdown of amino acids results in the production of ammonia which is then converted into urea by the liver before being excreted by the kidneys.

In order for the cells of the body to be able to utilise the products of metabolism, two hormones are needed – insulin and glucagon – which are secreted by the pancreas.

Insulin

Insulin is secreted by the β cells in the islets of Langerhans in the pancreas. It is a very large polypeptide and the main role of insulin is the maintenance of blood glucose by binding with large protein receptors in the cell wall. Table 5.9 reviews the action of insulin on the products of carbohydrate, fat and protein metabolism.

Glucagon

Glucagon is secreted by the α cells of the islets of Langerhans in the pancreas. It has the opposite action to insulin. The effects of glucagon include the increased breakdown of glycogen stores to form glucose, increased breakdown of fats and glucose synthesis.

For more information on metabolism refer to Chapter 7.

Growth of the infant and child

Growth only occurs when more nutrition is provided than is required to meet basic metabolic needs and have a balanced intake of both macronutrients and micronutrients. Macronutrients include carbohydrates, lipids and proteins. Micronutrients include minerals such as calcium, magnesium, phosphate, iron, zinc and copper. Micronutrients include electrolytes, water-soluble vitamins B and C and fat-soluble vitamins A, D, E and K.

It is expected that normal growth pattern would see an infant doubling its birth weight by 6 months, trebling birth weight by 12 months and quadrupling birth weight by 24 months. Sixty per cent of children's energy go to the major organs in order to maintain normal function. Basal metabolic rate reaches its maximum around the age of 2, then decreases with age.

Nutritional assessment

Nutritional assessment of the well infant and child is routinely carried out in general practice and in health care centres. Nutritional assessment of the child with high dependency needs is more difficult. Weighing patients may be difficult

Table 5.9 Effects of insulin on carbohydrate, fat and protein metabolism.

Nutrient group	Action of insulin
Carbohydrate metabolism	Insulin is important for the transport of glucose into the adipose cells, providing the glycerol portion of the fat molecule for the deposition of fat in these cells
Fat metabolism	Insulin decreases the utilisation of fat as a source of energy. It inhibits the action of lipase. In the absence of insulin, increased breakdown and utilisation of fat for energy occurs which leads to excessive amounts of acetoacetic acid being formed which cannot be metabolised by the body and leads to a buildup of acid systemically
Protein metabolism	Little is understood about the effects of insulin on protein synthesis and storage other than that insulin causes active transport of amino acids into the cells. Insulin has a direct effect on ribosomes by increasing the translation messenger RNA, so forming new proteins, and it inhibits the catabolism of proteins, decreasing the rate of amino acid release from cells

if attached to machinery and may not give a true indication of nutritional status if oedematous. Illness may alter or mask biochemical results. Enteral feeding in the highly dependent child needs to be commenced as soon as possible.

Types and methods of feeding

Children require more calories per kilogram due to a higher metabolic rate and any child who has an illness/disease will need additional calorific intake (Singh 1997). Nutrition including type, volume and administration of feed needs to be decided as early as possible to prevent deleterious physiological effects (Alexander 1999). Enteral feeding is the method best suited to achieving maximal nutritional status in the child with high dependency needs. There are obvious advantages of enteral feeding and these include the facts that it is efficient and economical, readily available, and the majority of nurses have the skills and expertise to administer feeds safely enterally. Enteral feeding maintains gut barrier structure and function. It is an important stimulus to mature the gut of a premature infant, maximise the immunological properties of the gut and minimise the risk of bacterial translocation.

However, for a number of reasons it may not be possible for children to receive their nutritional requirement by this method. These include recent gut surgery, small gut syndrome, paralytic ileus, non-absorption of feeds, severe breathlessness and respiratory distress. Another consideration of method and frequency of feeding is the age of the child. The volume capacity of the stomach alters with age (see Table 5.10) and this together with the condition of the child needs to be taken into account when considering method and frequency of enteral feeding.

Whenever possible intermittent oral feeding is the preferred method of feeding, and for the infant breast milk is the preferred feed. However, there are many situations where oral feeding may not be an option or indeed intermittent feeding may not be appropriate, e.g. endotracheal

Table 5.10 Stomach capacity by age.

Age	Capacity (in mL)
Newborn	10–20
1 week	30–90
2–3 weeks	75–100
1 month	90–150
3 months	150–200
1 year	210–360
2 years	500
10 years	750–900
16 years	1500
Adult	2000–3000

From Moules and Ramsey (1998).

intubation, absent or impaired swallowing reflexes, coma and severe breathlessness. In these situations enteral feeding can be administered by the use of naso-/orogastric, nasoduodenal or nasojejunal tubes, or in the situation where long-term tube feeding is anticipated, a gastrostomy or jejunostomy may be performed. Frequency of feeding can also be adapted from intermittent to continuous in order to meet the individual needs and condition of the child.

Stop and think

It is essential that when feeding by the nasogastric route the position of the tube is tested correctly. This must be done by measuring the pH value using indicator strips. The pH should read 5.5 or below. Alternatively or in addition, tube position can be checked by radiography. Tube position must not be checked by inserting air down the tube and listening for air in the stomach with a stethoscope, by testing for pH with litmus paper or by any other means.

Types of enteral feeds

Breast milk is universally advocated as the milk of choice for feeding infants. Current recommendations are for exclusive breast milk for

6 months and as a dietary supplement for up to 2 years (WHO 2005). Not surprisingly it is well tolerated even in seriously compromised guts. Approximately 50% of energy in breast milk is provided by fats whereas in infant formulae this equates to approximately 25%. Breast milk has protective properties, e.g. immunoglobulin A (IgA) has antibodies which are active against a wide range of bacterial, viral, fungal and parasitic antigens. Lactoferrin binds with free iron in milk and is thought to inhibit the growth of *Escherichia coli* and lysosome is present which attacks bacteria membranes.

Growth factors in breast milk may have a role in maintaining the protective nature of the intact gastrointestinal mucosa. Breast milk promotes the growth of normal gut flora. Breast-fed infants are less likely to experience bouts of infection compared to formula-fed infants, particularly where there are risks of unhygienic preparation and storage of the feed. For the infants of mothers unable to express breast milk or who are unable to express sufficient milk to feed their infants, donor milk is becoming more available again.

Most infant feeding formulae are based upon cows' milk which has been modified to resemble the nutritional composition of mature breast milk. Modified cows' milk feeds can be divided into three group:

- Whey dominant – whey to casein ratio similar to breast milk. Examples of whey-based infant formulae are Aptamil First™, Cow & Gate Premium™, Farley's First Milk™, SMA Gold™
- Casein dominant – whey to casein ratio similar to cows' milk. There is no scientific evidence to support the claim that a casein-dominant feed will help to satisfy a hungry infant
- Follow-on formulae for infants over 6 months of age (higher iron content)

The best enteral feed for the child

The type of enteral feed to be used should consider patient condition, availability of feed and parental

Table 5.11 Types of formula feed.

Age	Type of formula feed
Preterm below 2 kg	Nutriprem, SMA Low Birth Weight
Preterm above 2 kg	Nutriprem 2, Premcare
Full term and under 1 year	EBM, SMA Gold, Cow & Gate Premium or Plus, Aptimil, Farley's First Milk
1–6 years (8–20 kg)	Nutrini, Nutrini-Fibre, Nutrini-Energy, Multifibre
7–12 years (21–45 kg)	Tentrini Multifibre, Tentrini Energy with Fibre
13 years and above	Nutrison Multifibre

choice. Dieticians should be involved in ensuring that high dependency children are receiving the appropriate feed, including any additional supplements, in order to meet their growth and metabolic needs. Types of enteral feeds and diets available are listed in Tables 5.11 and 5.12 and a strategy by which the enteral feed can be commenced and built up is considered in Figure 5.1.

Parenteral nutrition (PN)

Parenteral nutrition means administering feed by any means other than the mouth. Giving nutrition directly into the blood circulation is common with highly dependent children. The infusion consists of a sterile prescription of water, amino acids, glucose, minerals and vitamins. Emulsified fats can also be administered. PN is hyperosmolar and must be infused slowly into a large vessel where there is a good circulating volume to dilute and buffer the infusion. The subclavian or the jugular veins are frequently used. These are major blood vessels, and to avoid ascending infection or loss of patency the line needs to be handled aseptically and kept flushed even during times when nutrition is not being administered. This is particularly important if the child is mobile or to emphasise to the parents who have children on long-term TPN and

Table 5.12 Types of enteral feed.

Type of feed	Usage
Oral supplements	Not complete diets but used as supplements to supply more energy
Polymeric diets	For children with normal/near-normal gut function. Contain protein, long chain fatty acids, complex carbohydrates, vitamins and minerals (e.g. Pediasure and Ensure)
Pre-digested diets	For children with severely impaired gastrointestinal function. Contain free amino acids, di- and tripeptides, short carbohydrate polymers and fat, as well as vitamins, minerals and essential fatty acids (e.g. Pregestimil)
Elemental diets	For patients with severe gastrointestinal dysfunction
Disease-specific diets	Diets specifically formulated for specific conditions such as renal failure and hepatic encephalopathy chylothorax
Modular diets	Individual components of a feed can be adjusted to achieve optimum diet

are being taught to administer this at home. If the requirement is going to be a long-term one a Hickman or a Broviac line may be surgically inserted.

The solution usually needs to be protected from light to prevent the formation of free radicals and should be stored in the fridge until preparation is being made for it to be infused. It is usually taken out of the fridge approximately 2–4 hours before use depending on bag size, to bring the temperature of the solution up to room temperature.

A number of standard PN 'recipes' are commercially available, but many pharmacies augment these according to the individual child's requirements. A number of feeding regimes are advocated; some try to replicate the normal peaks and troughs that would be experienced if the child was on a normal bolus diet, while others try to maintain a status quo.

A range of sophisticated infusion devices and filters are available for use with PN and these detect air emboli to prevent these from entering the child's circulation. If children are ambulant there are smaller battery-powered packs available.

Reasons why PN might be necessary

- A child is severely undernourished
- As support following extensive surgery, radiotherapy or chemotherapy

- In a hypercatabolic state following severe burns
- A child cannot absorb nutrients or suffers from chronic diarrhoea and vomiting
- The gut is too immature or insufficient
- The gut is paralysed, e.g. after major surgery
- The child is unconscious and gut feeding is not possible

Complications of PN

These are mainly preventable:

- Emboli, thrombosis and infection
- Swings in blood sugar
- Phlebitis
- Cholestasis

Emboli, thrombosis and infection

The reason for these are that the catheter remains in place for a relatively long time and the body has the capacity to recognise foreign materials and acts in a defensive manner, leading to fibrin deposits or blood clots obscuring the line. As these lines can be critical to the survival of these children these are serious complications.

For consideration of infection of the long line and septic shock readers are referred to Chapters 12 and 4. Children with long lines have a higher risk of sepsis, especially those who are already immuno-compromised.

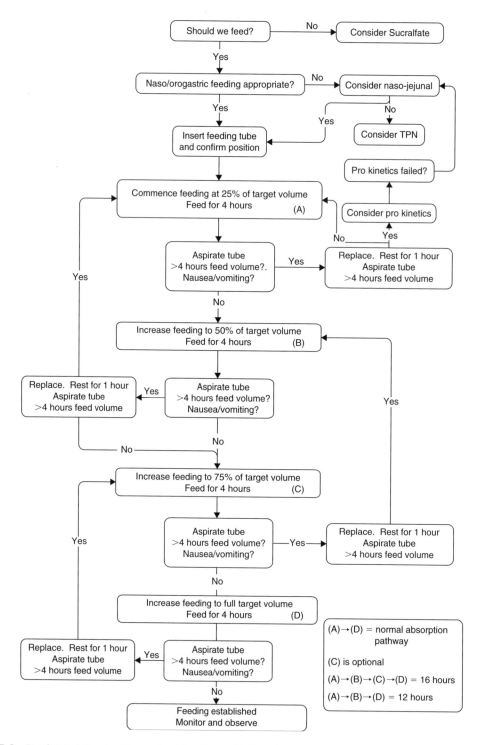

Figure 5.1 Paediatric Intensive Care enteral feeding guidelines (Martin and Cox 2001). Reproduced with kind permission.

Managing swings in blood sugar

Insulin may sometimes be added to the PN but more commonly is administered by a separate infusion. Sometimes a change in the way that the PN is administered can be effective. Sometimes the recipe might need to be changed.

Top tip

An unstable blood sugar level can be an indication of sepsis.

Phlebitis

Phlebitis is inflammation of the vein and is usually associated with blood clots, but with PN the lining of the veins may react to the chemical stimulus of the solution. The signs and symptoms are often non-specific. There may be redness along the track of the vein if a large peripheral vessel was used, burning pain or a low-grade fever. This is a serious complication.

Cholestasis

Bile is a secretary function of the liver. Cholestasis means that bile does not flow from the gall bladder into the intestine. This may be due to a lack of intestinal stimulus to trigger the release of bile. The metabolic complications of this are considered in Chapter 7.

Management of PN at home

The aim of domiciliary PN is to keep children alive and well and able to enjoy as normal a life as possible. They should, where possible, be independent and mobile between infusions. Success depends on the commitment of the family and a stable and secure family home. The parents need to have a reasonable understanding of the rationale behind asepsis and they need good communication skills to act as advocates for their child if needed. As the setting up of infusions can be fiddly they will need considerable manual dexterity.

Even given favourable circumstances, with excellent support and care, most children are readmitted to hospital because of some complication such as an infection, displacement or blockage of the catheter.

Future options

There are a range of surgical options to conserve or increase the surface area of the intestine for absorption. A specific strategy is the STEP procedure (see Chapter 7).

Blood and blood products

Blood components

The volume of blood varies greatly according to age (Table 5.2). Blood can be divided into two main components: plasma and cells. Approximately 45% of blood is made up of cells and 55% plasma. The cell component can be expressed by the haematocrit. Blood cells are made in the bone marrow. The bone marrow contains five different types of blood-forming cells: myeloblasts, lymphoblasts, monoblasts, erythroblasts and megakaryocytes. Table 5.13 illustrates the function of these cells.

Plasma

Plasma is the yellowish-coloured fluid in which the cells are suspended. Its main constituents are water, plasma proteins and electrolytes and all the substances that are being carried by the blood around the body. Plasma proteins consist of albumin and globulin, which are mainly produced by the liver. Plasma proteins can be used in times of starvation as a protein source, they play an important role in fluid distribution by exerting an oncotic pressure, they transport certain hormones, substances and drugs, they increase the viscosity of blood, thereby helping to maintain blood pressure, and they have the ability to act as a buffer by neutralising acids and alkalis in the blood. Table 5.14 illustrates typical

Table 5.13 Bone marrow cells and their function.

Type of cell	Function	Action
Myeloblasts	Produce white blood cells known as granulocytes. Granulocytes include neutrophils, basophils and eosinophils	Phagocytic, ingesting and dissolving foreign particles
Lymphoblasts	Produce lymphocytes	Production of antibodies to destroy antigens
Monoblasts	Produce monocytes	Phagocytic, ingesting and destroying foreign particles/bacteria
Erythroblasts	Produce red blood cells	Contain haemoglobin which is essential for oxygen transport
Megakaryocytes	Produce platelets	Important component in the clotting of blood

Table 5.14 Typical values of blood substances.

Substance	Normal values	Reasons for increased values	Reasons for reduced values
Hydrogen ions (H^+)	36–44 mmol/L	Acidosis	Alkalosis
Arterial oxygen (PaO_2)	11–14 kPa	Hyperoxia	Hypoxia, R→L shunt
Arterial carbon dioxide ($PaCO_2$)	4.7–6.0 kPa	Under-ventilation	Hyperventilation
Bicarbonate (HCO_3^-)	21–26 mmol/L	Compensation for respiratory acidosis or furosemide effect	Bicarbonate loss through kidney or gut
Base excess (BE)	+2 to –2	Excess alkali	Excess acid
Lactate	0.6–2.4 mmol/L	Anaerobic metabolism, reduced clearance in liver failure	
Chloride (Cl^-)	98–110 mmol/L	Usually too much NaCl IV causes metabolic acidosis	Increased↑ loss, e.g. due to vomiting, rare renal disease
Sodium (Na^+)	132–146 mmol/L	Dehydration, too much IV	Fluid overload, Na deficient, increased loss
Potassium (K^+)	3.5–5.5 mmol/L	Acute renal failure, acidosis, too much IV, tumour lysis	Alkalosis, K deficient, increased loss
Glucose	3.6–5.4 mmol/L	Stress, TPN, diabetes, steroids	Stress in newborns, metabolic disease
Urea	2.1–6.5 mmol/L	Dehydration, renal failure, GI bleed	Protein malnutrition
Creatinine	45–70 μmol/L	Renal failure	Protein malnutrition
Calcium total (Ca^{2+})	2.0–2.7 mmol/L	Hyperparathyroidism	Increased loss
Calcium ionised ($_iCa^{2+}$)	1.2–1.3 mmol/L	Too much IV	Increased loss, alkalosis
Phosphate (PO_4^{3-})	1.30–2.1 mmol/L	Acute renal failure	Sepsis, DKA, increased loss
Magnesium (Mg^{2+})	0.7–0.9 mmol/L	Too much IV	Increased loss

Table 5.14 Continued.

Substance	Normal values	Reasons for increased values	Reasons for reduced values
Bilirubin total (tBR)	Child: 0–24 μmol/L Newborn: 0–217 μmol/L	Jaundice: increased haemolysis, liver failure, TPN	
Bilirubin conjugated (cBR)	<10% of tBR	Obstructed jaundice	
Alkaline phosphatase (ALP)	275–875 IU	Renal failure, rickets, biliary obstruction	
Alanine transferase (ALT)	15–40 IU	Hepatitis, reduced liver perfusion	
Aspartate transferase (AST)	15–40 IU	Hepatitis, reduced liver perfusion	
Gamma glutamine transferase (γGT)	<40 IU	Increased ALP causing biliary obstruction, isolated in alcohol abuse	
Albumin	28–43 g/L		Protein malnutrition, increased loss
Ammonia (NH_3^+)	<50 mmol/L	Urea cycle disorders, Reye's syndrome, liver failure	
Amylase	8–85 IU	Pancreatitis, peritonitis	
Osmolality (serum)	270–295 mmol/kg	Dehydration, Diabetes insipidus, mannitol	SIADH (syndrome of inappropriate antidiuretic hormone)
Creatinine kinase (CK)	40–240 IU	Myoglobinuria	
Haemoglobin (Hb)	12–14 g/(dL)	Dehydration	Anaemia, haemolysis
Platelets (PLT)	150–400 × 10^9/L	Infection, inflammation	Consumption by pump, disseminated intravascular coagulation (DIC), clot
Haematocrit (HCT) (= 3×Hb)	0.45%	Dehydration	Blood loss
White cell count (WBC)	4 × 10^9–11 × 10^9/L	Infection, steroids	Infection, bone marrow suppression
Prothrombin time (PT)	11–14 seconds	Liver dysfunction, reduced vitamin K, warfarin, DIC	
Partial thromboplastin time (PTT)	25–40 seconds	Heparin, DIC	
Fibrinogen	1.6–4 g/L	Inflammation	DIC
C-reactive protein (CRP)	<1 gdL	Inflammation, infection	

Permission for use given from Duncan (2007, unpublished).

Table 5.15 Blood products and uses.

Product	Situations	Considerations
Whole blood or packed cells Whole blood, approximately 400 mL/unit Packed cells, approximately 220 mL/unit	Major blood loss, such as during trauma or surgery, severe anaemia, haemoglobinopathies	Always cross match if possible. In emergency, O negative blood can be used. Should be filtered. Use a blood-giving set. If giving rapidly, should be warmed using blood warmer only. Patient should be monitored for signs of incompatibility: signs may include rigor, tachycardia, fall in blood pressure, itching, back pain, sweating, rash, vomiting. Strict fluid balance. May require administration of diuretic halfway through transfusion to avoid fluid overload
Fresh frozen plasma (FFP)	Following cardiopulmonary bypass, abnormal coagulation, microvascular bleeding	Contains clotting factors, albumin and immunoglobulin. Usually given as 10—20 mL/kg but titrated to clinical condition. Should be administered as soon as possible but within 4 hours. Filtered through blood-giving set. Patient should be monitored for signs of anaphylaxis
Cryoprecipitate	Usually used to increase fibrinogen level	Administer as soon as possible through blood administration set, but within 30 minute. Patient should be monitored for signs of anaphylaxis
Platelets	Severe microvascular bleeding, conditions that lead to low platelet counts, e.g. bone marrow suppression/failure	Administer as soon as possible. Should be administered through a specific platelet-giving set
4.5% human albumin	Hypovolaemia, shock	Administer through fluid-giving set. Long half-life. Expensive

values of blood substances and possible reasons for increased or reduced values.

Blood/blood component transfusions

The highly dependent child, particularly in critical illness, may need transfusion therapy during a stay in hospital. Table 5.15 lists the main products available and the situations in which they may be given. It must be emphasised that the administration of any product must only be given by a suitably trained health care professional and that national and local guidelines and policies must be adhered to.

Chapter 6

THE CHILD WITH ACUTE NEUROLOGICAL DYSFUNCTION

Michaela Dixon and Janet Murphy

Introduction

The diagnosis and management of childhood neurological disorders can be very complex. Due to the varied nature and scope of conditions classified under this system children can present in a number of ways. Children may be affected acutely having no previous history, such as in meningitis or trauma. They may present with an acute exacerbation of a chronic condition such as epilepsy or with a gradual deterioration in their underlying condition, as may be the case with tumour. This chapter focuses primarily on the child presenting acutely who requires immediate assessment and management rather than the child who requires a more detailed and ongoing review and planning of care.

Children with acute neurological dysfunction of any aetiology account for 15% of all paediatric intensive care admissions. In children coma is caused by diffuse metabolic insult in 95% of cases and by structural lesions in the remaining 5% (APLS 2005). Seizures are one of the most common reasons for children presenting to the emergency department (Davis *et al.* 2005) and prompt management is important in reducing, where possible, the potential for long-term impairment. Head injury is the single most common cause of death in children aged between 1 and 15 years. Head trauma is a primary insult

about which little can be done; therefore the child's outcome is often determined by the severity of secondary insults relating to hypoperfusion and hypoxia. The early signs of raised intracranial pressure (RICP) are subtle in the young child and can be easy to miss.

Development of the brain and nervous system

The embryonic development of the brain and nervous system occurs at a very early stage of gestation. It is an extremely complex process and the very detailed nature of this could be the subject of a complete volume on its own. For that reason readers are guided through the major key stages only in Table 6.1. Further embryological development of the nervous system may be found in Chapter 9 or in the sources identified in the references.

Overview of children and their neurological development

The immaturity of the infant's neurological system is very evident as is their subsequent growth and development. The major portion of brain growth occurs in the first year of life along with completion of the myelination of the brain and

Table 6.1 Embryological development of the brain and nervous system.

Gestational age	Development
14–21 days	The developing nervous system appears in the third week of gestation which is a period of rapid embryonic development. There is differentiation of the three primitive germ layers: ectoderm, mesoderm and endoderm. The ectoderm layer gives rise to the central nervous system (CNS), the brain and the spinal cord as well as other structures such as the skin
	The notochord (a cellular rod) develops during this time and is responsible for the development of the neural plate which is a thickened area of the ectoderm (known as neuroectoderm) which overlies the notochord
	Around day 18, the plate widens and starts to fold inwards on itself to form a longitudinal groove – 'the neural groove'. The raised edges of the groove, known as neural folds, increase in height to the point at which they meet and form a tube which is the neural tube. The upper two thirds of the neural tube (the rostral end) is the area from which the brain develops, while the lower third or caudal end, as the name suggests, ultimately gives rise to the spinal cord
Week 4	**Formation of the neural crests:**
	Groups of neuroectoderm cells, which are found on the crest of each neural fold, separate from the neural tube and form a mass which is called the neural crest. This mass of cells differentiates to form:
	• Spinal nerves and the posterior root ganglia of spinal nerves
	• Ganglia of cranial nerves
	• Ganglia of the autonomic nervous system (ANS)
	• Adrenal medulla
	Development of the primitive brain:
	By week 4 and before complete fusion of the neural tube the upper portion of the neural tube develops three fluid-filled enlargements or vesicles which are the beginnings of the primitive brain. These three primary vesicles are:
	• Forebrain or prosencephalon
	• Midbrain or mesencephalon
	• Hind brain or rhombencephalon
	Closure of the neural tube:
	Fusion or complete closure of the neural tube occurs within the fourth week of gestation. The process of fusion begins in the centre of the tube, moving in an upward direction (towards the future brain) first and then about 2 days later moves downwards to complete closure
	The canal through the middle of the complete neural tube will become the ventricular system of the brain and the central canal of the spinal cord
	A failure of the tube to completely close at this point leads to neural tube defects. If the closure is not complete at the caudal end of the tube then congenital malformations affecting the spinal cord will develop, e.g. spina bifida occulta or a myelomeningocoele. If closure is not complete at the rostral or cranial end of the tube then congenital malformations affecting the brain will develop, such as anencephaly
Week 5	By the fifth week, the vesicular region has undergone several flexures and changes and the embryonic brain consists of five secondary vesicles:
	• The prosencephalon has divided into telencephalon and diencephalon (2 vesicles)
	• Rhombencephalon has divided into metencephalon and mylencephalon (2 vesicles)
	• Mesencephalon is unchanged (1 vesicle), total number = 5
	Cranial nerve nuclei start to appear in the brain stem during the fifth week
	The cells of the wall that encloses the neural tube differentiate into three types:
	• Outer layer – known as the marginal layer, develops into the white matter of the nervous system
	• Middle layer – known as the mantle layer, develops into the grey matter of the nervous system
	• Inner layer – known as the ependymal layer, forms the lining of the ventricles within the brain

Table 6.1 Continued.

Gestational age	Development
Week 6	Further differentiation and development of the five secondary vesicles refines the developing brain into the identifiable components seen in the adult brain. This is completed by the end of the sixth week: • Telencephalon – cerebral hemispheres/basal ganglia • Diencephalon – thalamus/hypothalamus/pineal gland • Mesencephalon – midbrain • Metencephalon – pons/cerebellum • Myelencephalon – medulla oblongata The cavities within the vesicles develop into the ventricles of the brain

Sources: Barker *et al.* (2003); MacGregor (2003); Neill and Knowles (2004); Levy *et al.* (2006).

nervous system. Motor function maturation proceeds in a cephalocaudal direction and is a succession of integrated milestones. Brain growth continues up to 15 years of age.

Primitive reflexes present in infants

- Palmar grasp (birth) – disappears by 3 months
- Plantar grasp (birth) – disappears by 9 months
- Moro reflex (birth) – disappears by 6 months
- Placing (4 days) – disappearance variable
- Stepping (0–8 weeks) – disappears before walking
- Fencing (2–3 months) – disappears by 6 months

The absence of these reflexes or their prolonged presence is a cause for concern and should prompt further investigation.

The fontanelles of the head

The ability of the skull of a child less than 2 years of age to accommodate increased volume relating to intracranial bleeds is due to the presence of open fontanelles. This means that there may be considerable blood loss and damage to brain parenchyma before overt clinical signs become apparent. The posterior fontanelle closes by 2 months of age and the anterior by 2 years of age.

Neurological assessment in children

Neurological assessment is important in children because:

- It is the only guide to neurological function in children who are unable to communicate due to age or cognitive ability.
- It has major importance in detecting deterioration in the acute unwell child.
- Prevention of secondary insult is vital in improving morbidity (and mortality).

Difficulties in assessing children's neurological function

- Inappropriate assessment scales
- Age of child/fear factor
- Individual interpretation
- Sedation/muscle relaxants used for scanning/ongoing care

Overcoming difficulties in assessing children's neurological function

- Age-appropriate tools (see assessment charts in the Appendix)
- Parental involvement
- Double checking your interpretation with that of colleagues

- If in doubt recheck, but trust your/parental instincts

Considerations for assessment

- Remember factors such as pain and fear which will affect the assessment
- Observe child from a distance before approaching
- Utilise parents
- Does your presence get a response (positive or negative)?
- Find out about the child's favourite toy/TV programme/pet – use that information to assist with assessment
- For infants – assess how the infant handles
- Remember to record exactly what you see, but note external factors such as sedation

Other clinical indicators as part of neurological assessment

- Heart rate/blood pressure/respiratory pattern
- Presence of photophobia
- Presence of neck stiffness (meningism)
- Assess fontanelles
- Glucose
- Pupils – size/shape and reactivity
- Speech clarity
- Cognition and comprehension
- Muscle tone and co-ordination; abnormalities may be unilateral or bilateral, may involve the upper or lower limbs/body

Management of the child with seizures

The brain has over ten million neurones whose function is to transmit information from cell to cell. This is achieved by the presence of chemical messengers which make the cells more or less excitable. During super-excitability, many cells fire together and the brain activity at a cellular level becomes out of control. The burst of excessive activity is known as an epileptic spike discharge and groups of these discharges, which are uninhibited, lead to epileptic fits or seizures.

Causes of seizures in children

- Fifty per cent of seizures have no identifiable cause
- Febrile convulsions
- Toxic ingestion – poisons/alcohol
- Metabolic disorders
- Pre-existing seizure disorder
- Trauma (head injury/birth trauma)
- Cerebral pathology – tumours/bleeds/abscesses
- Systemic disturbances – sepsis, hepatic or renal failure

Classification

There are a myriad of different types of seizure; however, most can be classified into one of two broad categories.

Generalised

These arise over a wide area of the brain and affect both sides of the body from the beginning.

The most common seizure within this group is the tonic–clonic seizure (Figure 6.1), but other seizure types include:

- Absences (may be known as petit mal seizures)
- Juvenile myoclonic epilepsy
- Drop attacks
- Infantile spasms

Partial

Partial seizures arise from a specific focus in the brain and may be termed either simple or complex.

Simple partial seizures originate from a focal point but may go on to spread throughout the brain. Auras are normally associated with this type of seizure and may be the only component of the seizure. Additionally there is not normally

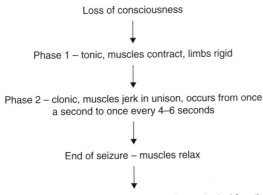

Loss of consciousness

↓

Phase 1 – tonic, muscles contract, limbs rigid

↓

Phase 2 – clonic, muscles jerk in unison, occurs from once a second to once every 4–6 seconds

↓

End of seizure – muscles relax

↓

Post ictal phase and gradual recovery of neurological function

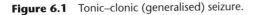

Figure 6.1 Tonic–clonic (generalised) seizure.

a loss of consciousness, but the child may be left with transient weakness and/or dysphasia. Complex partial seizures originate specifically from the temporal lobe.

Neonatal seizures

Many healthy babies will display fine tremors or startle-like movements when stimulated or make jerky movements during active sleep; however, seizure activity is usually unstimulated. Owing to the immaturity of the neonate's brain, clinical signs of seizure activity may well be subtle and can therefore be missed. This is particularly applicable in the pre-term infant population (Thalange *et al.* 2006; Lissauer and Clayden 2007). The causes of neonatal seizures differ slightly from those of children, although there are some identical causes (see below).

Causes
- Acquired sepsis
- Meningitis
- Metabolic causes – hypoglycaemia, hypo-/hypernatraemia, hypocalcaemia, inborn errors of metabolism
- Hypoxia
- Hypoxic–ischaemia encephalopathy (HIE)

- Drug withdrawal (from maternal source)
- Kernicterus (condition in which bilirubin is deposited in the brain tissue as a consequence of jaundice)
- Intracranial haemorrhage
- Congenital infections – group B streptococcus, hepatitis B and C, herpes simplex virus (HSV), cytomegalovirus (CMV)

Clinical signs
As noted above, the clinical signs may be subtle in this age group, and therefore frequent assessment of the infant is essential if there are concerns about the possibility of seizure activity.

- Movement of the mouth – either a chewing motion or lip smacking
- Grimacing
- Deviation of the eyes or staring
- Increased tone in one or more of the infant's limbs
- Hiccoughs not associated with feeds

Additionally there are other general clinical signs such as:

- Tachycardia
- Tachypnoea
- Bradycardia
- Apnoeas
- Posturing (abnormal flexion or extension of the limbs)

Management of neonatal seizures
The management of seizures within the neonatal population is related to the underlying cause(s). It is important to rule out hypoglycaemia and meningitis as primary causes. Investigations such as EEG and CT or MRI scan may be undertaken to exclude or identify causes.

Febrile Convulsions Febrile convulsions (a seizure which is usually associated with a body temperature of greater than 39°C in the absence of other causes) are common in children between the ages

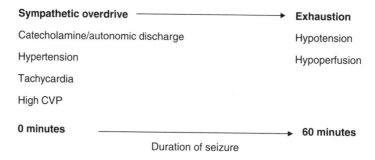

Figure 6.2 Systemic effects of seizures.

of 6 months and 6 years and are usually linked to a childhood illness such as tonsillitis, or coincide with teething. Between 3 and 5% of all children will experience one febrile convulsion and there is a genetic predisposition in children having a parent with a history of febrile convulsions of around 10%. Additional risk factors are frequent episodes of illness accompanied by high temperatures or having a first febrile convulsion with a temperature of less than 39°C.

Febrile convulsions may be termed either simple or complex:

- Simple are generally brief tonic–clonic seizures lasting a few minutes which are self-limiting
- Complex include those that are prolonged (lasting more than 15 minutes), focal seizures or those that reoccur within 24 hours

Febrile convulsions are not the same as epilepsy and for a child who has a simple febrile convulsion the risk of developing epilepsy is similar to that for the general child population, at around 1–2%. In a child who has had prolonged or more complex febrile convulsions there is a slightly higher chance of developing epilepsy than children in general, at between 4 and 12%.

Management of febrile convulsions is dependent upon the duration of the seizure episode, and the use of anti-convulsants is not indicated in most children. The majority of children require no intervention other than the general management

of their fever using appropriate antipyretics as directed, although there is no evidence to suggest that this will necessarily prevent further febrile convulsions (NICE 2007). For children whose seizures are of a prolonged nature the use of rectal diazepam or buccal midazolam may be indicated.

Status Epilepticus (SE) Such seizures can be life threatening and may result in permanent neurological injury if they are not managed in a timely manner. The systemic effects of prolonged seizure activity are shown in Figure 6.2. The outcomes for children presenting with SE is determined by a number of factors including the age of the child, the length of seizure activity and the aetiology.

Mortality from SE is approximately 4% and neurological injury occurs in 6% of children >3 years and 29% of children <1 year (APLS 2005).

Management of the child in SE The key to managing the child in SE is to stop the seizure activity, thereby minimising the risks associated with prolonged seizures.

Immediate steps employing a structured approach cover the essential considerations in any acutely unwell child as well as the specific considerations (Table 6.2).

It is important that practitioners are familiar with their local unit or Trust guidelines for the

Table 6.2 Initial management of the child in SE.

Primary intervention	Notes/considerations
Airway Ensure infant/child has patent airway	
Breathing Administer high flow oxygen therapy	Seizure activity increases the cerebral metabolic demands; therefore providing supplementary oxygen can reduce the risk of secondary hypoxia
Circulation Assess heart rate and pulse volume	At initial presentation full cardiovascular monitoring may be difficult to establish due to the child's seizure activity; therefore baseline observations are essential
Disability Stop seizure activity using local guidelines	Key medications involved in this will depend upon whether the child has intravenous access or not (see Table A1 in the Appendix)
Glucose Check the child's blood sugar level	Hypoglycaemia can cause seizures in children Seizure activity increases cerebral metabolic demands and the main source of energy for brain cells is provided by glucose

management of SE as there may be slight differences between them and the National Guidelines. Once the child's seizures have been controlled, ongoing assessment and management measures may be instituted (Table 6.3).

Meningitis

Meningitis (an inflammation of the meninges or membranes that cover the brain) is a relatively uncommon illness in children. The severity is usually dependent on the causative organism, viral or bacterial, but it should always be treated seriously.

Viral meningitis

This is the most common cause of meningitis; most cases are relatively mild and seldom fatal. Viral meningitis does not usually result in septicaemia and the risk of complications is minimal in contrast to the bacterial form of the disease.

Causes include adenoviruses, herpes viruses, Epstein–Barr virus and more rarely the mumps virus. Clinical signs may develop quite suddenly or over a period of days but are rather non-specific and mimic those seen in a flu-type illness.

- Fever
- Vomiting
- Severe headache

More specific signs include:

- Light sensitivity/photophobia
- Stiff painful neck
- Altered level of consciousness
- Seizures

Management of viral meningitis is essentially supportive, with the majority of children not being admitted to hospital. Home care involves rest and the use of appropriate analgesics to reduce the severity of the headaches. Occasionally, children will require admission for supportive therapy as there is no specific drug therapy available to treat the viral cause. Management is limited to IV fluids if vomiting has been severe enough to cause

Table 6.3 Ongoing assessment and management.

Ongoing interventions	Notes/considerations
Continuous monitoring once stable ECG, respiratory, non-invasive blood pressure and saturation monitoring	Full assessment of the child's clinical condition once seizure activity has been controlled is important to assess for: • Side effects of anti-convulsants • Ongoing effects of seizure activity
Neurological assessment Use of age-appropriate tool	Allows for assessment of recovery of normal neurological function or detection of any ongoing neurological impairment
Identify cause and treat where necessary Blood samples Lumbar puncture May require CT scan	Identification of cause will allow specific treatment strategies to be instituted
Gain history	Information can be gained from children themselves if they have appropriate understanding. Parents can provide valuable information to help identify possible cause of seizures. Communication is a two-way process and children and their parents need information about recovery or expected prognosis
Fluid management	Fluid restriction reduces the risk of the child developing cerebral oedema depending on the cause of the seizures.
Temperature management	Increased temperature can be a contributory factor in some children Fever also increases cellular metabolic demands and the use of glucose and oxygen supplies
Family care	First presentation of seizures in any child is an extremely stressful time for parents. Similarly in children with known seizure disorders, an increase in the level of seizure activity may represent deterioration in the child's condition which is also extremely stressful for the child and family

dehydration and regular analgesia. Recovery normally takes between 2 and 3 weeks although it will depend on the individual child.

Bacterial meningitis

This is less common than viral meningitis, but bacterial meningitis has an overall mortality of between 5 and 10%. Up to 10% of children affected will suffer some ongoing neurological impairment such as hearing loss, memory loss or altered mood patterns. The causative pathogens vary with age although there are some common causes across the age range seen in children's care (Table 6.4).

Table 6.4 Age-related bacterial causes of meningitis.

Age	Organism
Newborn (up to 3 months)	Group B streptococcus E. coli Listeria Haemophilus influenza type B (uncommon in this group)
Infants/young children	Neisseria meningitidis (meningococcal infection) Streptococcus pneumoniae (pneumococcal infection) Haemophilus influenza type B
School-age children	Neisseria meningitidis (meningococcal infection) Streptococcus pneumoniae (pneumococcal infection)

Unlike viral meningitis, the clinical signs of bacterial meningitis develop over a relatively short period of time, normally just a few hours. Early signs are very similar in nature to those found in viral meningitis, although the relative rapidity of their development may give a clue towards a bacterial cause in the acutely unwell child.

General signs include:

- Lethargy/drowsiness
- Irritability and poor handling in the neonate
- Poor feeding/nausea and/or vomiting
- Fever
- Headache

More specific findings include:

- Bulging fontanelle in infants
- Light sensitivity/photophobia
- Neck stiffness (may not be evident in infants)
- Positive Brudzinski's or Kernig's signs. These are physical signs which can be elicited when the spinal cord is stretched or flexed
- Decreased level of consciousness
- Seizures or other focal neurological signs
- Clinical indicators for shock

The presence of a non-blanching petechial rash in the acutely unwell child is indicative of septicaemia and must be acted upon immediately.

Management of the child with bacterial meningitis

Priorities of care for this group of children are geared towards treating the symptoms present and, where possible, preventing the child developing complications such as cerebral oedema (Table 6.5).

Complications
- Hearing loss
- Subdural effusions (particularly associated with pneumococcal meningitis)
- Cerebral abscesses which will require surgical drainage

- Seizures
- Hydrocephalus

Encephalitis

Encephalitis is a much rarer form of neurological illness than meningitis and refers to a more generalised inflammation of the brain tissue as well as possible involvement of the meninges. Encephalitis is normally viral in origin and only certain viruses have the capability to affect nerves and gain access to the Central Nervous System (CNS). Viral encephalitis can be either primary (where virus is present in the CNS) or post infectious, due to immunoallergic mechanisms. The differential diagnosis is difficult to make due to the similarity in initial clinical presentation. It may also be difficult to differentiate between encephalitis and meningitis in the early phase of illness, again due to the similarity of clinical symptoms. Viruses associated with encephalitis include enteroviruses, respiratory viruses and herpes viruses (e.g. *Varicella*), but in up to 50% of cases identification of the underlying organism is not possible.

General clinical signs

- Fever
- Uncharacteristic behaviour
- Confusion and/or altered level of consciousness
- Seizures

More focal neurological signs may be noted at initial presentation or they may become apparent as the illness progresses. These signs will be determined by the specific area(s) of the brain affected and will therefore vary from child to child. Management of encephalitis is essentially supportive and follows the same major principles detailed in Table 6.5.

As the cause is normally viral in origin, the use of antibiotics is normally limited, but Aciclovir therapy should be continued until there is either

Table 6.5 Management of a child with bacterial meningitis.

Intervention	Notes/considerations
Identify and treat cause Blood samples Lumbar puncture CT scan	The main treatment priority is the administration of appropriate IV antibiotics according to sensitivity of organism involved. Once samples have been obtained broad-spectrum therapy can be given until results are available Lumbar puncture is contraindicated in children who are demonstrating signs of possible Raised Intracranial Pressure (RICP) as the sudden release of pressure could cause herniation of the brain stem, coagulopathy or cardiovascular instability. CT scan may be required to determine presence of cerebral oedema in these children
Continuous monitoring ECG, respiratory, Non-invasive/invasive blood pressure and saturation monitoring	Full assessment of the child's clinical condition provides baseline information from which signs of improvement or deterioration may be detected
Neurological assessment Use of age-appropriate tool Hourly observations	Allows for assessment of recovery of normal neurological function or detection of any ongoing neurological impairment
Reduce stress and anxiety Promote a quiet environment	A calm quiet environment may help to reduce anxiety and promote trust for the child and family, encouraging the development of a therapeutic partnership of care
Fluid and electrolyte management Maintenance fluids at 70% of normal fluid requirements Monitor electrolyte levels and replace accordingly Monitor child's blood glucose levels and maintain within normal limits	Fluid restriction reduces the risk of the child developing cerebral oedema Maintaining electrolytes within normal limits can prevent fluid shifts and reduce the risk of the child developing cerebral oedema (see Chapter 5) Increased cellular activity increases the metabolic demands for glucose and other nutrients. Hypoglycaemia may cause seizures in children
Temperature management Maintain a neutral thermal environment Use of antipyretics	Maintaining a neutral thermal environment and the appropriate use of antipyretics can reduce the adverse effects of fever on the body Fever increases cellular metabolic demands and the use of glucose and oxygen supplies
Family care Provide full explanation of treatment plans and regular updates for parents/care-givers and child (where appropriate)	The diagnosis of meningitis is obviously a major cause of concern to parents. This is not helped by the term, which is often misused in the media and by the public to describe a child with meningococcal septicaemia. It is important that parents (and the child) are kept fully informed with factual information rather than being left to imagine worst-case scenarios

confirmation of the viral organism involved or there has been exclusion of the herpes simplex virus (HSV) as the cause.

HSV is one of the least common causes of encephalitis, but it can have devastating consequences if not managed correctly, with a mortality rate of more than 70% if untreated and ongoing neurological impairment in many of the children who survive. It may occur either as a primary infection or due to reactivation of latent infection especially in the neonatal population.

Clinical presentation is normally associated with a history of fever and malaise in addition to which there may have been disturbances of memory or behaviour. The illness progresses with reduced levels of consciousness and seizures which are often focal and ongoing. HSV causes necrotic lesions, typically in the temporal lobes, but these can be widespread and even involve the brainstem. There is raised ICP and papilloedema in approximately 15% of cases and these children will normally require intensive care admission.

As well as infective causes of encephalopathy there are a number of other causes including hepatic encephalopathy (see Chapter 7) and inborn errors of metabolism.

The child with meningococcal disease

Meningococcal infection is the most common infectious cause of death in childhood in developed countries (Ninis *et al.* 2005; Hart and Thomson 2006). It is an illness that causes significant mortality, the rate of which has remained relatively static at around 10% despite advances in terms of both recognition and early management as well as advances in intensive care treatment strategies. Additionally it is a disease that causes a significant degree of long-term challenges due to the severity of complications suffered by a number of the children affected. The cause of meningococcal septicaemia is the *Neisseria meningitidis* organism which is also the commonest cause of bacterial meningitis.

Approximately 50% of meningococcal infection presentations are as meningitis alone, 10% are septicaemia alone and the remaining 40% are mixed presentations with clinical signs of both meningitis and septicaemia (Welch and Nadel 2003). In children who present with meningococcal septicaemia, it may not be possible to confirm the presence of meningitis, as lumbar puncture is contraindicated, but it must be a consideration in management plans.

The exact mechanism that leads to some children developing fulminant septicaemia while others develop meningitis only is not clear although it is thought that genetic factors, the presence of underlying immune insufficiency and environmental factors all contribute to its development. The impact this illness has on both the child and the family should never be underestimated by the healthcare professionals involved in caring for these children, even if the child appears to be suffering from a less severe form of the disease.

Neisseria meningitidis is an encapsulated bacteria and it is the properties of the capsule that determine the sero-group of the infection. Common sero-groups in the UK were group B and group C until the introduction of the MenC vaccine against the group C sero-group in 2000, which reduced the number of cases with that specific sero-group by more than 90%. Currently there is no vaccine against group B available, but a number of organisations are working towards this and are at various stages in the research and development process.

Clinical presentation

The general signs of meningococcal septicaemia are very non-specific and it can easily be mistaken for mild-to-moderate viral illness in the early stages.

Non-specific or early signs

Infants
- Drowsiness
- Irritability – distress on handling
- Poor feeding
- Fever
- Macular rash (may be the only form of rash present throughout illness)

Older children
- Vomiting
- Backache
- Joint pains
- Fever
- Macular rash (may be the only form of rash present throughout illness)
- Headache

The virulent nature of the disease means a quick progression to specific clinical signs including:

- Development of a petechial rash (non-blanching spots whose colour remains when pressure is applied to the skin using a clear glass tumbler). This may progress to large areas of skin becoming discoloured and necrotic. This is known as purpura fulminans
- Cardiovascular compromise – tachycardia, low blood pressure, prolonged central capillary refill time, poor pulse volume
- Development of a coagulopathy – prolonged clotting times
- Coma

In addition to these clinical signs there are a number of ongoing physiological processes which contribute to the severity of the illness. These processes occur partially as a consequence of endotoxin release by the bacteria as the antibiotics take effect.

Specific physiological processes in meningococcal septicaemia

- Deranged cellular and metabolic function
- Myocardial dysfunction and depressed cardiac contractility
- Endothelial injury
- Increased vascular permeability
- Disseminated intravascular coagulopathy (DIC)

Factors involved in the management of meningococcal septicaemia

- Early recognition of the signs and prompt administration of antibiotics (normally Benzylpenicillin) even before the child reaches hospital. It is estimated that, at current levels of disease incidence, GPs may only see one case during their career (Hart and Thompson 2006) but will see thousands of children with viral illness and the non-specific signs previously identified
- Prompt resuscitation and stabilisation when the child reaches the Emergency Department, which includes seeking specialist advice early on in the child's admission
- Appropriate hospital management of both potential illnesses present
  - Septicaemia and circulatory failure (see Chapter 4)
  - Meningitis and possible RICP

The use of the Glasgow meningococcal septicaemia prognostic score (Table 6.6) is advocated by many of the published guidelines available. A score of greater than 8 is deemed to be significant in terms of predicting mortality.

Public health measures

- There is compulsory notification by law of all meningococcal cases whether they are meningitis or septicaemia.

Table 6.6 Glasgow meningococcal septicaemia prognostic score.

Criteria	Indicators	Score
Systolic BP	<75 mmHg if <4 years or <85 mmHg if >4 years	3
Core–skin temperature gap	If >3 degree difference	3
Modified CSS	If initial score >8 or deterioration of 3 or more points at any time	3
Deterioration	Ask parents/nurses – if yes	2
Neck stiffness	If absent	2
Extent of purpura	Widespread ecchymoses or extending lesions on review	1
Base deficit	If >8	1

- The Public Health Laboratories Services (PHLS) are responsible for collation of national data and treating potential hotspots.
- Chemoprophylaxis is necessary for close contacts of the affected child. This is usually oral Rifampicin for 2 days; however, Ciprofloxacin can be used as an alternative (e.g. in pregnant women).
- It is not usual for staff involved in caring for the child to require any form of chemoprophylaxis, but if uncertain then advice should be sought from the Infection Control Team within the hospital or the PHLS team involved in the child's care.

Resource box

Health Protection Agency (HPA) – www.hpa.org.uk/infections (epidemiological data and surveillance information)

Meningitis Research Trust – www.meningitis.org/disease-info (general information)

Meningitis Trust – www.meninigits-trust.org (general information)

Meningitis Trust – www.inmed.co.uk/resources (resources for healthcare professionals)

Complications of meningococcal septicaemia

Most children will survive meningococcal septicaemia, which has a mortality rate of around 8%. The complications and their after-effects can be complex, requiring a multidisciplinary approach to ensure ongoing optimal care for the child and family. Complications include:

- Long-term neurological impairment including hearing loss, behavioural difficulties or the development of an ongoing seizure disorder
- Need for amputation of digits and/or limbs
- Need for skin grafts following significant areas of skin involvement

Top tip

Children admitted with meningococcal disease should be referred to the plastic surgery team as soon as possible if there are areas of skin involvement.

The child with Raised Intracranial Pressure (RICP)

The brain occupies a rigid container (the skull) with a fixed volume (once the fontanelles have closed). It shares the space with the two other components that together make up the contents of the intracranial vault:

- Brain (80%)
- Cerebrospinal fluid (10%)
- Blood (10%)

The pressure within the skull is known as intracranial pressure (ICP) and a normal ICP in healthy individuals is less than 10 mmHg. This is not a static measurement as it will vary with exercise, position of the individual and everyday activities, e.g. ICP will rise very transiently when a person coughs or sneezes but returns to normal values almost instantaneously. As the contents of the skull are essentially non-compressible, if there is a sustained change in the volume of any of the three component parts then there must be a reciprocal change in one or more of the others to compensate. The ability to do this is a protective mechanism to avoid RICP. Normal ICP is maintained through a balance between CSF production and CSF absorption. (Normal CSF volumes = 80–150 mL in the CNS at any one time.)

The ability of the brain to accommodate changes in the ICP is described in the Monro–Kellie hypothesis and is achieved through:

- *Elastance* – which relates to the tightness or stretchiness of the intracranial compartments

- *Compliance* – the ability to tolerate an increase in volume without a corresponding compromise in function

If the brain develops poor compliance and high elastance, owing to pathological processes it will no longer have elastic properties.

Causes

- Trauma
- Tumour – primary/secondary
- Hypoxia – ischaemic encephalopathy
- Hyper-metabolic states – seizures, hyperpyrexia
- Metabolic disorders – liver failure, DKA, severe hypoglycaemia
- Infection – encephalitis, meningitis
- Vascular – subarachnoid haemorrhage, infarction

Once the brain is stretched to its maximum and there is additional increase in volume from any cause there will be increased or RICP present (see Table 6.7).

Clinical signs of acute RICP

The clinical signs can be divided into early and late signs. Some signs may be relatively subtle initially; therefore careful assessment and the use of appropriate monitoring tools are important in detecting changes in the child's condition.

Early signs:

- Drowsiness, leading to altered level of consciousness

Table 6.7 Definition of raised ICP measurements.

Status	Measurement
Normal	<10 mmHg
Abnormal	Sustained level >15 mmHg
Moderate	Between 21 and 40 mmHg
Severe	>40 mmHg

- Motor weakness, abnormal muscle tone in neonates and infants
- Irritability – general agitation, high-pitched cry in infants
- Bulging fontanelle in neonates and infants
- Nausea and vomiting
- Headache – if child is able to self report
- Pupillary changes – pupils may react more sluggishly than previously or become unequal in size
- Seizures – may be generalised or focal

Late signs:

- Coma
- Altered posture: decorticate/decerebrate
- Cushing's triad: hypertension, bradycardia, respiratory irregularity

Cerebral perfusion pressure (CPP)

RICP affects cerebral blood flow and, as a consequence, may worsen cerebral ischaemia, causing secondary brain injury.

One method of reducing or minimising the possible ongoing damage is to ensure that the brain continues to receive adequate blood flow even in the presence of RICP.

Cerebral perfusion pressure or CPP is an estimate of the pressure gradient between the carotid artery and the subarachnoid veins and is therefore the driving force of blood flow into the cerebral circulation. A minimum CPP of 50 mmHg is thought to be necessary to maintain effective brain perfusion in the infant and younger child; however, the value increases with age, so in adolescents the aim would be a CPP of 70 mmHg.

Calculation of CPP

This is determined by the following equation:

CPP = mean arterial pressure (MAP)
minus intracranial pressure (ICP)

Example:

If MAP = 70 mmHg
ICP = 15 mmHg

Then CPP = 70–15 = 55 mmHg.

In order to accurately measure CPP the child requires invasive monitoring and the insertion of an arterial line and an ICP monitor. This is not normally carried out in the high dependency setting. However, even without both of these invasive measurements, steps may be taken to limit the potential ongoing ischaemic damage by maintaining a good blood pressure in the child. This will be indicated by measuring and monitoring the child's MAP.

Management of the infant or child with RICP is aimed specifically at reducing or minimising the secondary damage that may occur as a consequence of hypoperfusion and/or hypoxia (Table 6.8).

Table 6.8 Specific management of the child with RICP.

Intervention	Notes and considerations
Maintain oxygenation If not intubated administer high flow oxygen therapy If intubated ensure high percentage of oxygen delivered by ventilator	Secondary brain injury occurs as a consequence of either hypoperfusion or hypoxia. Maximising oxygen availability will ensure that cells receive enough oxygen to match their demands, allowing normal metabolism to occur
Maintain serum glucose levels within normal limits Monitor blood glucose levels 4 hourly as a minimum	It is important to meet the needs of the cells to maintain normal metabolic function
Administration of glucose in the presence of hypoglycaemia Administration of insulin in the presence of hyperglycaemia	There is a growing evidence base supporting tight control of blood glucose levels, with recognition that hyperglycaemia is as much of phenomena of concern as hypoglycaemia
Maintain CPP Use of inotropes to maintain mean arterial blood pressure once normovolaemia is restored	Ensures that there is sufficient pressure present even if ICP is elevated to drive blood through the cerebral circulation
Prevent intracranial hypertension Use of mannitol (osmotic diuretic) and/ or hypertonic saline (3 or 5% saline) to reduce free water	Intracranial hypertension contributes to overall increase in pressure within the cranial cavity which will increase the degree of hypoperfusion present
Prevent/control seizures Use anticonvulsants as prescribed	Seizure activity will increase the cellular metabolic demands and leads to further increases in ICP
Maintain normothermia where possible Use of warming or cooling strategies as indicated to maintain normothermia In children with persistently raised ICP, cooling to below normothermia may be beneficial	Fever increases the metabolic demands made by the cells which may not be adequately met due to degree of RICP and hypoperfusion Wide variations in core body temperature cause significant alteration in both cardiovascular and neurological function Cooling strategies which lower the body temperature to around 35.5°C reduce the metabolic needs of the cells. In conjunction with auto-regulation of regional cerebral blood flow this can reduce the volume of blood needed in the cerebral circuit without reducing the delivery of essential oxygen and nutrients

External ventricular drains (EVD)

Reasons for insertion

In some circumstances children with neurological disease or neurological trauma may develop RICP. One temporary method of preventing and treating this is by the insertion of an EVD under general anaesthesia. A specifically designed catheter is inserted into the ventricle of the brain and then attached to a closed and sterile system which will allow the drainage of cerebro-spinal fluid (CSF) from the ventricles of the brain. The mechanism for controlling the amount of CSF drained is by controlling the level of the drip chamber. To achieve the correct level the chamber needs to be level with the foramen of Monro. This can be estimated by the midpoint of a line drawn from the outer corner of the eye to the external auditory canal (or top of the child's ear). The CSF then drains by gravity. An EVD may be used in the following circumstances:

- Head injury
- Neurosurgical surgery
- Blockage of the flow of CSF
- To divert infected CSF from the brain, allowing the administration of antibiotics directly into the CSF
- Obstructive hydrocephalus

Management

There needs to be specific local guidelines on the nursing care and management of children with EVD. These children should only be cared for in ward areas or on high dependency units where the nursing and medical staff are competent in caring for them. Key management issues are shown in Table 6.9.

Table 6.9 Key management issues in caring for children with EVD.

Intervention	Consideration
Moving	The drain must be clamped if there is any movement of the child, e.g. sitting up, lying down and getting out of bed. Once in the new position the position of the drain should be re-measured and then unclamped. Failure to do so could lead to abnormal quantities of CSF drainage
Patient monitoring	Strict hourly recording of CSF drainage. Colour should also be noted. If there is no drainage then check that the tubing is not clamped or kinked. If still no drainage, report to senior doctor The patient's temperature, heart rate and blood pressure should also be monitored frequently for signs of infection or RICP Frequent neurological assessment
Safety	Children with EVD should only be cared for by appropriately trained medical and nursing staff. The device should be safely secured both to the patient and the drip stand. The drainage system must not be put over cot sides as this can alter the amount of CSF drainage The system needs to be clearly labelled. The bag should only be changed when necessary. The level of the chamber must be decided by the consultant or other appropriate senior doctor Intrathecal drugs must only be given by medical staff. Local policies and guidelines *must* always be adhered to
Laboratory investigations	Samples of CSF may be taken by medical staff. The patient's blood count should be closely monitored according to condition, in particular electrolyte values

EVD are usually only used for short-term management until the problem is resolved or more permanent treatment is instigated. The removal of EVD is always by a doctor. This is achieved by removing the sutures and then gently pulling on the tube. The tip of the catheters is usually sent to the laboratory for culture (see Charts A1 and A2 in the appendix).

Appendix

See Table A1 for drugs and their methods of delivery and also the observation charts.

Table A1 Common drug therapies.

Drug	Method of delivery	Points of note
General anti-epileptic drugs (AED's): **Phenobarbitone** • Adjusts the threshold at which seizure activity may occur by increasing the intracellular concentrations of chloride thus altering the resting membrane potential of the cell *Adverse effects:* Hypotension, respiratory depression, drowsiness, lethargy, depression, ataxia	Intravenous infusion – should be diluted with water and infused over 20 min Oral – available in tablets or liquid form	• Used in the management of tonic–clonic, partial seizures and neonatal seizures • Rebound seizures can occur if treatment is stopped rapidly • Rarer side effects include hepatic impairment, thrombocytopaenia and skin reactions • It is common practice to measure serum concentrations
Phenytoin • Primary site of action is the motor cortex where it acts to reduce the electrical conductance among brain cells by stabilising the inactive state of voltage–gated sodium channels *Adverse effects:* Hypotension, respiratory depression, cardiac arrhythmias leading to cardiac arrest if administration is too rapid	Intravenous infusion – should be administered over a period of 20–30 min with continuous ECG and BP monitoring in place Oral – available in tablets or liquid form	• Effective in the management of tonic–clonic, partial seizures and neonatal seizures • Oral administration – discontinue enteral feeds for at least 1 h before and after giving Phenytoin. If possible give with water to enhance absorption • It is common practice to monitor the serum concentrations
Fos-phenytoin • Is the pro-drug of Phenytoin which is converted into the active compounds of Phenytoin in the body *Adverse effects:* Are similar to those of Phenytoin but it produces less cardiovascular instability	Intravenous infusion May be given IM but this is not common practice and efficacy is not proven	• Conversion into the active Phenytoin compounds takes up to 15 min making it a second-line medication in the treatment of status epilepticus • The prescription may be confusing as 1 mg of Fos-phenytoin *does not equal* 1 mg of Phenytoin, therefore, careful attention must be paid to ensure correct dose is prescribed and administered

Benzodiazepines:

Diazepam

- Binds to a specific subunit on the Gamma amino butyric acid (GABA) cell receptor known as the $GABA_A$ which is distinct from the general GABA receptor site
- The $GABA_A$ receptor is an inhibitory channel which when activated decreases neuronal activity thus reducing hyperexcitability and possible seizure activity
- The anticonvulsant properties of diazepam and other benzodiazepines may be in part or entirely due to binding to voltage-dependent sodium channels rather than benzodiazepine receptors however this has not been definitively established

Adverse effects:
Respiratory depression, drowsiness and or confusion, hypotension

Intravenous as a bolus dose
Intramuscular injection
Rectal
Oral – available in tablet and liquid form

- Has a high lipid solubility which means it gets absorbed with equal speed whether given intravenously, orally or rectally (non-intravenous routes being convenient in non-hospital settings)
- This means it does not remain in the vascular space but soon redistributes into other body tissues and so it may be necessary to repeat diazepam doses to maintain anticonvulsant effects, resulting in excess body accumulation

Lorazepam

- Actions are very similar to those noted for Diazepam

Adverse effects:
Respiratory depression, drowsiness and or confusion, hypotension

Intravenous – bolus dose
(For the management of seizures)
Oral

- Lorazepam has a low lipid solubility which makes it relatively slowly absorbed when administered by any route other than intravenously
- Once given IV it does not get significantly redistributed beyond the vascular space, therefore unlike Diazepam, the anticonvulsant effects of Lorazepam are more durable, reducing the need for repeated doses

(Continued)

Table A1 Continued.

Drug	Method of delivery	Points of note
Midazolam Is a short-acting, water-soluble benzodiazepine with Gamma amino butyric acid (GABA) enhancing actions in the central nervous system, notably the spinal cord, hippocampus, cerebellum and cerebrum At all these sites Midazolam reduces neuronal activity therefore reducing the hyperactivity of cells and seizure activity *Adverse effects:* Respiratory depression, apnoea, hypotension (at large doses or rapid IV administration), bradycardia, drowsiness, confusion. *Intranasal* – burning sensation and irritation of nasal mucosa	Intravenous – may be given as bolus dose or continuous infusion Buccal Oral Intranasal Intramuscular injection	Buccal Midazolam is easy to administer to children without IV access presenting with seizures. Evidence suggests that it is more effective than rectal diazepam in controlling seizures It is also being offered to parents rather than rectal diazepam for home management of prolonged seizures (defined as lasting longer than 5–10 minutes)
Paraldehyde • Acts to increase the effects of the neurotransmitter Gamma amino butyric acid (GABA) which regulates cell excitability • Decreases the effect of other neurotransmitters such as glutamate that excite nerve activity and may contribute to hyperexcitability *Adverse effects:* Rashes, sterile abscesses at injection sites, irritation of rectal tissue	Rectal administration Intramuscular injection	• For rectal administration it is common to give the dose diluted ml for ml with olive or sunflower oil. It is also possible to dilute with 0.9% Saline but this will increase the volume to be administered • Ready mixed solutions for rectal administration are available • Regular rotation of injection sites if the IM route is being used should reduce risk of abscess formation • Paraldehyde is corrosive when in contact with plastic and rubber therefore immediate administration once dose is drawn up is essential

Note: It is the responsibility of the individual practitioner to check prescribed medications against recognised National Formularies such as the British National Formulary (BNF) for Children (2007).

Observation charts

<table>
<tr><td colspan="2">

ADDRESSOGRAPH LABEL

Name : ....
Date of Birth : ....
Hospital No : ....
Ward/Hospital : ....

</td><td colspan="2">

Modified Paediatric Coma Score
Adapted by Tatman, Warren, Powell, Whitehouse & Noons 1997, Birmingham Children's Hospital NHS Trust
Coma Score (Infant - < 4yrs)

Ward Area: ....
Patient's Weight: .... in kilograms (kg)
Patient's Height: .... in centimetres (cm)

</td></tr>
</table>

DATE:				
TIME:				
NEURO OBSERVATIONS:				

COMA SCALE

Eyes Open

Spontaneous	4
To verbal stimuli	3
To painful stimuli	2
No response to painful stimuli	1
Eyes closed – swelling/bandages	C

Best Motor Response

Obeys commands or normal spontaneous movements	6
Localises to painful stimuli or withdraws to touch	5
Withdraws to painful stimuli	4
Abnormal flexion to pain	3
Abnormal extension to pain	2
No response to pain	1
Not applicable	NA

Best Verbal OR Grimace Response

Verbal

Alert, babbles, coos, words/ sentences to normal ability	5
Less than usual ability or spontaneous irritable cry	4
Cries inappropriately	3
Occasionally whimpers &/ or moans	2
No response	1
Silent or mute	S
Intubated	T

Grimace

Spontaneous normal facial/oro-motor activity	5
Less than usual spontaneous ability or only response to touch stimuli	4
Vigorous grimace to pain	3
Mild grimace to pain	2
No grimace to pain	1
Not applicable	NA

Total Coma Score (out of 15)

PUPIL SCALE IN mm

1 mm	2 mm	3 mm	4 mm	5 mm	6 mm	7 mm	8 mm	9 mm

PUPIL

Right	Size	
	Reaction	
Left	Size	
	Reaction	

+ = Reaction   − = No Reaction   S = Sluggish   C = Eyes Closed

LIMB MOVEMENTS

Arms	
	Normal power
	Mild weakness
	Severe weakness
	Spontaneously
	Painful stimuli
	No response

Legs	
	Normal power
	Mild weakness
	Severe weakness
	Spontaneously
	Painful stimuli
	No response

Record right (R) and left (L) separately if there is a difference between the 2 sides.   P = Paralysed   # = Fracture

Chart A1 Neuroassessment chart for children under 4 years of age. *Source:* University Hospitals of Bristol NHS Foundation Trust – Bristol Royal Hospital for Children.

DATE:

TIME:

NEURO OBSERVATIONS:

COMA SCALE	**Eyes Open**	Spontaneous	4
		To verbal stimuli	3
		To painful stimuli	2
		No response to painful stimuli	1
		Eyes closed – swelling/bandages	C
	Best Motor Response	Obeys verbal commands	6
		Localises to painful stimuli	5
		Withdraws to painful stimuli	4
		Abnormal flexion to pain	3
		Abnormal extension to pain	2
		No response to pain	1
		Not applicable	NA
	Best Verbal OR Grimace Response — Verbal	Orientated (person, place, etc)	5
		Confused	4
		Inappropriate words	3
		Inappropriate sounds	2
		No response	1
		Silent or mute	S
		Intubated	T
	Grimace	Spontaneous normal facial/oro-motor activity	5
		Less than usual spontaneous ability or only response to touch stimuli	4
		Vigorous grimace to pain	3
		Mild grimace to pain	2
		No grimace to pain	1
		Not applicable	NA
		Total Coma Score (out of 15)	

PUPIL SCALE IN mm

1 mm	2 mm	3 mm	4 mm	5 mm	6 mm	7 mm	8 mm	9 mm

PUPILS	Right	Size
		Reaction
	Left	Size
		Reaction

+ = Reaction   – = No Reaction   S = Sluggish   C = Eyes Closed

LIMB MOVEMENTS	Arms	Normal power
		Mild weakness
		Severe weakness
		Spontaneously
		Painful stimuli
		No response
	Legs	Normal power
		Mild weakness
		Severe weakness
		Spontaneously
		Painful stimuli
		No response

Record right (R) and left (L) separately if there is a difference between the 2 sides.   P = Paralysed   # = Fracture

Chart A2 Neuroassessment chart for children between 4 and 15 years of age. *Source:* University Hospitals of Bristol NHS Foundation Trust – Bristol Royal Hospital for Children.

Chapter 7

CARE OF A CHILD WITH A HEPATIC OR METABOLIC DISEASE

Graham Gordon, Doreen Crawford, Debra Teasdale
and Michaela Dixon

Introduction

The liver is one of the key organs in the maintenance of homeostasis within the body. Dysfunction may occur for a number of reasons and can have devastating and/or fatal consequences. The nurse's role is paramount in recognising early signs of liver malfunction, assessing for deterioration and preventing irreversible progression of the disease. In addition the nurse acts as a key conduit for ensuring that parents have the information they require to ensure sound decision making.

Development of the liver and pancreas

The primitive gut can be divided into three segments: the foregut, midgut and hindgut. Each segment gives rise to specific gut and gut-related structures in the newborn, as shown in Table 7.1.

Although a 'snapshot' perspective is provided, it must be emphasised that the process of embryo development and fetal development is continuous. The development of the liver and pancreas is intertwined with the development of the GIT.

Overview of anatomy and physiology

Anatomy of the liver

The liver is the largest gland in the body. The adult liver weighs between 1200 and 1800 g (gender dependent) and accounts for approximately 2% of body weight. The newborn liver is approximately 5% of body weight. The liver is subdivided into smaller and smaller functioning units:

Liver → four lobes → lobules → hepatic
plates → hepatocytes

The hepatocytes are responsible for performing many of the functions. Blood flows into the liver lobules from the branches of portal vein and hepatic artery to enter exchange areas called sinusoids. Within the sinusoids oxygen is extracted from arterial blood, oxygen and nutrients are absorbed from venous blood and foreign material is removed. Blood is drained from sinusoids via central veins that unite to form sub-lobular veins and hepatic veins. Hepatic veins enter the inferior vena cava below the level of the diaphragm.

Table 7.1 Embryological and fetal development of the liver and pancreas.

Gestational age	Development
Weeks 2–3	The liver and pancreas will form from the rudimentary gastrointestinal tract (GIT) which arises from the endoderm of the trilaminar embryo. The rudimentary GIT extends as a continuous tube from the buccopharyngeal membrane to the cloacal membrane
Week 4	There are now three distinct portions to the embryo GIT: the foregut, midgut and hindgut. These extend the length of the embryo and will contribute different components of the tract. The large midgut is generated by lateral embryonic folding which 'pinches off' a pocket of the yolk sac; the two compartments continue to communicate through the vitelline duct
Week 5	The liver originates from the hepatic plate transverse septum at a junctional region where foregut and midgut meet. The transverse septum then differentiates to form the hepatic diverticulum and the hepatic primordium, and these two structures will go on to form components of the liver and the gall bladder
	Rapid proliferation of cells. These hepatoblasts are bipotential in that they can differentiate as either hepatocytes or cholangiocytes (bile duct cells)
	The foregut/midgut junction at the septum transversum generates two pancreatic buds – the dorsal and ventral endoderm – which will fuse to form the pancreas. The dorsal bud arises first and generates most of the pancreas. The ventral bud arises beside the bile duct and forms only part of the head and uncinate process of the pancreas
Weeks 6–8	The pancreatic buds develop an internal network of ducts which, when the buds fuse, interconnect with each other to form the pancreatic ducts. The proximal end of the pancreas joins with the bile duct. The pancreas, originally a midline fetal structure, is deviated from this axis as the stomach distends and rotates. With further rotation, owing to growth and migration of the developing stomach and intestines, the pancreas becomes a retroperitoneal structure
	Explosive developmental spurt of cells forming liver tissue means that the outline of the organ can be seen on the surface anatomy of the embryo. Internally the liver is competing for space with the heart. From the eighth week of gestation the site of the production of fetal erythrocytes shifts from vessels within the yolk sac to the liver sinusoids
Week 9	As the embryonic period gives way to the fetal period the structural framework of the GIT is in place; cells continue to differentiate, but the system organisation is in place. In the fetal period, islet cell clusters differentiate from pancreatic bud endoderm. These cell clusters form the acini and the exocrine ducts. On the edge of these cell clusters the pancreatic islets form
Weeks 10–15	Alpha cells differentiate first (glucagon), delta (somatostatin) and beta (insulin) cells differentiate after
	Islets of Langerhans present, and insulin secretion begins by week 12 and has a likely role in fetal growth and development. Glucagon is detectable in fetal plasma by week 15
	At 12 weeks' gestation hepatocytes begin to produce bile and this is excreted into the intestine in small amounts during fetal life, resulting in dark green meconium after birth. By week 14 the liver is increasingly metabolically active and produces sufficient quantities of bile containing bile salts, cholesterol and inorganic salts which the gall bladder stores. Towards the end of this period the liver begins to synthesise antibodies
Week 22	Digestive enzymes such as amylase begin to be produced by pancreatic exocrine cells
Week 33	Haematopoiesis in the liver is beginning to regress and the primary site is now the bone marrow
Week 37 to term	The liver and pancreas sufficiently mature to function independently, although further maturation of the GIT continues for several years postnatal

From Chamley *et al.* (2003) and Moore and Persaud (2003).

The porta hepatis is a fissure where the hepatic artery, portal vein and hepatic duct enter and exit the liver. These make up the portal triads or tracts and divide and follow septa through the liver. The hepatic artery contains blood rich in oxygen carrying approximately 25% of the total hepatic blood supply. The portal vein carries blood rich in nutrients absorbed from the GIT and supplies 75% of the hepatic blood flow. The venous blood from the stomach, spleen, intestines and pancreas flows from the capillary beds into small veins, and these combine to form large veins which drain into the hepatic portal vein.

The hepatic biliary system synthesises and transports bile composed of bile salts, bilirubin pigment (an iron-free degradation product of old red blood cells), cholesterol, phospholipids, haemoglobin and other toxins to the gall bladder. Bile is synthesised by liver hepatocytes and is secreted into bile canaliculli (spaces between the rows of hepatic cells empting into terminal intra-lobular bile ducts) and then into a specialised part of the bile duct known as the gall bladder; here storage can occur until secretion of bile into the duodenum is stimulated. Terminal bile ducts drain into the right and left hepatic ducts. The right and left hepatic ducts join to form the common bile duct. The common bile duct and major hepatic duct merge at the ampulla of vater and empty into the duodenum.

The adult liver produces 0.5 L/day of bile and proportionally less in infants and children. Most flows directly into the duodenum. Bile salts are reabsorbed passively in the whole of the bowel but actively in the terminal ileum. The liver reconjugates primary bile salts and rehydroxylates secondary bile salts which result from bacterial action in the gut. Fat in the duodenum stimulates bile release through the excretion of cholecystokinin from the intestinal mucosa. The excretion of bile is essential for emulsification of fat and activation of pancreatic lipase. This leads to intestinal absorption of fat and fat-soluble vitamins (A, D, E and K).

Kupffer cells are tissue macrophages (reticuloendothelial cells) that line the walls of the sinusoids, which are involved in the breakdown of old haemoglobin. They are very effective in removing intestinal and foreign bacteria in addition to other toxins. The lack of bacteria from the gastrointestinal tract reaching the general circulation demonstrates the filtering effectiveness of Kupffer cells.

Functions of the liver

In addition to the synthesis and excretion of bile, the liver has many metabolic, maintenance and storage functions. Metabolism involves the catabolism (breakdown of substances) and anabolism (buildup of substances).

Metabolism of fats

The role of the liver in fat metabolism starts when fat has been absorbed from the intestine in the form of triglycerides and fatty acids. The liver converts triglycerides to many substances that are essential for body functioning and regulation. Fatty acids can be converted to form ketone bodies in the liver. Ketone bodies can then be used to produce metabolic energy via the citric acid cycle in the cells. Lipoproteins formed in the liver are released into the blood stream and then deposited in adipose cells for storage. Storage fat in this form is also synthesised from carbohydrate and protein by the liver. Phospholipids and cholesterol which are manufactured in the liver are required for production of plasma membrane components, bile, steroid hormones and vitamin D.

Metabolism of carbohydrates

The liver has a key role in carbohydrate metabolism. It regulates blood sugar levels by conversion and storage of glycogen from glucose (glycogenesis), conversion of glucose into fat for storage, release of glucose during hypoglycaemia and take-up of glucose during hyperglycaemia. When glycogen stores have been used, the liver converts amino acids from protein and glycerol from fat into glucose, a process called gluconeogenesis (formation of new sugar).

Metabolism of proteins

The liver manipulates amino acids and in the process ammonia is released. This is a process called deamination. It then converts ammonia to urea which is passed into the blood, carried to the kidneys and then excreted in the urine. The liver also breaks down amino acids to ketoacids such as pyruvic acid, which are then converted into fatty acids for fat synthesis or storage or used for the production of metabolic energy for the liver cells by the citric acid cycle. The liver has a key role in the maintenance of blood volume and plasma colloid osmotic pressure via synthesis of albumin and other plasma proteins, which form a concentration gradient that draws water via osmosis into the blood vessels to maintain a dynamic equilibrium. Haemostasis is maintained through the manufacture of clotting factors such as fibrinogen and prothrombin. Immunity is enhanced via synthesis of most globulins. Synthesis of non-essential amino acids and serum enzymes occurs in the liver (transamination).

Detoxification

The detoxification of drugs occurs in the liver. Endogenous substances such as steroids and hormones and exogenous substances such as alcohol or barbiturates are altered to make them less harmful unless biologically active. This process is called metabolic detoxification. It prevents excessive accumulation and adverse effects by reducing the amount of substances reabsorbed and promoting excretion from the intestine or the renal tubules.

Storage

The liver stores fat, glycogen, minerals such as iron and copper and vitamins A, B_{12}, D, E and K. The length of time stored depends on the substance and the needs of the body.

Heat production

These metabolic processes require energy and produce heat. The temperature of venous blood leaving the liver is higher than body temperature.

Signs of liver dysfunction

The function of the liver can be affected by a variety of causes including congenital causes (genetic or iatrogenic), trauma and other disease processes. The impact can be wide-ranging (see Table 7.2).

Liver function tests

To determine the underlying cause of liver dysfunction, liver biochemical indices have been grouped into categories of enzymes, bilirubin, coagulation and proteins. The review of each liver function test will include a description, paediatric reference values and enzyme specifics relevant to interpretation. Reference values are institution specific and are variable depending on the methods of laboratory testing. There are no hard and fast rules as to what represents mild versus moderate versus severe elevations (see Table 7.3 for normal values).

Enzymes

Enzymes are catalysts that enhance reactions and exist for nearly all bodily metabolic reactions. Enzyme presence in the blood indicates changes have occurred allowing the enzyme to move into the extracellular fluid; thus enzyme presence reflects normal metabolic function. However, abnormal values may reflect a disease state. Many of the liver enzymes are measured in international units. One international unit equals the amount of the enzyme that will catalyse transformation of one millimole of the substrate per minute. Efforts to standardise the study of enzymes have lead to the development of new terminology for enzymes. Some liver-specific enzymes are described below.

Alanine aminotransferase (ALT). ALT catalyses the reversible transfer of an amino group between the amino acid alanine and alpha ketoglutamic acid. Hepatocytes are the only cells with high amounts of ALT; however, other cells including heart, kidney and skeletal muscle contain

Table 7.2 Functions of the liver and assessment of dysfunction.

Function	Effect of dysfunction	Assessment
Metabolism of carbohydrate Metabolism of fat	Loss of glucose homeostasis Fat accumulation in hepatocytes	Hypoglycaemia on fasting/stress High/low cholesterol Raised lactate Increased ratio FFA:BOH Raised acyl carnitines Organic aciduria
Metabolism of protein	Increased catabolism	Low BCAA, urea Increased ammonia Raised Tyr, -phe, -met
Synthesis of albumin	Loss of muscle mass	Low albumin Protein energy malnutrition
Synthesis of coagulation factors	Coagulopathy	Prolonged PT/PTT
Degradation of drugs	Prolonged drug effect, e.g. sedation	Clinical
Degradation of oestrogens	Telangectasia Gynaecomastia	Clinical
Degradation of toxic products	Encephalopathy	Abnormal EEG/clinical signs
Bile synthesis and excretion	Cholestasis Fat malabsorption Fat-soluble vitamin deficiency Pruritus Malnutrition	Increased conjugated bilirubin Increased GGT, Increased ALP, Increased cholesterol Anthropometry

Modified from Kelly (2004).

ALP, alkaline phosphatase; BOH, beta-hydroxybutyrate; BCAA, branched chain amino acids; EEG, electroencephalogram; FFA, free fatty acids; GGT, gamma glutamyl transpeptidase; met, methionine; phe, phenylalanine; PT, prothrombin time; PTT, partial thromboplastin time; tyr, tyrosine.

moderate amounts of this enzyme. Presence of this enzyme is a sensitive index of liver damage indicative of cell injury or increased turnover.

Aspartate aminotransferase (AST). AST catalyses the reversible transfer of an amino group between the amino acid aspartate and alpha ketoglutamic acid. Large amounts of this enzyme are found in the liver and myocardial cells. However, smaller but significant amounts are found in skeletal muscle, kidneys, pancreas and brain. The specificity of AST for liver function test increases with an increase in the enzyme level. Primary hepatocyte damage is indicated with laboratory values 10 times the upper limit of reference values.

Top tip

ALT and AST are often described as transaminases in the clinical setting. The transaminases can be elevated with rejection of the transplanted liver. However, isolated increases are more characteristic of hepatitis.

Alkaline phosphatase (ALP)

Enzymes that remove phosphate from compounds with a single phosphate group are called phosphatases. Phosphatases are optimally active at a pH equal to 9 and are grouped under the name of ALP. Liver, bones and intestines are the major sources of ALP. The hepatic isoenzymes are believed to largely derive from the epithelium of the intra-hepatic bile ducts rather than from the hepatocytes. ALP values are highest in disorders that cause obstruction or inflammation of the hepatobiliary tract.

Gamma glutamyl transpeptidase (GGT)

GGT is found in hepatobiliary tissues, renal tubules and pancreatic epithelium. GGT catalyses the transfer of glutamyl groups among peptide and amino groups. Serum levels are mainly attributable to the liver; therefore hepatobiliary aetiology should be considered with increased levels. Pronounced increases may reflect hepatobiliary obstruction, whilst modest increases indicate hepatocellular destruction. Increased ALP and GGT values together suggest increased ALP of liver origin.

Bilirubin

Bilirubin is the by-product of the breakdown of the haemoglobin molecule. Fat-soluble bilirubin binds to albumin as indirect (pre-hepatic/unconjugated) bilirubin for transport to the liver. In the liver fat-soluble bilirubin is detached from albumin and conjugated with glucuronic acid, rendering bilirubin water soluble. Direct (post-hepatic/conjugated) bilirubin is excreted into the hepatic ducts and eventually into the intestinal tract. Direct and indirect bilirubin are terms derived from the method of testing used in the past. Total bilirubin is the sum of the direct and indirect bilirubin. An increase in indirect (unconjugated) bilirubin levels will result as the liver is not able to conjugate the bilirubin with impaired synthetic function. Impaired excretion of direct (conjugated) bilirubin into the bile ducts will result in increased levels of conjugated bilirubin by increased re-absorption into the blood. Impaired synthetic function and obstruction increases total bilirubin (both conjugated and unconjugated bilirubin), resulting in jaundice – the yellow coloration of the skin and sclera of the eye.

Top tip

The yellow discoloration of jaundice can be upsetting for parents and for older children who do not want to stand out. It can be camouflaged to some extent by avoiding strong green, brown and yellow clothing and bedding, and opting for pastels, pinks and blues.

Coagulation studies

Prothrombin time (PT) measured in seconds is a laboratory measure of the time required for a firm clot to form after tissue thromboplastin (factor 3) and calcium are added to the sample. The liver synthesises many coagulation factors. The half-life of these varies from hours to days. Prothrombin time (PT) allows the clinical evaluation of the extrinsic pathway of the coagulation cascade. PT is often expressed as *INR* (the international normalised ratio). It is the ratio of PT to the control, with normal being 1.0–1.2. This allows for direct comparison when individual laboratory normal values may vary. Prothrombin time is vitamin K dependent. With liver disease, prolonged PT reflects poor utilisation of vitamin K due to parenchymal disease or low levels of vitamin K due to obstructive jaundice. Therefore prolongation of more than 3 seconds after intravenous administration of vitamin K suggests loss of synthetic function. Obstructive liver disease is indicated if the PT is normal after vitamin K administration. Partial thromboplastin time (PPT) clinically evaluates the intrinsic and common pathways of the coagulation cascade. This laboratory value represents the time required for a firm fibrin clot to develop after phospholipid reagents are added to the specimen. PPT will be prolonged with liver dysfunction.

Proteins

Proteins are composed of amino acids linked by peptide bonds. Fibrinogen, albumin and 60–80% of the globulins are synthesised by hepatocytes. With acute liver disease due to immune dysfunction, an increase in a patient's total protein may be observed; however, with other types of liver disease this value is generally decreased. Albumin is the major circulating protein and is responsible for maintaining plasma oncotic pressure. A patient's albumin value reflects one component of the liver's synthetic function. Despite the presence of normal or increased rates of albumin synthesis, hypoalbuminaemia may present as protein leaks into lymphatic or other extracellular components. The half-life of albumin is 21 days and therefore with chronic liver disease a decrease in serum albumin levels may be observed.

Stop and think

Albumin levels must be carefully interpreted as other factors may affect the laboratory values. For example, decreases may be observed with inadequate protein intake and increased losses from the gut and kidneys, and increases with albumin administration.

Ammonia

Ammonia is formed from the deamination of certain amino acids during protein metabolism and is also a product of the degradation of proteins by colonic bacteria. The liver converts ammonia into urea and then to glutamine. The kidneys use glutamine as a source for synthesising ammonia for renal regulation. Increased ammonia levels indicate decreased hepatocellular function due to cirrhosis or hepatitis.

Glucose

The liver's role in glucose homeostasis is linked to pancreatic hormones, insulin and glucagon. When blood sugar level rises after the ingestion of food, insulin release facilitates the movement of glucose into the cells, where it is used to create cellular energy. Blood glucose that is extra to requirements is converted into glycogen and stored within the liver. When blood glucose levels fall and the body reaches a state of fasting, glucagon is released from the pancreas, causing the stores of glycogen within the liver to break down into glucose, which then raises the blood sugar level. This constant balance means that in health glucose levels are maintained despite fasting. Abnormalities of glucose levels occur in acute and chronic liver failure, metabolic disease (e.g. diabetes; see later) and hypopituitarism.

Interpretation of liver function tests

The interpretation of liver function tests is an art not a science. There are a battery of tests in which patterns of abnormalities can be identified. Characteristic patterns of change have been associated with clinical conditions. The patient's liver function test, like other laboratory findings, cannot be considered in isolation from other clinical findings and diagnostic tests. When interpreting tests, the first consideration is whether the patient's values fall within normal reference ranges. Determining whether the value reflects synthetic or hepatobiliary function is the next step. AST, ALT, glucose, ammonia and PT reflect hepatic function. Gamma GT and ALP reflect hepatobiliary function. Bilirubin can be categorised as synthetic, biliary or both depending on the patient's clinical profile. The child's clinical condition must always be considered to ensure accurate interpretation. Reference ranges are shown in Table 7.3.

Neonatal liver disease

Unconjugated hyperbilirubinaemia

Bilirubin is the major waste product of haemoglobin degradation which mainly takes place in the spleen. A raised bilirubin level in the blood is called hyperbilirubinaemia. The causes of this can be split into two main groups: unconjugated, caused by increased red cell breakdown, and conjugated, caused by impairment in bilirubin excretion as in liver disease. Haemolytic

Table 7.3 Reference ranges for liver function tests.

Biochemical indices		Age range	Child	
Alanine aminotransferase (ALT) (U/L)			<40	
Aspartate aminotransferase (AST) (U/L)		1–5 days	<120	
		6–14 days	<100	
		14 days–1 year	<80	
		1–3 years	<60	
		>3 years	<50	
Alkaline phosphatase (ALP) (U/L)		Neonate	150–700	
		1 month–9 years	250–1000	
			F	**M**
		10–11 years	250–950	250–730
		12–13 years	200–730	275–875
		14–15 years	170–460	170–970
		16–18 years	75–270	125–720
Gamma glutamyl transpeptidase (GGT) (U/L)		5–14 days	<250	
		14–28 days	<150	
		1–2 months	<115	
		2–4 months	<80	
		>4 months	<30	
Bilirubin	Total (μmol/L)	Neonate	<200	
		Child	<15	
	Conjugated (μmol/L)	Neonate	<30	
		Child	<2	
Albumin g/L		Neonate	25–45	
		1 month–3 years	34–42	
		4–6 years	35–52	
		7–19 years	37–56	
Ammonia (μmol/L)		Preterm/sick neonate	<150	
		Term neonate	<100	
		Child	<40	
PT (seconds)		>6 months	9–13	
		<6 months	11–15	
PTT (seconds)		>6 months	26–35	
		<6 months	30–38	

Reference values from Birmingham Children's Hospital Paediatric Laboratory Medicine Handbook (August 2001). F = female; M = male.

hyperbilirubinaemia is usually associated with unconjugated or indirect bilirubin. It is common among premature infants and indeed in some term babies. The main causes are listed in Table 7.4.

Management

Low-level unconjugated hyperbilirubinaemia in the neonate does not need active intervention other than support to establish effective feeding, since jaundice causes sleepiness in the infant.

Table 7.4 Causes of unconjugated hyperbilirubinaemia.

Cause	Aetiology
Physiological jaundice	Owing to excessive RBC breakdown at birth and functional immaturity of the conjugation processes in the liver Term babies treated with phototherapy if bilirubin greater than 300 µmol/L
Breast milk jaundice	Persistence of fetal mechanisms (e.g. β-glucuronidase) causes low-level continued jaundice in some infants. This can be exacerbated by poor feeding techniques leading to dehydration. Surveillance is required by doctor if lasts over a month
Systemic disease Rhesus and ABO incompatibility Glucose-6-phosphate dehydrogenase Sickle cell disease Thalassaemia Spherocytosis Hypothyroidism Upper-intestinal obstruction Sepsis Hypoxia/acidosis Galactosaemia Fructosaemia	All cause increased haemolysis, which is particularly problematic if encountered in the newborn period, exacerbating jaundice levels because of liver immaturity
Iatrogenic Trauma at birth Blood transfusion Administration of certain drugs	Bruising → breakdown of RBC Administration process can damage RBC Some drugs displace bilirubin from albumin, thus increasing the free component, for example, diazepam, hydrocortisone, gentamycin, cefalosporins, digoxin
Inherited disorders Crigler–Najjar syndrome (type 1 and type 2) Gilbert's syndrome	Deficiency in enzyme uridine diphosphate glucuronosyltransferase (UDPGT). Type 1 is total and needs phototherapy long term. Type 2 is partial and may ultimately be treated with enzyme inducers such as phenobarbitone Mild transient jaundice that needs no treatment, only reassurance

The 97th centile for bilirubin in the well term baby varies between 210 and 250 µmol/L depending on whether the baby is breast or bottle fed. Treatment may be started at 80 µmol/L on day 1, increasing to 300 µmol/L on day 3 for well term babies, with treatment thresholds being significantly reduced for sick or preterm babies. For those at risk of kernicterus, phototherapy, exchange blood transfusion and occasionally medication are indicated.

Stop and think

Excessively high levels of unconjugated hyperbilirubinaemia in the first 24 hours of life should be investigated as should persistent levels above 200 µmol/L. These neonates are at risk of kernicterus which occurs when free bilirubin crosses the blood–brain barrier and binds with the basal ganglia, causing a yellow discoloration. This causes bilirubin encephalopathy and permanent brain damage.

Phototherapy

Phototherapy is the application of fluorescent lights to convert unconjugated bilirubin (fat soluble) into a pigment that is soluble in water, facilitating bilirubin excretion. Threshold levels are presented above but local guidance should dominate decision making.

Key considerations for nurses

- Nurses play an important role in the identification and assessment of jaundice; however, judgement can be impeded by poor environmental conditions. Always observe the child in daylight. In non-Caucasian infants/children this can be particularly problematic; however, careful inspection of the sclera of the eyes and mucous membranes allows successful assessment.
- As a rule of thumb, jaundice progresses cephalo-caudally, and serum testing should be considered if jaundice extends down to the umbilicus.
- The infant requires maximum skin exposure to the phototherapy lights so should be undressed to receive treatment. Consequently, a judgment must be made to determine the appropriate environment of care – basinette or incubator – and the appropriate surrounding environment (away from draughts, windows, doors, sunlight, etc.).
- Temperature must be monitored hourly until stable – Perspex cot lids may be useful, but any such barrier between the light and infant will reduce the efficiency of the treatment.
- The infant's eyes must be covered and checked to ensure covers remain *in situ*. Eye care should be provided.
- Phototherapy, although non-invasive, can result in the infant producing dark green loose stools (due to the pigments causing 'intestinal hurry') and a pin prick rash may develop. Parents must be informed of this prior to commencing the treatment to minimise anxiety levels.
- Skin care is important to remove acidic urine and stools; however, skin creams, oils or ointment must be avoided as the heat produced by the lights will result in skin burns.
- The nurse needs to negotiate with parents to ensure that visits and feeding (if appropriate) continue whilst the infant remains under treatment for the maximum time possible.

Stop and think

The infant will require regular monitoring of bilirubin levels. When blood sampling is taking place, phototherapy lights should be turned off to reduce any risk of reducing the bilirubin lights in the sample, i.e. preventing erroneous results. Often blood for analysis is obtained via a capillary sample. It is important that the sample is free flowing and the heel not 'squeezed' as haemolysis increases bilirubin results.

Exchange transfusion

This involves removal of the child's blood and simultaneous replacement with fresh blood or packed red blood cells. The result is that the overall load of bilirubin in the blood is reduced, so reducing the risks of kernicterus. This technique is also useful in reducing symptomatic polycythaemia (excessive numbers of RBC) after birth and to reduce antibody loads in rhesus haemolytic disease. Exchange transfusion is indicated at bilirubin levels greater than 380 µmol/L in the term baby, 350 µmol/L at 35–38 weeks' gestation, 280 µmol/L at 31–34 weeks and 240 µmol/L below 30 weeks' gestation.

Top tip

If you are assisting in an exchange transfusion, total concentration is required. Before commencing make sure that *you* have eaten, attended to calls of nature and have a comfortable seat.

- Ideally any exchange transfusion should be performed in a single room – cardio-respiratory monitoring must be *in situ*, as hyperkalaemia and hypocalcaemia can result. As a result, in addition to resuscitation equipment, many practitioners have ampoules of 10% calcium gluconate to hand.

- Venous and arterial catheters must be appropriately secured and aseptic technique applied.
- Consent is required from parents.

Stop and think

If there are any concerns regarding the infant's genetic make-up, a sample of blood must be taken prior to the transfusion as the replacement of RBC will prevent genetic analysis for ~3 months.

- Blood products are warmed and the exchange is accomplished through a continuous cycle of withdrawal and infusion of blood.
- The routes chosen will vary and depend on the infant's age; however, the umbilical artery allows effective withdrawal and the umbilical vein allows replacement in infants in the first week. In older infants, two venous catheters or a venous and arterial catheter may be used.
- Commonly double volume exchanges are performed for those at greatest risk (birth weight × 85 × 2); the total volume must be agreed prior to the transfusion and recorded clearly on the fluid chart to prevent overload.
- Using a closed system, 5–10 mL of the blood is aspirated slowly by the medical practitioner from the circulation and then discarded via a three-way tap in the closed system into a waste bag. An equivalent volume of transfusion blood is then slowly administered back into the circulation. Each cycle takes ~3–5 minutes. This cycle of aspiration/infusion may last between 3 and 6 hours depending on the volumes to be replaced.
- The nurse's role is to track total volumes carefully and to monitor the child's systemic perfusion, temperature and vital signs. Samples

of haemoglobin, bilirubin and electrolyte balance should be obtained prior and post transfusions. Some practitioners advocate that all blood packs undergo similar testing.

- Feeding is generally withheld during the exchange transfusion, so blood sugar monitoring is required. In well infants the timing of the exchange will determine the need for IV infusion support. In the ill infant, IV access and 10% dextrose infusion should be in place in order to keep blood glucose levels within normal ranges.
- Although many infants are sleepy, occasionally some will become fractious, so the expeditious use of a soother may be required (providing parental consent has been obtained).

Conjugated hyperbilirubinaemia

Elevated conjugated bilirubin mostly commonly results from obstructive liver disease, but can be seen in many types of liver disease which affect hepatocyte function. Conjugated hyperbilirubinaemia is said to be present when >20% of the total plasma bilirubin is conjugated or when the total conjugated level is greater than 20 mmol/L. Total and conjugated bilirubin levels are measured in the laboratory and the level of unconjugated is the difference between the two. The ratios of types of bilirubin can be helpful in diagnosis of the cause. In hepatobiliary disease, the total and conjugated will be raised. Total and unconjugated will be raised in hepatic disease. A split bilirubin (total and conjugated) should be performed on any baby who remains jaundiced after 2 weeks of life (3 weeks for preterm infants). If the conjugated fraction is raised as defined above then investigations for possible liver disease should be started. Liver disease in the newborn can present as:

- An ill infant with liver failure (deranged clotting unresponsive to intravenous vitamin K)
- Neonatal hepatitis syndrome
- Biliary obstruction

Management

General practitioners, neonatologists and paediatric gastroenterologists would typically perform first line tests of jaundiced babies before or during on-going discussions with a specialist unit (see below). It is vital that sick infants and those with abnormal stools are discussed early with a liver unit while awaiting the results of first-line investigations. In some cases direct referral to a supra-regional liver unit is appropriate to exclude the diagnosis of biliary atresia as quickly as possible. Second-stage investigations will be undertaken according to indications from history, examination and laboratory findings and/or discussion with a specialist consultant. An overview of specific treatment against cause can be seen below; however, the most significant cause of conjugated hyperbilirubinaemia is biliary atresia.

First-stage investigation for prolonged conjugated jaundice

- ALT, AST, ALP, GTT
- Albumin and total protein
- Glucose, cholesterol and triglyceride
- Prothrombin time (if prolonged give 300 µg/kg of IV vitamin K and repeat 12 hours later. If still prolonged contact a liver unit)
- Partial thromboplastin time
- Fibrinogen
- Full blood count
- Reticulocyte count
- Group and Coomb's test

Infection

- Bacterial culture of blood and urine
- Viral culture of urine (CMV)
- TORCH screen (IgM to CMV, toxoplasma, rubella and herpes)
- Hepatitis A, B, C if history is suggestive

Radiology

- Abdominal ultrasound after 4-hours fast to see if gall bladder present and to see if choledochal cyst is present

Metabolic investigations

- α_1-antitrypsin level + phenotype
- Immunoreactive trypsin (up to 8 weeks or sweat test), plasma amino acids galactose 1 phosphate uridyl transferase, Free T4, TSH levels of cortisol after a 4 hour fast. If low short Synacthen test
- Urine-reducing substances
- Protein
- Organic acids
- Amino acids and succinylacetone
- Consultant to examine stool colour
- T4, thyroxine; TORCH, toxoplasma, rubella, cytomegalovirus, herpes simplex; TSH, thyroid-stimulating hormone

Overview of neonatal liver disease (See Table 7.5)

Table 7.5 An overview of neonatal liver disease specific treatments.

Disease	Strategy
Infection	
Toxoplasma	Spiramycin
Cytomegalovirus	Ganciclovir
Herpes simplex	Aciclovir
Syphilis	Penicillin
Bacterial infection	Appropriate antibiotics
Tuberculosis	Quadruple antitubercular therapy (not ethambutol)
Giant cell hepatitis	Nutritional, vitamin and cholerectic support

Table 7.5 Continued.

Disease	Strategy
Endocrine	
Panhypopituitarism (septo-optic dysplasia)	Corticosteroids, thyroxine, growth hormone
Structural	
Extra-hepatic biliary atresia	Kasai portoenterostomy
Choledochal cyst	Surgical resection
Choledocholithiasis	Surgical removal
Spontaneous perforation of CBD	Surgical repair
Metabolic	
$\alpha1$ anti-trypsin deficiency	Nutritional, vitamin and cholerectic support
Primary disorders of bile acid synthesis	Bile acid supplements
Toxic	
PN-associated liver disease	Enteral feeding, metronidazole and ursodeoxycholic acid
Immune	
Neonatal hepatitis with autoimmune haemolytic anaemia	Immunosuppression
Syndromes	
Alagille syndrome	Nutritional, vitamin and cholerectic support

CBD, common bile duct; PN, parenteral nutrition.

Biliary atresia

Biliary atresia is a progressive disease, usually present at birth, which leads to cholestasis, hepatic fibrosis and cirrhosis. It is the commonest surgical cause of jaundice in neonates. Late diagnosis may result in irreversible liver damage and the need for liver transplantation in the first year of life. The frequency is 1 per 16 000 live births, there is usually no family history, but a slight female preponderance exists. The aetiology is unknown; however, 10% have extra-hepatic abnormalities (polysplenia, situs inversus, interrupted inferior vena cava, preduodenal portal vein and cardiac defects). This is called biliary atresia splenic malformation syndrome.

Stop and think

All infants who have conjugated jaundice after 14 days of age should be investigated to exclude biliary atresia.

Referral to a specialist centre is mandatory for suspected cases in order to facilitate early surgery. Clinical presentation includes conjugated hyperbilirubinaemia, dark urine, pale (acholic) stools and hepatomegaly.

Birth weight and gestation are usually normal and infants feed and thrive appropriately at first. The lack of fat-soluble vitamin K absorption may result in coagulopathy and rarely in a bleed (possibly intracranial). Older infants may have ascites and splenomegaly.

Diagnosis is by exclusion of other medical causes (e.g. alpha 1 antitrypsin deficiency) and by identifying the characteristic histological appearance of a percutaneous liver biopsy. Abdominal ultrasound will exclude other surgical causes such as choledochol cyst and inspissated bile syndrome. Other relevant signs include an absent or contracted gall bladder after fasting. Radionuclide hepatobiliary imaging will show failure of bile excretion into the bowel within 24 hours. Infants less than 60 days old with a high suspicion are recommended for surgery utilising the Kasai portoenterostomy. Bile drainage is achieved in 60% of infants, but complications include malnutrition, ascending bacterial cholangitis, cirrhosis and portal hypertension.

Post-operative care
- Normal post-operative surgical care
- Intravenous antibiotics followed by oral prophylactic antibiotics
- Intravenous fluids with early return to feeding with medium chain triglyceride-based feed
- Epidural analgesia
- Steroids for 2 weeks
- Choleretics (phenobarbitone or ursodeoxycholic acids)

Key nursing responsibilities include educating parents in correct administration of medication, nutritional therapy, and vitamin and mineral supplements. On occasion tube feeding may be needed to supplement oral intake (Hockenberry 2003).

Discharge is common by the seventh post-operative day; however, fat-soluble vitamins (A, D, E and K) are required for up to 1 year. A normal vaccination schedule is advised which should include, Pneumovax® and influenza. Despite this relatively good outcome, biliary atresia remains the most common indication for paediatric liver transplantation (up to 50%).

The acutely ill infant with conjugated hyperbilirubinaemia

Some infants will present as acutely ill to their local paediatric unit.

Initial investigations in the acutely ill infant

An asterisk below means store plasma, serum and urine samples for further investigation. The following is taken from McKiernan (2004).

Blood*
- Bacterial culture
- Prothrombin time, partial thromboplastin time, fibrinogen, D-dimer
- Bilirubin, alkaline phosphatase, transaminases, albumin, GGT
- Acid–base balance
- Lactate
- Ammonia, amino acids
- Full blood count and film
- Urea, creatinine, sodium, potassium, chloride, calcium, phosphate, magnesium
- Acylcarnitine profile

Urine*
- pH
- Microscopy and culture

- Reducing substance
- Ketones
- Organic acids
- Amino acids

CSF (if coagulation and neurological state allow)
- Gram stain and culture
- Protein, glucose
- Lactate

Radiology
- Chest and wrist X-ray
- Echocardiography

The tests identified previously for investigation into prolonged conjugated hyperbilirubinaemia should be completed. Contact should be made with a liver unit for advice on what further tests should be done locally and to assess the need for transfer. Management of specific conditions is described in Table 7.6.

Liver disease in the older child

The clinical presentation of liver disease in the older child will vary.

Asymptomatic onset:

- Incidental detection of abnormal liver enzymes
- Screening of someone at risk from family members of a hepatitis B/C virus carrier
- Patient with an associated disorder such as inflammatory bowel disease
- Recipient of a known toxic agent such as methotrexate

Insidious onset characterised by gradual onset of:

- Fatigue, anorexia and weight loss
- Abdominal discomfort
- Intermittent jaundice

Table 7.6 Management of specific conditions.

Condition	Management
Galactosaemia	Exclude lactose from diet, monitor for life-long complications. Neonatal screening available in some areas
Tyrosinaemia type 1	NTBC (1 mg/kg/day), phenylalanine- and tyrosine-restricted diet, monitor amino acids, regular α-fetoprotein, abdominal ultrasound, hepatic MRI for hepatocellular carcinoma, consider liver transplantation for unresponsive children or for life-threatening complications. Neonatal screening available in areas of high incidence
Neonatal haemochromatosis	Risk increases with each pregnancy, managed in neonatal intensive care in transplant centre, antioxidant cocktail (n-acetylcysteine, selenium, α-tocopherol, prostaglandin E, desferrioxamine), liver transplantation likely to be needed, antenatal diagnosis of subsequent siblings, may respond to maternally given immunoglobulins
Disorders of mitochondrial energy metabolism	Supportive management of acute liver failure may be *the* only therapy, liver transplant if defect only confined to liver
Urea cycle disorders	Withdraw dietary protein, sodium benzoate IV, arginine in 10% dextrose, consider dialysis, maintain on low protein diet and oral sodium benzoate, liver transplantation may be considered.
Defects in fatty acid oxidation	Avoid fasting and suppress lipolysis, with overnight nasogastric feeding or nocturnal uncooked corn starch in older infants
Organic acidaemias	10% dextrose IV, sodium bicarbonate, dietary protein restriction, carnitine (200 mg/kg/day) and metronidazole (20 mg/kg/day) help to detoxify and decrease propionate, sodium benzoate may be needed for hyperammonaemia, maintain with low protein, high calorie diet with overnight tube feeding and carnitine. Outlook is poor and liver transplantation has had limited success

Acute onset:

- Acute illness

Investigation

The principles of investigation should be to establish a diagnosis, stage the disease and detect complications and associated conditions (see Table 7.7). The history should take into account ethnic origin, recent transfusions of blood, piercing, tattoos, birth and infancy history, vaccination status, allergies, previous illness, family history, potential drug abuse, foreign travel and recent school performance. A careful history is invaluable in considering a wide range of disorders.

Chronic hepatitis

Hepatitis occurs when the cells of the liver are altered by inflammation, fibrosis, degeneration and necrosis. As a result hepatocyte structure may be altered, resulting in abnormal function. Although hepatitis can be self limiting as liver cells may regenerate without scarring, in some instances normal liver function is never restored without liver transplantation. Table 7.8 summarises the common causes and required management of chronic hepatitis.

Wilson's disease

Copper is an essential nutrient and is present in food and drinking water. Normally excess

Table 7.7 Diagnostic investigations of liver disease in the older child.

Diagnostic area	Methods employed
Autoimmune markers	ANA, SMA, LKM, AMA, GPC Immunoglobulins
Wilson's disease markers	Copper, caeruloplasmin, urinary copper, C3, C4 Ophthalmology Full blood count and haemolysis
Viral serology	Epstein–Barr virus Hepatitis A, B and C
Metabolic	α1-antitrypsin level and phenotype
Drug levels	
Histology	Liver biopsy for • histology • electron microscopy • enzyme analysis • immunohistochemistry • culture
If splenomegaly present	Endoscopy Endoscopic ultrasound
Radiology	Abdominal ultrasound

AMA, antimitochondrial antibodies; ANA, antinuclear antibody; C3, C4, complement components 3 and 4; GPC, general parietal cell antibodies; LKM, liver/kidney microsomal antibodies; SMA, smooth muscle antibodies.

copper is passed into bile and excreted; however, an abnormality on chromosome 13 prevents this normal process so copper builds up in the liver and then spills over, increasing serum copper levels. This excess is toxic and is known to build up in other areas – the brain, cornea and renal system.

Manifestations may be of almost any variety and severity, but liver disease is an early sign. Presentation includes insidious onset of vague symptoms:

- Liver failure (acute hepatitis, fulminant hepatic failure with haemolysis, portal hypertension with bleeding varices and ascites, decompensated cirrhosis)
- Neurological symptoms (odd type of tremor in the arms, slowness of movement, difficulty with speech, writing problems, difficulty swallowing, an unsteady walk, headaches, seizures)
- Psychological symptoms (depression, mood swings, inability to concentrate)
- Opthalmic symptoms (copper may build up in the cornea, causing characteristic brown Kayser–Fleischer rings)

Diagnosis is indicted by low plasma caeruloplasmin, raised urinary copper particularly after penicillamine, raised liver copper and mutation analysis.

Nursing priorities aim for compliance with treatment, since without management the disease can be fatal. Treatment aims to reduce copper levels initially and then prevent recurrence of high copper levels. Chelating agents, e.g. penicillamine, cause excess copper to be excreted in urine. Initial high doses can be reduced to maintenance doses after ~1 year. Zinc supplements prevent copper from being absorbed from the gut and are useful if diagnosis is early. Nutritional management also requires education for both parents and child; high copper foodstuffs may need to be avoided, for example nuts, chocolate, mushrooms, organic meats and shellfish.

Stop and think

Wilson's disease is an autosomal recessive disorder; thus other family members make be carriers or sufferers. Genetic testing should be offered to all family members and strongly advised if further pregnancies are being considered.

Liver transplantation may be required for cases where liver damage is severe.

Acute liver failure (ALF)

Acute necrosis of a previously normal liver is called acute liver failure. Table 7.9 shows the causes of ALF in children. Liver failure not only produces

Table 7.8 Causes and management of chronic hepatitis.

Disease	Management
Chronic viral hepatitis	
Hepatitis B	Identification of natural resolution of chronic carriage, early identification of progressive liver disease, consideration for immune modulatory therapy or antiviral therapy, detection of hepatocellular carcinoma, support and education of whole family regarding transmission, screening and immunisation of family members
Hepatitis D	Prevention of hepatitis B infection and eradication of chronic hepatitis B will prevent the disease associated with hepatitis D
Hepatitis C	Monitor viraemia and detect resolution of infection, assess liver dysfunction and its progression, consider prognostic factors, consider optimal timing of antiviral therapy
Autoimmune liver disease	
Autoimmune hepatitis Type 1 (ANA and/or SMA) Type 2 (LKM)	Responsive to anti-inflammatory and immunosuppressive therapy in both fulminant and cirrhotic presentations. Needs liver biopsy to confirm diagnosis, monitor for effectiveness of treatment and early indications for liver transplant. May be associated with autoimmune disorders particular in the gut in type 1
Overlap syndrome/autoimmune sclerosing cholangitis	Features of biliary disease associated with type 1. Responds to immunosuppression but additional treatment of ursodeoxycholic acid is added
Drug-induced liver disease	
Paracetamol	Treatment with *n*-acetylcysteine IV and supportive measures
Non-steroidal anti-inflammatory drugs	Can occur within weeks of starting treatment, avoid in known liver disease
Aspirin	Usually mild but can be associated with Reye's syndrome
Antimicrobials (erythromycin, flucloxacillin, tetracycline)	Idiosyncratic and dose unrelated with features of hypersensitivity
Antituberculous Isoniazid Rifampicin Pyrazinamide	Frequently associated with liver dysfunction, needs withdrawal of treatment and use of alternative Associated with cholestatic liver dysfunction, withdrawal of drug Dose-related hepatotoxicity
Anticonvulsants (phenytoin, carbamezepine, valproic acid)	An underlying metabolic abnormality may be the precipitating factor and the cause of the underlying neurological disease

clinical and biochemical evidence of failing liver function but also can result in the development of hepatic encephalopathy with decreased level of consciousness and possible signs of increased intracranial pressure (ICP) – see Chapter 6. This is called fulminant liver failure (FLF). Diagnosis in the newborn is problematic due to difficulty in detecting encephalopathy. It is associated with an extremely high mortality and rarely improves without liver transplantation.

Initial management

Figure 7.1 shows a scheme for initial local management of children with ALF, dependent on underlying aetiology.

Management will depend on the symptoms the child presents with or develops. The section on 'Pruritus' identifies the general management of acute liver failure. Specific treatments can be started when a main cause is found – see Table 7.10.

Table 7.9   Causes of ALF in children.

Aetiology	Disease	Incidence
Neonates		
Infectious	Herpes viruses, echovirus, adenovirus, HBV	Frequent
Metabolic	Galactosaemia[a], tyrosinaemia[a], neonatal haemochromatosis[a], mitochondrial disease	Moderately frequent
Ischaemic	Congenital heart disease, cardiac surgery, myocarditis, severe asphyxia	Rare
Older children		
Infectious	HAV, HBV, NA-G, herpes viruses, sepsis[a], other	Frequent
Drugs	Valproate, isoniazid, paracetamol, carbamazepine, halothane	Moderately frequent
Toxins	*Amanita phalloides*, carbon tetrachloride, phosphorus	Rare
Metabolic[a]	Hereditary fructose intolerance[a], Wilson's disease[b]	Rare
Autoimmune	Hepatitis	Rare
Ischaemia	Congenital heart disease, cardiac surgery, myocarditis, severe asphyxia, Budd–Chiari syndrome	Rare
Other	Malignancy	Rare

Modified from Whittingham and Alonso (2004).

[a] Diseases do not fulfil definition of fulminant liver failure.
[b] Rare under 3 years of age.

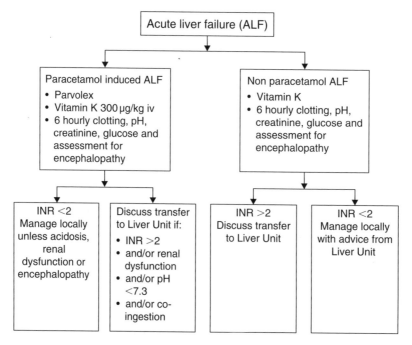

Figure 7.1   Initial management – aetiology dependent.

Table 7.10 Specific therapies in ALF in children.

Therapy	Explanation
Paracetamol ingestion	Emergency management of ingested poisons. *N*-acetylcysteine (150 mg/kg/day within 24 h of ingestion and continue until liver failure resolves
Amanita phalloides poisoning	Benzylpenicillin (10^7 U/kg/day) with thiocetic acid (300 mg/kg/day) IV infusion. Haemofiltration
Hepatic support	
Molecular absorbent recirculating system (MARS)	Albumin cleaning as bridge to transplant
Hepatocyte transplantation	Early stage of research
Liver transplantation	Considered for all children who reach stage III or IV hepatic coma without a contraindication
Family support	Devastating effect on family especially if self poisoning in adolescents. Need psychological support and counselling. Patient information on ALF is available from Children's Liver Disease Foundation

From Whittingham and Alonso (2004).

Ongoing management

No sedation except during procedures. Minimal handling but monitor:

- Heart and respiratory rate
- Arterial BP, CVP
- Core–toe temperature
- Neurological observations
- Gastric pH (<5.0)
- Blood glucose (>4.0 mmol/L)
- Acid–base
- Electrolytes
- PT, PTT

Fluid and electrolyte balance:

- 75% maintenance
- Dextrose 10–50%
- Sodium (0.5–1.0 mmol/L)
- Potassium (2–4 mmol/L)
- Maintain circulating volume with colloid/FFP. Give coagulation support only if required.

Drugs:

- Vitamin K
- H_2 antagonist
- Antacids
- Lactulose
- N-acetylcysteine
- Broad-spectrum antibiotics
- Antifungals

Nutrition:

- Enteral feeding (1–2 g/kg of protein/day).

It needs to be recognised that there are potential ongoing clinical issues which the nurse should consider when undertaking assessment of the child with ALF. These include:

- Hypoglycaemia
- Coagulopathy and haemorrhage
- Encephalopathy
- Cerebral oedema
- Electrolyte and acid–base disturbance
- Renal dysfunction
- Ascites
- Cardiovascular and pulmonary complications
- Respiratory problems
- Secondary bacterial and fungal infection
- Pancreatitis
- Aplastic anaemia

Supporting the family

The nurse's role in supporting the family is first one of assessment of family functioning, need for information and ability to cope with the changes that liver disease brings. The nurse will seek to meet the immediate needs of the family from the facilities available within the ward and hospital. These will relate to a place to sleep, taking regular breaks and meals and understanding how the ward and hospital function. The nurse will be able to meet many of the immediate information needs as to nursing care and immediate medical investigation and treatment. The skills of the wider multidisciplinary team will need to be utilised to provide specialist information, in-depth family support and professional psychology support. Some liver specialist units have web information available for download for families.

Resource box

http://www.childliverdisease.org/
http://www.biliary-atresia.com/
http://www.wilsonsdisease.org/
http://www.kidshealth.org/

The child with chronic liver disease

The primary aims of management are to:

- Minimise or prevent progressive liver damage by treating the cause, if possible
- Anticipate, prevent or control the complications
- Predict outcome in order to offer liver transplantation at optimum time

Malnutrition and nutritional support

The liver has a central role in digestion and utilisation of absorbed nutrients. The key to nutritional therapy is a multidisciplinary approach including a paediatric dietitian, nurse specialist, feeding psychologist and the local clinician.

Pruritus

This is a distressing symptom caused by cholestasis or abnormal bile acid metabolism. It ranges from mild to severe and can affect daily living activities and disturb sleep. It may be an indication for liver transplantation in itself. The cause is unknown, but high levels of bile acids and other retained wastes normally excreted in bile may damage hepatocyte membranes, releasing agents that interact with nerve endings in the skin. Treatment is by trial and error and generally is unsatisfactory for the child and family. The management should be escalated gradually through local skin treatments to careful use of different drug groups, giving adequate time for proper evaluation and only changing one aspect at a time. An itch scale and diary should be kept by the child or the family. Skin care should include the liberal use of emollients and evening primrose oil in combination with avoidance of soap.

Portal hypertension

Portal hypertension is an increase in the portal venous pressure above 5–10 mmHg. It is caused by obstruction of blood flow through the portal system, hepatic sinusoids or the hepatic veins. The main result of portal hypertension is congestion of the splenic and mesenteric circulation, the development of collateral vessels and sequestration of blood in the gut and spleen that normally drains into the portal vein. Stasis of blood in the spleen causes hypersplenism and damage to blood cells, producing anaemia (rare), thrombocytopenia and neutropenia. Collaterals develop between the systemic and portal system. These are particularly evident around the stomach, the oesophagus and occasionally around the rectum. Around the oesophagus they are called oesophageal varices and may be a source of sudden haemorrhage.

The diagnosis is confirmed on clinical history, abdominal ultrasound and endoscopy. Nursing and medical management need to focus on priorities:

- Bleeding is the most severe complication and requires urgent volume resuscitation.
- Ball tamponade with a Sengstaken tube may be effective in the management of severe bleeding, but it can produce complications such as oesophageal necrosis and perforation.

Stop and think

Sengstaken tubes must be stored in the refrigerator and a manual sphygmomanometer must be available within the locality to allow inflation. Because of the risks of aspiration, ideally this procedure should be carried out in a paediatric (or adult) intensive care unit; however, if this is not possible the child must be intubated to protect the airway.

- Suppress hydrochloric acid production with medication such as omeprazole or ranitidine, gastric cytoprotection with sucralfate and use of vasoconstrictors given intravenously such as octreotide.
- Further advice for on-going management should be obtained from the regional liver centre.

Ascites

Ascites is the accumulation of free fluid in the peritoneal cavity. It is often associated with oedema, portal hypertension resulting from cirrhosis, severe congestive cardiac failure or other obstructive vascular conditions. It is nearly always a sign of advanced chronic disease. It may be associated with diseases that result in sodium and water retention such as nephrotic syndrome. In rare situations it may occur as a response to irritation of the peritoneum such as in a bile leak.

Nursing and medical management aims to control symptoms:

- Strictly record fluid input and output plus daily or twice daily weights.
- Take regular abdominal girth measurements over a marked point.
- Monitor physiological parameters, e.g. central venous pressure (CVP) to evaluate circulating blood volume (see Chapter 2), and observe for tachypnoea and increased oxygen requirement, tachycardia, peripheral vasoconstriction, decreased or absent urine output and high urine specific gravity. Circulatory and respiratory support may be required.
- Position child with elevated head of bed.
- Diuretics may be given intravenously first and then orally (intravenous frusemide and then oral spironolactone) with albumin infusions to improve oncotic pressure.
- Paracentesis (drainage of peritoneal fluid) may be performed for diagnostic reasons (culture for infection and analysis for cause).
- Limit fluid and salt intake.
- Monitor for signs of infection or sepsis (spontaneous bacterial peritonitis). In some cases broad-spectrum antibiotics may be given prophylactically.
- Transjugular intra-hepatic portal-systemic shunting (TIPS) can lower portal pressure and successfully treat ascites resistant to other treatments, but TIPS is invasive and may produce complications, including portal-systemic encephalopathy and worsening hepatocellular function.

Hepatic encephalopathy

This is a clinical condition in which there is altered/impaired neurological function secondary to liver failure. For further information see Chapter 6. Hepatic encephalopathy in children with chronic liver failure is often precipitated by gastrointestinal bleeding, large ingestion of protein, and excessive use of diuretics, sepsis or the administration of sedatives.

Specific management includes the reduction of ammonia levels by limiting the child's protein intake (between 1 and 2 mg/kg/day) and the administration of lactulose (1 mg/kg/dose) as many times a day as needed to produce a loose stool (this works by acidifying colonic contents, promoting ammonium ion excretion).

Coagulopathy

This is commonly found in the child with hepatic failure due to a combination of underproduction of clotting proteins (e.g. prothrombin) plus the failure of the liver to remove anti-thrombolytic proteins from the circulation. In the presence of portal hypertension, thrombocytopenia may contribute to the bleeding tendency as a result of hypersplenism.

The nurse is key to observing important clinical signs, e.g. petechiae, increased bleeding from puncture sites or from damaged mucosal membranes.

Nursing and medical priorities focus on restoring normal clotting mechanisms:

- Blood components such as fresh frozen plasma, platelets and cryoprecipitate may be given to reduce the bleeding tendency, particularly if an invasive procedure is needed.
- Administration may be avoided, particularly if decisions about listing for transplant are being considered, as coagulation trends are useful in this situation.
- Every effort must be made to prevent damage to mucosal surfaces.

Pulmonary complications

Chronic liver disease and cirrhosis have a number of potential pulmonary complications such as hepatopulmonary syndrome and pulmonary hypertension. Advice should be sought from the regional centre.

Bacterial infections

These are common in chronic liver disease and may precipitate other complications such as encephalopathy, ascites and hepatorenal failure. Prevention of pneumococcal, meningococcal and *Haemophilus influenzae* disease early in the disease process by vaccination is to be recommended as is vigorous nutritional support to maintain optimum physical condition.

Hepatocellular carcinoma

This is a rare complication of cirrhosis in the context of chronic liver disease. It is commonest in the setting of hepatitis B and tyrosinaemia type 1. It may only be found as an incidental finding at liver transplantation.

Transplantation

Paediatric liver transplantation has dramatically improved the outlook for children dying of end-stage liver failure. It is now well accepted therapy due to the improvements in survival that have occurred in the last 20 years. These improvements have been due to:

- Better pre-operative management of hepatic complications and nutritional support
- Innovative surgical techniques to expand the donor pool
- Improvements in post-operative immunosuppression

As a result the range of indications has expanded to include hepatic tumours and metabolic liver disease. A range of transplants involving the kidney and intestine are now available for children who meet the criteria.

Referral

Referral for transplantation should be made at an early stage to allow for a period of assessment and to allow sufficient time for finding an appropriate donor if listing goes ahead. In the child with chronic liver failure this should be ideally before the child develops signs of end-stage disease. In the child with acute liver failure this should be facilitated when coagulopathy is present (and not amenable to correction with vitamin K and other treatments) and before the development of encephalopathy which would make transfer difficult.

The transplant process involves pre-transplant evaluation, the liver transplant surgery itself, post-operative care and management, recovery and discharge, and life after transplant.

Glucose homeostasis

The primary source of energy for all cells in the body is glucose. Secondary sources of cellular energy include fats and protein. Two major hormones, insulin and glucagon, both of which are produced by the pancreas, are primarily responsible for the regulation and maintenance of blood glucose levels. Other hormones involved to a lesser extent in the maintenance of blood glucose levels and/or meeting cellular energy demands are adrenaline (epinephrine), growth hormone and cortisol (a glucocorticoid).

The role of insulin and glucagon in glucose regulation

Insulin and glucagon are counter-regulatory hormones that work in opposition to each other to maintain steady blood glucose levels. In normal healthy individuals, when one hormone is needed the other is usually not (see Figure 7.2). The relationships between insulin, glucagon and the nutrients they act upon is complex and beyond the remit of this chapter. It is important that practitioners understand the key actions of both and how the absence of one or the other may affect the child.

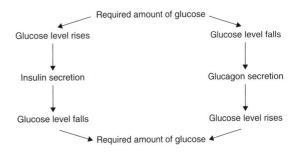

Figure 7.2 Glucose homeostasis.

Primary action of insulin
Insulin has an overall anabolic (the building of larger molecules from smaller ones, requiring energy, e.g. making fat from fatty acids and glycerol) effect in the body. The role of insulin in cellular uptake of glucose is to bind with a large receptor protein in the cell membrane (see Figure 7.3). It is the activated receptor, not the actual insulin, that causes the subsequent effects that promote the entry of glucose into the cell.

Additionally insulin exerts the following actions:

- It decreases the utilisation of fat as a source of energy.
- It inhibits the action of lipase (responsible for the release of stored fatty acids).
- It causes active transport of many amino acids into the cells.
- It has a direct effect on ribosomes by increasing the translation messenger RNA (ribonucleic acid), thus forming new proteins.
- It inhibits the catabolism (the breakdown of large complex molecules into smaller ones releasing energy) of proteins, thus decreasing the rate of amino acid release from the cells.

Primary action of glucagon
Glucagon has an overall catabolic effect and its purpose is to restore the serum glucose levels to normal. It achieves this in a number of ways, primarily through stimulating the production of

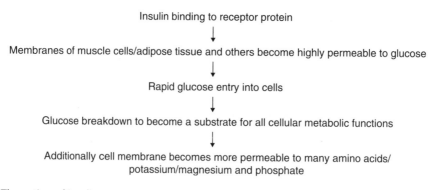

Figure 7.3 The action of insulin.

new glucose molecules from glycogen stores in the liver. This process is known as hepatic glycogenolysis. Glucagon also causes gluconeogenesis (the production of glucose from non-carbohydrate precursors) secondary to an increase in the breakdown (oxidation) of fats (lipolysis) into fatty acids and keto acids. In addition to being released in response to hypoglycaemia, glucagon release is stimulated by the neural impulse pathways associated with the stress response (Costanzo 2006; Levy *et al.* 2006).

The child with hypoglycaemia

The amount of glucose stored as hepatic glycogen varies according to age. In a healthy child glycogen stores are sufficient to maintain blood glucose levels for up to 8 hours of fasting. Infants due to their immaturity have limited stores lasting between 4 and 6 hours. Once glycogen stores are exhausted, the body becomes reliant upon gluconeogenesis to provide glucose sources for the cells (Curley and Moloney-Harmon 2001).

Primary isolated hypoglycaemia is an unusual presentation in the acutely unwell infant or child as hypoglycaemia tends to occur as a secondary consequence of systemic illness and exhaustion of glycogen stores in such children. There are a number of conditions/diseases in which hypoglycaemia which is not resolved through the usual measures may be a presenting

symptom, such as inborn errors of metabolism (e.g. carnitine deficiency, disorders of fatty acid metabolism, galactose intolerance, glycogen storage disorders), hypopituitarism and adrenal insufficiency.

Additionally a condition known as congenital hyperinsulinism in which there is an overproduction and inappropriate production of insulin (not related to actual blood glucose levels) by the β cells leads to episodes of hypoglycaemia in children suffering with the disorder. (Further information is available from http://www.hi-fund.org.)

Management
The consequences of hypoglycaemia are primarily found within the central nervous system – headache, altered level of consciousness and seizures are all complications associated with hypoglycaemia. The management of the child is related to the specific nature of any underlying disorder such as those identified above, but the general principles for the care of the acutely unwell child still apply (see Table 7.11).

The child with Diabetes Mellitus

Diabetes mellitus (DM) is a chronic and progressive disease whose prevalence is increasing in all age groups within the UK. It is estimated that over 2 million people are currently diagnosed with DM, 90% of whom have type 2 DM (non-insulin

Table 7.11 Management of the child with hypoglycaemia.

Assessment/intervention	Notes/considerations
Airway Ensure patent and protected If child is comatosed consider Guedel airway	If child has altered level of consciousness secondary to hypoglycaemia he/she may lose ability to maintain own airway
Breathing Assess respiratory effort	Reduced respiratory effort may occur as a consequence of reduced cerebral metabolic function
Circulation Assess circulatory status HR/BP/capillary refill time	Hypoglycaemia causes stimulation of the adrenergic receptors causing tachycardia and diaphoresis (cold clammy sweat)
Disability Assess using AVPU/GCSS (age appropriate)	Neurological consequences of hypoglycaemia can be severe, resulting in seizures
Glucose Monitor and record sequential blood glucose levels Administer dextrose as prescribed Evaluate effectiveness of therapy through frequent reassessment.	

dependent) while the remaining 10% have type 1 DM (insulin dependent). There are a number of sub-types of DM but it is broadly divided into the two types identified above. The incidence of type 1 DM is increasing amongst the under 5s, with 1 child in every 700–1000 developing the disease. This equates to approximately 25 000 children and adolescents living with type 1 DM in the UK (DH 2007).

There are an enormous number of discussion points relating to the care of children living with DM which are outside the remit of this book. The challenges faced by children vary according to their age and stage of cognitive development as with most chronic conditions. Further information and guidance regarding general care for these children may be found from the following:

Resource box

British Society for Paediatric Endocrinology and Diabetes (BSPED) (2004) Recommended DKA Guidelines, www.diabetes.org.uk/sharedpractice.

Department of Health and Department for Education and Skills (2004) National Service Framework for Children, Young People and Maternity Services.

Department of Health (2007) Making Every Young Person with Diabetes Matter: Report of the Children and Young People with Diabetes Working Group.

National Institute for Health and Clinical Excellence (NICE) (2004) Clinical Guidelines CG15: Diagnosis and Management of Type 1 Diabetes in Children, Young People and Adults.

Management of a child with Diabetic Ketoacidosis (DKA)

This section focuses on the care and management of the acutely unwell child presenting with diabetic ketoacidosis. The guidelines used within are those published by the BSPED (2004) which are recommended by the Department of Health. There may be some small local differences in policy and therefore it is important that practitioners are familiar with their individual clinical guidelines.

Diabetic ketoacidosis (DKA) is one of the commonest metabolic disorders seen in the paediatric

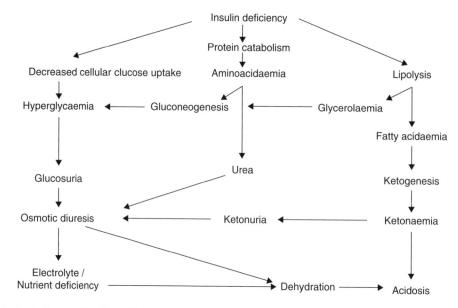

Figure 7.4 End effects of insulin deficiency in the body.

population. It has a mortality of 9% in paediatric patients and child deaths from DKA account for approximately 2% of all diabetic deaths. DM arises from inadequate insulin effects within the body, and in children almost always occurs as a result of inadequate amounts of insulin being available. The initial and key event in DKA is therefore insulin deficiency (see Figure 7.4); however, many of the physiological processes seen are mediated by increased levels of counter-regulatory hormones such as:

- Glucagon
- Adrenaline (epinephrine)
- Noradrenaline (nor-epinephrine)
- Growth hormone
- Cortisol

The clinical features of DKA occur as a consequence of:

- Hyperglycaemia
- Ketogenesis
- Hyperosmolality

- Dehydration
- Electrolyte imbalance

The management of the child with DKA is centred on the correction of these clinical features in combination with the early detection and/or prevention of possible complications. The clinical presentation of the child will vary slightly from individual to individual and those children with previously diagnosed DM may present earlier on in the DKA picture than those undiagnosed, due to their familiarity with the acute episode. A child presenting before diagnosis normally demonstrates the clinical signs/indicators shown in Table 7.12.

The guidelines discussed here are for the management of the child who has the following:

- Hyperglycaemia (BG >11 mmol/L)
- pH <7.3 on blood gas analysis
- Bicarbonate <15 mmol/L
- >5% dehydrated

The child may also be vomiting, drowsy and clinically acidotic, though these signs may be absent.

Table 7.12 The clinical signs/indicators of DKA.

Non-specific (high index of suspicion of DM with DKA)	Specific to DKA presentation
History of polydipsia/ polyuria Presence of acidotic breathing Drowsiness/altered level of consciousness Dehydration Abdominal pain/vomiting Weight loss	High blood glucose on dextro-stix testing Presence of ketones in the urine Marked metabolic acidosis with attempted compensation indicated by a significantly low PCO_2 (see Chapter 2, section on 'Blood gas analysis')

Management priorities can be divided into two sections: initial management on presentation to the Emergency Department (ED) (see Table 7.13) and then the ongoing management of the child in the HDU. Not all children presenting with DKA will require HDU care, but they do merit very close observation which may only be possible when provided by a designated HDU area with appropriate staffing levels. There are also a small but significant number of children for whom admission to a paediatric intensive care unit (PICU) is necessary straight from initial presentation in the ED. As recommended by the BSPED (2004) children within this group include:

- Those with severe acidosis with a pH <7.1 and marked hyperventilation
- Very young children (under the age of 2)

Table 7.13 Initial management of the child with DKA.

Assessment/intervention	Notes/considerations
Airway Ensure patent and protected If child is comatosed consider Guedel airway and nasogastric tube insertion	Intubation and ventilation are rare in children with DKA unless there is concern about the presence of cerebral oedema and raised intracranial pressure
Breathing Assess respiratory effort	Children with DKA present with Kussmaul respirations (deep, laboured and rapid respiratory pattern), a compensatory mechanism in which the body attempts to reduce its acid load by excreting excessive amounts of CO_2
Give 15 litres O_2 via face mask	Although the child is normally well oxygenated with good saturations, the underlying pathophysiology of DKA is an acidosis and inadequate tissue perfusion, resulting in a relative tissue hypoxia
Circulation Monitor ECG (observe for elevated T waves) Assess circulatory status HR/BP/capillary refill time Insert two peripheral IV cannulae Take bloods for FBC, U+Es and formal glucose Monitor arterial blood gas level If the child is clinically shocked give 10 mL/kg 0.9% saline as a bolus Repeat as necessary up to 30 mL/kg (×3 volume boluses)	Elevated T waves are indicative of hyperkalaemia and if present the child should not receive potassium replacement in maintenance/replacement fluids at this point A complication of DKA is the development of cerebral oedema, the rationale for which is not clear BSPED guidelines (2004) recommend slow rehydration to reduce the risk of developing cerebral oedema In children with DKA therefore the volume bolus is 10 mL/kg not the usual 20 mL/kg and it is practice to include the fluid boluses given when calculating the child's fluid requirements

From British Society of Paediatric Endocrinology and Diabetes (2004) Recommended DKA Guidelines V (2004).

- Those with significantly decreased levels of consciousness
- Those suffering severe dehydration with shock

Fluids

Individual fluid prescriptions will be decided by the medical staff responsible for the child's care according to initial serum glucose levels and electrolyte values elicited from formal laboratory results. The values gained from a blood gas machine are fairly reliable but should always be checked against the formal results. A typical fluid strategy is available in the BSPED (2004) guidelines; however, the most important consideration for nursing staff is ensuring that the child receives the correct volume of fluid over the correct period of time, again to reduce the risk of the child developing cerebral oedema. The child will need two fluid infusions, one to replace fluid deficit and a second to provide maintenance fluids.

Replacement fluids are calculated based upon the degree of dehydration present and are normally prescribed to run over a 48-hour period. It is the practitioner's responsibility to ascertain the required period of time and ensure it is clearly prescribed to effect good communication. If you are uncertain recheck with the member of medical staff responsible for the prescription and the senior nurse.

Maintenance fluids (if following BSPED guidelines) are prescribed at different volumes to those normally encountered and are based on age rather than weight *per se*. Maintenance fluid requirements for the child with DKA are as follows:

0–2 years	80 mL/kg/24 hours
3–5 years	70 mL/kg/24 hours
6–9 years	60 mL/kg/24 hours
10–14 years	50 mL/kg/24 hours
>15 years	30 mL/kg/24 hours

The total fluids required by the child will therefore be:

48-hour maintenance + deficit − resuscitation fluid (boluses) given

To calculate the hourly infusion rate, divide the total by 48.

Caution must be taken with rehydration in certain groups of children and may be undertaken over 72 hours rather than the usual 48 hours:

- Young children (under 2 years of age)
- Children with very high serum sodium levels
- Children with very high initial blood glucose

Insulin infusion

Children with DKA will require intravenous insulin to restore control of serum glucose levels and reverse the consequences of inadequate insulin availability.

> **Stop and think**
>
> Never switch an insulin infusion off while dextrose is being infused because the insulin is required to switch off ketone production.

The usual insulin used for continuous infusion is a human-soluble insulin preparation (Actrapid is the commonest brand name in use) which has a very short half-life of about 5 minutes and an effect that disappears within 30 minutes of therapy stopping (British National Formulary for Children (BNFC) 2007). It is common practice to make up a standard solution of 50 U of Actrapid in 50 mL 0.9% saline which equates to 1 U insulin/mL. Insulin infusions normally commence at 0.1 U/kg/h which is 0.1 mL/kg/h and guidelines suggest the following steps to manage the child's infusion rate.

Suggested steps to manage insulin infusions in DKA

- Run at 0.1 U/kg/h.
- Once serum glucose is down to 12 mmol and fluids have changed to those containing dextrose, reduce the infusion to 0.05 U/kg/h.
- If serum glucose falls below 7 mmol add extra dextrose to the replacement fluid.

• If serum glucose falls by >5 mmol/h reduce insulin infusion to 0.05 U/kg/h.

Electrolyte replacement

As with the fluids it is the responsibility of the medical staff to prescribe appropriate electrolyte replacements as required by the child based on actual blood values. Potassium replacement is nearly always required by children with DKA because they tend to have lost a lot of potassium with the ongoing diuresis. Potassium is the main intracellular ion, but as insulin is required to facilitate the movement of potassium into the body's cells, in its absence potassium remains in the extracellular fluid spaces where it can be easily excreted by the renal system.

Raised serum potassium on initial presentation is not an uncommon finding in a child with DKA, but once an insulin infusion is started potassium moves rapidly back into the cells and serum levels will fall quickly. Most children will therefore be prescribed maintenance and replacement fluids containing potassium. There are two notable exceptions to this rule:

• Children who are anuric (if anuric they will be unable to regulate their potassium levels through the renal system to meet their body's needs)
• Children who have elevated T waves on their ECG (elevated T waves are indicative of high serum potassium levels which could trigger cardiac dysrhythmias)

Neurological observations

One of the complications of DKA is the development of cerebral oedema and consequently raised intracranial pressure. The exact mechanisms that trigger the development of cerebral oedema in some children but not in others have not been identified and are subject to ongoing discussion. Changes to fluid resuscitation and ongoing fluid management strategies have been made to address concerns; however, cerebral oedema is still seen in children with DKA and is a significant cause of morbidity (25%) when present (BSPED 2004).

It is essential therefore that practitioners are alert to this possibility and carry out thorough and frequent neurological assessment as part of their care. The use of the Glasgow Coma Scale Score (GCSS) or the Modified GCSS for children aged 4 and under is advocated and the use of this tool is discussed in more detail in Chapter 6.

Ongoing general cares

In addition to the specific areas highlighted, other general cares are required by the child and family as follows:

• Continued ECG/sat monitoring
• Strict fluid balance
• Replacement of fluid losses as prescribed
• Regular urinalysis
• Hourly blood glucose monitoring
• Regular formal bloods – common practice is 2 hours after commencing therapies and 4 hourly as a minimum thereafter
• Care of venous and arterial accesses (see Chapter 2, section on 'Blood pressure monitoring' for further information)
• Comfort cares such as oral hygiene and eye care

Psychological care for child and family

For any child (and family) the need for admission into hospital is a distressing time. Regardless of whether the child has been previously diagnosed with DM or not, contact should be established with the diabetes clinical nurse specialist as soon as possible. The majority of preparation for discharge home will probably not occur in the HDU, but the child (depending on his or her age) and parents/care-givers will need full explanation of the illness and treatment, which may need to be reinforced on a number of occasions. This communication starts from the minute the child presents to the ED and will need to include clear explanations of:

• Blood glucose monitoring
• Insulin administration

- Management of hypo-/hyperglycaemia
- Impact of diagnosis on child and family

Complications of DKA

As noted above, one of the major complications associated with DKA is the development of cerebral oedema. Other complications such as cardiac dysrhythmias, hypoglycaemia and hypokalaemia are largely preventable with careful monitoring and management of the child and infusions. Good communication between the nursing and medical staff is therefore essential and advice and support from senior staff should be sought whenever there are uncertainties or concerns about the child's condition or his/her response to therapies.

Chapter 8

RENAL

Kathryn Summers and Debra Teasdale

Introduction

This chapter will provide nursing staff who are confronted with a child in acute renal failure (ARF) with sufficient theory and practical support to facilitate safe and effective nursing care. The development and function of the kidneys is presented, selected renal conditions are reviewed and predisposing clinical situations that may induce ARF in children are considered.

The kidney

Embryological and fetal development
The development of the mature kidney occurs in three distinct stages during fetal life, with the origins of the blood supply progressively changing (see Table 8.1).

The function of the kidney

These relatively small organs produce urine to allow the excretion of waste but have a multitude of other functions, including promoting the production of erythrocytes, maintaining blood pressure, acid–base buffering capacity, maintaining appropriate blood volume and promoting blood electrolyte homeostasis (Lote 2000). Effective function relies on complex interactions between hormones, other body systems and renal processes.

The secretion of erythropoetin by the kidney stimulates bone marrow to produce erythrocytes.

In times of acute blood loss this secretion and stimulation increases as part of the compensatory mechanisms. The role of the kidney includes responses to deal with long-term deviations in blood pressure (BP). Concurrent physiological responses are seen as the hypothalamus monitors the BP and stimulates the pituitary gland to either increase or decrease secretion of anti-diuretic hormone (ADH). In the kidney, the specialist area known as the juxtaglomerular apparatus (JGA), which is located at the junction of the afferent vessels, efferent vessels, distal convoluted tubule and glomerular capsule, also monitors BP. ADH alters the permeability of the tubules, increasing or decreasing water reabsorption into the bloodstream (see water reabsorption below). The JGA responds by initiating a cascade of events across body systems known as the rennin-angiotensin cycle. The combined result is either a reduction in circulating fluid and vascular vasodilatation so BP is lowered, or an increase in circulating volume and vascular vasoconstriction so BP increases (Mader 2007).

The management of fluids and electrolyte within the kidney is crucial for survival. The key processes involved are summarised below – use Figure 8.1 to identify the different anatomical features.

Simple filtration
Blood delivered into the glomeruli undergoes non-selective filtration (i.e. it is not modified according to body requirements) within the

Table 8.1 Summary of embryological development of the kidneys.

Focus	Timing	Function
Stage 1 Pronephroi	Appear ~21 days	Located in cervical region Non-functioning, main structures degenerate by day 25 but ducts remain to be utilised by mesonephroi
Stage 2 Mesonephroi	Appear ~28 days	Elongated structures that utilise duct remnants; they contain primitive tubules and glomeruli. Blood is delivered to these structures and urine is produced. Act as functioning interim kidneys Degeneration occurs at 10 weeks' gestation, but some tubules and ducts remain **In the male:** Tubules → efferent ductules of the testes Ducts → epididimus, ductus deferens, ejaculatory duct **In the female:** Ducts mostly disappear Tubules retained near uterus and broad ligament
Stage 3 Metanephroi	Starts development early in 5th week	These originate from two embryonic sources which develop in partnership to form the functioning definitive kidneys: • Metanephric diverticulum → ureter, renal pelvis, calices, collecting tubules • Metanephric blastema → creates the nephrons, the basic functional unit of the kidney (the glomerular apparatus – a capsule that surrounds the glomeruli – a knot of blood capillaries, tubules and collecting duct) As the nephrons continue to grow during fetal life the tubules continue to elongate, forming the proximal tubule, the loop of Henle (LOH) and the distal tubule. In week 10 the ends of distal tubules connect and join to form the collecting tubule or duct. The metanephroi produces urine from week 11–13 onwards
Ongoing internal development	By week 15 10–32 weeks	Medulla and cortex visible as two distinct regions; both areas fully formed by 36/40 Glomerular apparatus, proximal and distal tubules are found within the cortex Collecting ducts + LOH grow down into the medulla. Length increases after birth which increases kidney size Numbers of nephrons increase during fetal life until birth. when full complement in place Postnatally glomeruli also increase in size, so rates of excretion increase progressively
Location		The location of each set of kidneys alters primarily due to the rapid growth of the tail section of the embryo which gives the impression of the kidneys migrating upwards during fetal life. Alongside this ascent, the kidneys undergo a 90° rotation to face the midline
Blood supply		External structures alter; ureters increase in length to provide the route to the bladder for urine storage, and the origin of the blood supply shifts The first source is the common iliac artery, but as the embryo grows, flow is derived from new branches off the aorta. Ultimately all previous blood supply routes degenerate as the renal arteries become the key supply route. Once blood is delivered into the kidney the renal arteries progressively subdivide, delivering blood into the glomerular capsule via the afferent arteriole (where simple filtration takes place) Blood flows away from the glomeruli via the efferent arterioles which become the peritubular capillaries surrounding the tubules in the cortex – (so allowing selective reabsorption, tubular secretion). Ultimately the peritubular capillaries drain into the renal vein and blood flows away from the kidney. All these vessels have thin semi-permeable walls to allow movement of solutes and electrolytes to and from the blood and nephron

Adapted from Lote (2000), Moore and Persaud (2003), Chalmley *et al.* (2005), and Hockenberry *et al.* (2003).

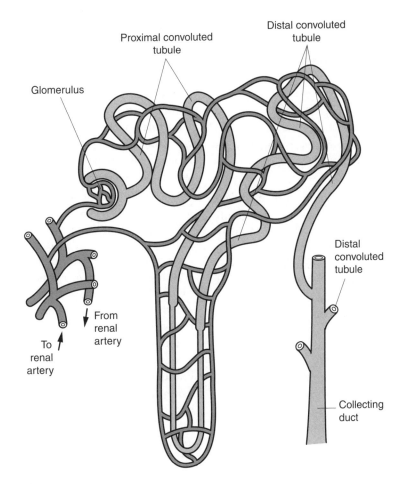

Figure 8.1 The nephron.

glomerular apparatus. This is due to the unique structure of the glomerular filtration surface, which is composed of three layers:

- The endothelial lining of the glomerular capillaries
- The glomerular basement membrane
- The epithelial cells of the Bowman's capsule

The layers fuse together and act as a barrier to the filtration of large molecular weight molecules such as proteins. In addition, the glomerular basement membrane emits a negative charge, which prevents molecules such as albumin from crossing into the filtrate (Lote 2000). As a consequence only molecules of a certain size pass through into the tubule (water, minerals, amino acids, glucose, hormones, creatine, urea, toxins and some drugs) to create the glomerular filtrate. Normally leucocytes, RBC, platelets and plasma proteins are too large and remain in the blood so their presence in the glomerular filtrate and subsequently the urine is suggestive of renal dysfunction or pathology. Three forces control simple filtration: the hydrostatic pressure in glomerulus (+ve pressure pushing components across the membrane), the osmotic pressure in blood (−ve pressure holding molecules in

Table 8.2 Glomerular filtration rates.

Age	Rate mL/min/1.73 m²
25 weeks' gestation	2
28 weeks' gestation	10
Term	20
Adult	80

Adapted from Kenner and Lott (2003) and Merenstein and Gardner (2003).

the blood) and the hydrostatic pressure inside the capsule. The rate of filtration across the glomerular apparatus is known as the glomerular filtration rate (GFR), which increases with age (Table 8.2) and in turn increases urinary output. However, variations in blood pressure, renal vascular resistance and renal blood flow can significantly impact the efficiency of the process.

Selective reabsorption

According to the body's needs, molecules leave the proximal convoluted tubules and return to the blood. This process can be facilitated by simple passive diffusion (i.e. substances that move from a high to a low concentration, e.g. sodium and chloride) or it may require active transport mechanisms which require energy to allow molecules to move back into the blood (amino acids, glucose, sodium, calcium, potassium, phosphate). The amounts selectively reabsorbed back into the bloodstream are influenced by hormones, e.g. aldosterone, parathormone and calcitonin.

Tubular secretion

Since the time within the glomerular apparatus is short, tubular secretion allows substances that failed to move across from blood during simple filtration to be removed. It occurs in the distal convoluted tubule (DCT), where blood vessels are in close proximity. Molecules move from blood to DCT via active transport mechanisms. It is particularly important for hydrogen ion excretion (so is important in acid–base balance) and for ammonia, creatinine and drug excretions.

Water reabsorption

The major sites of water reabsorption from the nephron into the bloodstream are the proximal convoluting tubule and the descending loop of Henle (120 mL water into kidney, 119 mL reabsorbed in adult); however, secondary sites are available in the ascending loop of Henle and the collecting ducts. Generally, the larger the loop of Henle the greater capacity to reabsorb water. Water reabsorption is controlled in two ways. Within the PCT and descending loop of Henle, the movement of sodium molecules is influenced by aldosterone and exerts an osmotic pull on water molecules, drawing them back into the blood. In the ascending loop of Henle and collecting duct, water reabsorption is controlled by ADH. This alters membrane permeability, so when levels of ADH increase more water is returned to the blood, and when levels of ADH fall more water is retained in the tubule.

Excretion

The collecting ducts progressively join to become a single ureter within each kidney which then delivers urine to the bladder for storage until micturition occurs. Urine is a sterile body fluid but can become contaminated by bacterial invasion through the urethra. Normally the act of micturition cleanses the urethra and prevents bacterial overgrowth.

Key differences in renal function in the infant and child

- At birth the change from a relatively hypoxic environment to an environment rich in oxygen causes erythrocyte production to be switched off in the newborn – erythropoietin, the enzyme that stimulates production of erythrocytes in the bone marrow, is only secreted when levels fall significantly. Infants under 3 months of age who suffer from a significant blood loss are less able to mount a physiological response to increase erythrocyte concentration to within normal limits.

- At birth the immature kidneys are less efficient. The loop of Henle is short in the newborn, so limiting the ability to reabsorb sodium and water. In consequence sodium disturbances are common, which is exacerbated as there is a concurrent inability to excrete water at sufficient rates. This increases the risk of oedema, which can be made worse when receiving infusions of normal saline.
- Conversely in situations where sodium losses are increased, e.g. vomiting or diarrhoea, the kidney will not be able to reabsorb sufficient sodium to redress the losses.
- Infants who become significantly hypoxic or who experience hypoperfusion of the kidney may suffer acute renal tubular necrosis, and in addition experience an associated surge of ADH. This exacerbates fluid overload, which can be seen as the infant becomes progressively more oedematous. Where the oncotic pressure is low due to low levels of plasma protein this increases the risk.
- Infants commonly produce very dilute urine so easily become dehydrated; however, tubular growth continues into the cortex, so by 3 months of age concentration ability is equal to that of the adult.
- Infants do not tolerate high glucose loads well. Glycosuria can quickly lead to dehydration.
- When the infant experiences renal disturbances, an output of <1 mL/h is cause for concern since the solute load is likely to be high and causes obstruction at the neck of the bladder, preventing efficient micturition. Catheterisation should be considered.
- In the infant, the synthesis and excretion of urea is also poor; however, rapid growth during the first few months of life means the burden is minimised since large amounts of nitrogen and electrolytes are retained to support growth. However, the production of urea from the breakdown of nitrogen contributes to the efficiency of the concentration mechanism – so low levels of urea contribute to the poor ability to concentrate the urine.
- Low rates of hydrogen ion excretion and low levels of plasma buffering agents in the first year contribute to the quick escalation of blood gas disturbances where metabolic acidosis is common.
- Urinary stasis due to shock, dysfunctional voiding, incomplete emptying or anatomical abnormalities allows bacterial multiplication. Antibiotics alter commensals, allowing increased ease of colonisation of the urethra. Extrinsic factors such as tight clothing, poor hygiene, the use of essential oils in baths, hot tubs and whirlpools, and increased sexual activity within adolescent all contribute to the increased risk of urinary tract infections (UTI), which ultimately may transcend the bladder and infect and scar the kidney. In the neonatal period males are most at risk of UTI. This trend is reversed in females who are 10 times more likely to have UTI between 2 and 6 years.

Compiled from Hockenberry (2003), Kenner and Lott (2003), Merenstein and Gardner (2003), and Chamley *et al.* (2005).

Acute renal failure (ARF)

ARF is a common medical condition which can affect between 5 and 7% of all hospitalised children (Singri *et al.* 2003). The integrity of the kidney depends upon adequate perfusion of the glomeruli producing glomerular filtrate, which is modified during its passage along the nephrons by the tubular cells and excreted by the drainage system consisting of ureters, bladder and urethra (Pocock and Richards 2006). ARF may occur due to disruption of any of these functions.

In some children there is obvious inadequate renal perfusion, and prompt replacement of blood volume or an increase in the cardiac function can restore renal function to normal. In other children there is obstruction to the urinary tract, which, once relieved, is similarly associated with a return to normal. In the majority of children, however, the syndrome consists of an initiating event which causes disruption of normal tubular activity and subsequent death of the tubular cells. The renal failure that ensues usually lasts 10–20 days, followed by a recovery phase and a return to normal function (Rees *et al.* 2007). This syndrome may be precipitated by numerous factors and can occur at any age. It presents the children's nurse with a challenging diagnostic and therapeutic problem, but as the majority of those who recover return to normal renal function, it is always worthy of treatment. The complexity of the illness in many children requires a multidisciplinary team approach for both investigation and management, particularly with high dependency nursing care.

Definition

ARF can be defined as a rapid and severe decline in the function of both kidneys, which results in a buildup of nitrogenous waste products, leading to uraemia over days or weeks. This is frequently associated with an identifiable precipitating cause.

Oliguria is usually present, where:

Urine output <1 mL/kg/hour in a neonate
Urine output <0.5 mL/kg/hour in a child.

Polyuria can also occur, where:

Urine output >600 mL/day in an infant
Urine output >1100 mL/day in a child
Urine output >1500 mL/day in adolescents.

There is an associated steady increase in plasma urea and creatinine. The child is unable to regulate fluid, electrolyte and acid–base balance. The condition is potentially reversible (Hockenberry *et al.* 2003; Glasper *et al.* 2007; Rees *et al.* 2007).

Top tip

When assessing urine output volumes, consideration must be given to the effects of any medication that the child is currently receiving, e.g. diuretic therapy.

The majority of children have preceding normal renal function, but increasingly it is recognised that acute or chronic renal failure can occur due to some superimposed insult in a child who has already-damaged kidneys. In the majority of children, it is usually reversible or self limiting. The renal damage is initiated by a primary insult which leads to disruption of normal tubular cell function. This is followed by a phase of established renal failure, and then recovery of structure and function and a return to normality.

Causes

ARF may be divided into three major categories in which each category has a physiological location of the insult:

- Pre-renal refers to ineffective perfusion of the kidneys which are structurally normal.
- Intra-renal is where there is damage to the renal parenchyma, sometimes secondary to pre-renal problems.
- Post-renal is where there is disordered urinary drainage of both kidneys or of a single functioning kidney (Metheny 2000).

Pre-renal ARF

This refers to the ineffective perfusion of the kidney (see below), resulting in the retention of excessive amounts of nitrogenous compounds in the blood. No actual parenchymal damage occurs and it can be reversed on correction of the underlying cause. Renal hypoperfusion causes intense vasoconstriction, which results in the initial decrease in GFR but with protection of the tubular function. If adequate perfusion is not restored rapidly, pre-renal uraemia may progress to intrinsic renal failure. It may be possible to prevent this stage if renal perfusion can be adequately restored before structural damage occurs.

Causes of decreased blood supply
- Hypotension
- Diminished cardiac output
- Inappropriate vascular volume (septicaemia, endotoxin and anaphylactic shock)
- Hypovolaemia
- Haemorrhage
- Gastrointestinal loss (diarrhoea, vomiting, aspiration)
- Loss to extravascular space (burns, severe nephritic syndrome)
- Urinary loss (diabetes insipidus, excessive diuretic therapy)
- Vascular disease
- Arterial thrombosis

Clinical features
- Glomerular filtration decreased
- Urine output decreased
- Urine sodium <10 mmol/L (<20 mmol/L in neonates)
- Urine osmolarity >500 mOsm/kg (>400 in neonates) suggests pre-renal failure
- Blood pressure decreased
- Central venous pressure (CVP) decreased
- Dehydration as evidenced by drowsiness, confusion, weakness, dry mucous membranes, loss of skin turgor, thirst

Top tip

Urinalysis and urine electrolytes are extremely helpful in distinguishing pre-renal from intra-renal causes of ARF. The urinalysis is a mirror of the structural integrity of the renal tubules, and the urine electrolytes reflect the functional ability of the renal tubules.

Urinary sodium <10 mmol is indicative of pre-renal cause, while urinary sodium >40 mmol

would suggest an intra-renal cause (Marshall 2002). However, urinary sodium concentration and osmolarity can be misleading, especially for those children taking diuretics or receiving dopamine, as both increase urinary sodium.

The importance of early recognition and treatment of pre-renal failure prevents the condition progressing to renal failure and a degree of parenchymal damage.

Intra-renal ARF
Intra-renal ARF is referred to as parenchymal/intrinsic or intra-renal failure and is associated with structural damage to the glomeruli/vessels and renal tubules. Generally the GFR falls due to hypoperfusion of the glomerular apparatus as a result of afferent arteriole vasoconstriction. Failure of the GFR to recover is common and is generally attributed to obstruction of the tubular lumen by debris and casts, interstitial oedema or release of intra-renal vaso-constrictive substances (Marshall 2002). Here the episode of ARF may run a lengthy duration and can often lead to chronic renal failure.

The clinical cause of intrinsic renal failure is often complex and, depending upon underlying disorders, the recovery may be prolonged for up to 6 weeks. Table 8.3 highlights the wide variety of causes of intrinsic renal failure, which may involve multi-system disease or originate from a primary renal disorder.

Post-renal ARF
Post-renal refers to the obstruction of urine drainage, either above or below the bladder, causing an increase in hydrostatic pressure in the kidneys. If this is prolonged, it can lead to secondary tubular damage.

Clinical features include:

- Loin pain
- Alternating oliguria, polyuria or complete anuria

Table 8.3 Causes of intra-renal failure.

Location	Common cause
Glomerular nephritis:	Acute post-streptococcal Systemic lupus erythematosus Haemolytic uraemic syndrome Good pasture's syndrome
Vascular	Renal artery stenosis Vasculitis Haemolytic uraemic syndrome
Tubular	Acute tubular necrosis Drug/toxic injury
Interstitial	Drug-induced Interstitial nephritis

Adapted from Armitage and Thompson (2003) and Singri *et al.* (2003).

Causes of post-renal ARF include:

- Obstruction of solitary kidney
- Bilateral ureteric obstruction
- Urethral obstruction, i.e. clot
- Posterior urethral valves
- Neuropathic bladder.

Adapted from Glasper *et al.* (2007).

Signs and symptoms

The signs and symptoms of ARF are outlined in Table 8.4. Children who have had ARF for a short period of time may not present with any symptoms, as there may not have been sufficient biochemical and fluid imbalance to cause any physiological effects.

Stop and think

It is important to interpret biochemical changes and fluid balance alongside considering the child's underlying condition – the significance of this increases with the newly admitted child.

Investigation to establish the diagnosis

Table 8.5 provides vital information to assist in diagnosis.

Prevention and management

Management of children with ARF requires a multidisciplinary approach. ARF is a complex disease process. Children's nurses are usually the first to observe deterioration in a child's condition and initiate further medical assessment of the child. On admission, it is important to assess the child's condition quickly with observations of:

- Blood pressure
- Pulse
- Respirations
- Central and peripheral gap
- Weight
- Jugular venous pressure
- Oedema

Key nursing points

Fluid resuscitation

For the child who is hypovolaemic or in septic shock, the prime objective is to re-establish normal haemodynamics in an effort to restore renal perfusion. However, fluid replacement should be guided by an assessment of the child's medical condition, in particular his or her cardiac status and circulating volume. Careful fluid replacement in the form of crystalloid (e.g. intravenous saline) or colloid (e.g. human albumin) may be given without delay not only to prevent shock but also to maintain and expand plasma volume and to improve renal blood flow. Careful fluid replacement must incorporate close monitoring of the child. Careful measurement of blood pressure, pulse, respirations and core-peripheral temperature gap plus accurate fluid balance are important in monitoring fluid status and jugular venous pressure (JVP). See Table 8.6 for additional information.

Direct measurement of central venous pressure (CVP)

If a central line is present this will help manage fluid replacement. The CVP will be low in

Table 8.4 Signs and symptoms of ARF.

Symptoms	Signs
Decreased urine output Weight gain	Anuria or oliguria (NB: Children's urine output = 1–3 mL/kg/hour). However, care must be taken as the quality of urine is clearly more important than the quantity Raised urea and creatinine – serum creatinine gives the most reliable indication of renal function as the blood urea will be more affected by such factors as protein intake and increased protein catabolism as a result of infection Peripheral or systemic oedema
Uraemic symptoms of: Nausea and vomiting – caused by accumulation of toxins Pruritis – caused by high phosphate level or uraemia Pericarditis Altered immunity	Weight loss Poor diet intake Dry, flaky skin
Thirst/dry mouth Breathlessness Fever Ankle swelling	Raised blood pressure may indicate fluid overload leading to pulmonary and peripheral oedema Lowered blood pressure may indicate dehydration or sepsis Abnormal, irregular pulse may indicate cardiac arrhythmias Increased respirations may indicate metabolic acidosis Raised temperature is a sign of infection
Confusion Twitching Irritability Convulsions	Depressed level of consciousness or seizures Electrolyte imbalance

Table 8.5 Diagnostic tests and investigations for ARF.

Test	Abnormality	Possible cause
Blood: urea and electrolytes	Raised creatinine level above normal levels of 70–120 mmol/L Reduced sodium below normal levels of 135–145 mmol/L Raised urea above normal levels of 2.5–6.4 mmol/L Raised potassium above normal levels of 3.5–8.5 mmol/L	All causes of ARF
Blood: complete blood count and coagulation studies	Raised white cell count >1% of total leucocytes Platelet consumption Red cell damage	Acute interstitial nephritis, haemolytic uraemic syndrome
Urinalysis and microscopy	Haematuria Proteinuria White cell casts Specific gravity ~1.010	Rapidly progressive glomerulonephritis Acute pyelonephritis Pre-renal insult Acute tubular necrosis
Renal ultrasound scanning Chest X-ray Renal biopsy	Identifies size of kidneys Pulmonary oedema Abnormality in renal tissue	Intra-renal or post-renal obstruction Fluid overload Intra-renal cause

Table 8.6 Assessment and management of hydration.

Hydration status	Clinical features	Initial management
Dehydration	Tachycardia Cool hands, feet and nose Core – peripheral temperature gap >2°C Prolonged capillary refill time Low BP (late sign) Dry mucous membranes Sunken eyes	Fluid resuscitation 10–20 mL/kg normal saline IV over 30 minutes Assess urine output and repeat if necessary
Euvolaemic		Fluid challenge 10–20 mL/kg normal saline over 1 hour, with furosemide 2–4 mg/kg IV
Intravascular overload	Tachycardia Gallop rhythm Raised JVP and BP Palpable liver	Furosemide 2–4 mg/kg IV dialysis if no response NB: must observe for urine output post administration of furosemide

Adapted from Rees *et al.* (2007).

volume depletion (normal CVP right atrium = 0–5 mmHg); with careful fluid replacement the aim would be to elevate this (refer to Chapter 2 for further information regarding CVP measurement). Further boluses of crystalloid and/or furosemide should be given as indicated by hydration and urine output. Ongoing management after initial fluid resuscitation should be as follows:

- Replace insensible losses (400 mL/m² /day or 30 mL/kg/day) plus urine output and other ongoing fluid losses. This can be given as feed if tolerated or IV normal saline (half normal if hypernatraemia).
- Replace 100% of urine output if euvolaemic.
- Restrict to 50–75% urine output if intravascularly overloaded to allow a negative fluid balance (Rees *et al.* 2007).

Inotropic agents

Dopamine and dobutamine increase renal blood flow and are sometimes prescribed at a renal dose to increase renal perfusion and urine output. It is important to monitor that the child's vital signs remain within the appropriate range for his or her age; normal skin colour, turgor and temperature; a relaxed body posture and behaviour; and a cardiac rhythm and rate that is consistent with the child's fluid and electrolyte status.

Hourly measurement of fluid input and output

Nursing staff should ensure that fluid balance charts are recorded accurately for children with ARF and those at risk of ARF. It is critical to record urine output accurately as it can be used to assess deterioration or improvement in renal function. Weigh twice daily or more frequently as condition dictates.

Stop and think

Nurses caring for children must ensure that fluid balance is reviewed regularly and be aware of trends towards either a positive or a negative balance.

Appropriate urine output is between 1 and 3 mL/kg/hour.

The Critical Care Outreach Report (DH 2003) recommends that diligent skilled monitoring of children's physiological vital signs, with timely and appropriate response to abnormalities, is fundamental to the pre-emptive care of children with established or potential critical illness.

Physiological observation

Toe–core temperature, pulse, respirations, blood pressure and oxygen saturation should be carried out at hourly intervals. Carry out 6-hourly blood glucose monitoring as disease may affect blood sugar (e.g. haemolytic uraemia syndrome (HUS)). Metabolic waste accumulation in the blood can cause neurological changes in a child's condition such as confusion, agitation and seizures (Campbell 2003). Neurological assessment should be recorded on a paediatric neurological assessment tool, such as the modified Glasgow scale, hourly. Nurses can enlist the support of family members to monitor and report any deterioration in the child's neurological condition.

Infection control

Children with ARF tend to be immunosuppressed because of uraemia, and as a result are at greater risk of developing infections. Good hand hygiene techniques will help to minimise hospital-acquired infections (see Chapter 11).

Nutritional support

Children with ARF generally have metabolic acidosis because of an abnormal biochemistry and frequently experience malaise, nausea, loss of appetite and sometimes vomiting. ARF is a catabolic state and children can become nutritionally deficient at this time. Children's nurses must involve the dietician in the multidisciplinary approach in managing these children. If children are extremely unwell and cannot tolerate oral food or fluids, they may require parenteral or enteral nutrition. Table 8.7 provides additional information.

Personal care

Keeping the child's skin intact is an important aspect of nursing care. Caring for oedematous

Table 8.7 Nutrition guidelines for the child with ARF.

Boys and girls	Energy (EAR) (kcal/day)	Protein (RNI) (g/kg)
0–6 months	95–115	1.5–2.1
6–12 months	95	1.5–1.6
1–3 years	95	1.1
4–6 years	1460–1810	1.1
7–10 years	1680–2040	28
11–14 years	1845–2220	42
15–18 years	2110–2755	Boys: 55 Girls: 45

Modified from Rees *et al.* (2007).

EAR, estimated average requirement.
RNI, reference nutrient intake, i.e. amount of protein needed for maintenance and growth.

skin is essential to prevent skin breakdown. The use of pressure-relieving mattresses is important for the immobile child. Providing regular mouth care can often help children to tolerate oral fluids. For those children who are on restricted fluid intake, mouth care can help to alleviate bad tastes, prevent dry oral mucosa and the development of oral infections.

Medications

The use of nephrotoxic drugs such as NSAIDS and amino-glycosides should be avoided in children at risk of renal impairment or in those with established ARF. Alternative medications need to be prescribed and administered if a child requires analgesia or antibiotic treatment during his or her stay. (If unsure seek the advice of a paediatric pharmacist.) See further information in the section on 'Drug prescribing'.

Treatment options

There are many options available to treat ARF and these are dependent on factors such as biochemical changes, fluid overload and symptoms of uraemia. The following treatment options provide a brief overview of current practices.

Table 8.8 Emergency management of hyperkalaemia.

Method of action to lower serum potassium (K⁺)	Treatment	Dose	Side effects
Reduce toxic effect of K⁺ by stabilising the myocardium	10% calcium gluconate IV	0.5–1 mL/kg over 5–10 minutes	Bradycardia, hypercalcaemia
Shift K⁺ into cells	Salbutamol nebuliser	2.5 mg if <25 kg or 5.0 mg if >25 kg maximum 2 hourly	Tachycardia
	Salbutamol IV	4 µg/kg over 10 minutes	Hypertension
	Sodium bicarbonate 8.4% IV	1–2 mmol (mL) kg over 10–30 minutes	Hypernatraemia reduces ionised calcium
	Glucose and insulin IV	0.5–1.0 g/kg/hour dextrose (2.5–5.0 mL/kg/hour 10% dextrose) and insulin 0.1–0.2 U/kg as a bolus or continuous infusion of 10% dextrose at 5 mL/kg/hour (0.5 g/kg/hour) with insulin 0.1 U/kg/hour	Hypoglycaemia (monitor blood glucose every 15 minutes during bolus, then at least hourly)
Remove K from the body	Calcium resonium orally or per rectum with oral lactulose	1 g/kg every 4 hour 2.5 mL if <1 year; 5 mL if 1–5 years; 10 mL if >5 years	Effect is slow Large doses can become impacted in the gut if given orally

Adapted from Rees *et al.* (2007).

Hyperkalaemia

This is a significant risk factor for children with ARF and prompt treatment needs to be initiated to protect the heart and lower the serum potassium concentration. Children in the early stages of ARF can be treated successful within the HDU setting with a variety of medications (see Table 8.8).

> ### Stop and think
>
> K > 6.5 mmol/L is an indication for emergency treatment until dialysis or urine output has been established.

Hypertension

This is usually due to fluid overload, although it is important to be sure that it is not due to intense vasoconstriction because of hypovolaemia. First Line treatment is furosemide. Failure to respond is an indication for dialysis, although it is usual to consider other first-line agents in addition (e.g. calcium channel blockers, and labetolol if severe hypertension with signs of encephalopathy), particularly since it usually takes several hours to establish emergency dialysis. If dialysis is adequate but hypertension persists, nifedipine is the first choice, with a starting dose of 250 µg/kg tds (three times daily). Maximum daily dose is 3 mg/kg/day. Referral to nephrologists should be made early on in the course of the disease; transfer may only be necessary to a paediatric renal unit if the child's condition deteriorates and dialysis treatment is required. Renal replacement therapy will be necessary if the child has any of the complications listed in the following section.

Indications for renal replacement therapy

- Persistent hyperkalaemia plus other treatment options that have not been successful in lowering the potassium or when the level of potassium in the blood is life threatening

- Severe metabolic acidosis, hypo- or hyperna-traemia
- Volume overload and pulmonary oedema which has not responded to diuretic therapy
- Severe uraemic symptoms – urea >40 mmol/L (>30 mmol/L in neonate)
- Pericarditis
- Encephalopathy.

Modified from Riegel (2003).

Renal dialysis

Options are peritoneal dialysis, haemodialysis or haemofiltration. Most children requiring intensive care are managed with continuous renal replacement therapy.

Haemodialysis

This is a method of removing excess water and solute from the blood in order to maintain a stable environment for cell function. Blood is pumped out of the child from suitable vascular access into the haemodialysis machine. It passes through a haemodialyser (the artificial kidney), where solutes and water are removed, before the blood is returned to the child. This cycle repeats continuously until enough blood is processed to ensure adequate dialysis.

The haemodialyser is composed of a semipermeable membrane enclosed with a casing. It is split into two compartments, the blood compartment and the dialysis solution compartment, which are separated by the membrane. Blood flows on one side of the membrane and the dialysis solution flows in the opposite direction on the other. The process of ultrafiltration causes fluid removal with diffusion effecting solute removal. Ultrafiltration is defined as the movement of fluid through a membrane by a pressure gradient (Van Stone and Duagirdas 1994). In haemodialysis, this pressure gradient is achieved by differences in hydrostatic pressure on each side of the membrane. A positive pressure in the blood compartment will push water across the membrane and a negative pressure in the dialysis compartment will pull water across. The machine manipulates the total pressure on the membrane to actively control fluid loss.

Diffusion is defined as the movement of solute from an area of high solute concentration to an area of low concentration (Pocock and Richards 2006). The dialysate contains physiological levels of solutes (sodium, potassium, magnesium, calcium chloride, glucose, bicarbonate) but has no urea or creatinine. So, e.g. urea will move from the blood (the higher concentration) across the membrane and into the dialysate (the lower concentration), therefore lowering the child's serum urea level (Wright 2004).

Haemodialysis is the preferred option if vascular access is needed for plasma exchange. If the urea is very high, a short session (2 hour) with mannitol will be necessary. Thereafter daily dialysis is likely to be needed until the biochemistry improves, when it can be weaned accordingly.

Paediatric peritoneal dialysis

The construction of the visceral and peritoneal layers of the peritoneal membrane, the blood supply to and the lymphatic drainage from each of these layers are functionally the same as adults. The major difference between the peritoneal membrane of the child and the adult is its size. The difference in size is one of the principal reasons that peritoneal dialysis is the preferred route of treatment for children. It is generally accepted that the peritoneal membrane of a child is functionally different from that of an adult and that normal growth and development results in alterations to the transport characteristics of the peritoneal membrane (Alexander *et al.* 1999).

The success of peritoneal dialysis (PD) in children depends greatly on the technique of catheter placement and the level of expertise of the surgeon. The catheters available for acute dialysis include the Trocath® paediatric catheter with stylet, Cook® paediatric catheter and

Tenckhoff® paediatric single-cuff straight and curled catheters. Although the choice of a temporary catheter depends largely on the paediatric nephrologists, the most commonly used is the Trocath® which has been renowned for its excellent flow characteristics and fewer complications (Debeukelaer *et al.* 1999).

The temporary catheter can be placed quickly and easily by the paediatric nephrologists under local anaesthetic, although sedation is often used. This eliminates the risks and delays associated with an anaesthetic and a surgical procedure. The common disadvantage of the percutaneous catheter is poor function due to the omentum enveloping and blocking the catheter (Alexander 1996). The catheter size is determined by the size of the child.

The dialysis prescription

In the acute situation where the child requires dialysis as soon as the catheter is inserted, flush the catheter until the effluent is clear of blood and debris. Use continuous 24-hour cycling, initially with 20–30 minutes cycles (10 minutes fill, 10 minutes dwell, 10 min drain), then varying according to response. Dialysis is initiated with very small volumes; it is usual to start with 1.36% dialysate 10 mL/kg fill volumes/exchange, but this can be increased if fluid removal is inadequate. The volumes of exchange are increased gradually to a maximum of 40 mL/kg exchange. The exchange is only increased when dialysate leak has been excluded. During the immediate post-operative period it is very important to keep the child quiet and comfortable, because crying and moving around can increase the intra-abdominal pressure, increasing the risk of leakage around the exit site.

Continuous renal replacement therapy (CRRT)

CRRT is a technique used in the PICU for the management of ARF. In the commonest type, blood is pumped from a vein, through the filter and back to a vein (continuous veno-venous haemofiltration (CVVH), but an artery to a vein can also be used (CAVH). Solute movement is principally by convective flow, so high filtration rates are needed. Ultrafiltration is the process whereby water is moved across the membrane by the convective flow of water down a pressure gradient, which is created by degenerating a transmembrane pressure within the dialyser (either negative to the dialysate or positive to the blood compartment). Large molecular weight molecules are removed better by convection than diffusion. A counter-current circuit can be used to haemodialyse too, thereby adding in diffusive solute clearance. The ultrafiltrate (UF) contains electrolytes in a concentration similar to that of plasma, so the larger the UF volume the greater the clearance. The UF is returned as replacement fluid, which is designed to correct abnormal biochemistry. The proportion of the UF that is replaced is adjusted in order to achieve or maintain euvolaemia. Slow continuous UF can be used to remove fluid (UF) in smaller quantities such that replacement is not required.

Advantages

- It is best for children with cardiovascular instability as it allows slow fluid removal so that major fluid shifts do not occur.
- Episodes of hypotension are less likely to occur with HD, decreasing the risk of further ischaemic insult if the kidneys are recovering.
- Therapeutic drug levels are more easily maintained than with HD.

Disadvantages

- Clearance is less than for HD, but can be increased by maximising blood, UF and/or dialysate flow rate, depending on type of CRRT.
- Potassium and phosphate losses may be excessive but can be replaced in the replacement fluid or IV

(Gregory *et al.* 2004, pp. 567–585).

Survival and renal recovery depends on the cause of ARF. Long-term follow-up is necessary, with the exception of children with pre-renal ARF, in order to detect the development of proteinuria, hypertension and chronic renal failure.

Nephrotic syndrome

Nephrotic syndrome is a triad of clinical features caused by abnormal, excessive loss of protein in the urine:

- Hypoproteinaemia
- Massive proteinuria
- Oedema

There are four subgroups of nephrotic syndrome which are all different in treatment, prognosis and presentation. This section concentrates on the commonest type – idiopathic or minimal change nephrotic syndrome.

Idiopathic nephrotic syndrome

As the name suggests there is no known cause, but this represents about 90% of all cases of nephrotic syndrome in children, although it can sometimes be related to a viral illness some weeks earlier which suggests that an immunological factor may be involved. It occurs more commonly in boys (2:1) and the commonest age of onset is 1–8 years old. A familial incidence is sometimes seen, but it is not hereditary (Bell 2002).

Signs and symptoms
- Oedema of dependent parts is the most common presenting factor. In babies up to 1 year it is most evident around the eyes with peri-orbital oedema. In toddlers and older children the oedema is found in the legs or scrotum and labia
- Urine – frothy with musty smell
- Lethargy and irritability
- Pallor
- Diarrhoea and vomiting
- Anorexia

Pathophysiology

In a healthy child the amount of protein lost in the urine is negligible. This is due to the unique structure and function of the glomerular filtration surface, which acts as a barrier to the filtration of large molecular weight molecules such as proteins (Lote 2000). In minimal change nephrotic syndrome there is a disturbance in the functioning of the glomerular basement membrane, which makes it increasingly permeable to plasma proteins and allows them to pass freely into the urine. This process is still not fully understood (Broyer et al. 1998). The resulting heavy proteinuria is the cause of all the presenting signs and symptoms listed above.

The proteinuria is in excess of 2 g/day, where the normal is 150–300 mg/day. It is a nonselective proteinuria, but it is mostly albumin as this is the smallest in molecular weight and size and can pass through the malfunctioning glomerulus most easily. The lack of plasma proteins leads to a reduced plasma oncotic pressure and this allows the plasma water to leak from the capillary vessels into the surrounding tissues, giving rise to the oedema of nephrotic syndrome.

As the water is lost from the circulation the intravascular volume is reduced and the blood pressure falls. Pressure receptors inside the kidney note this decrease in pressure and respond by secreting rennin which sets off a cascade of events, which result in increased blood pressure in order to maintain renal perfusion and increased sodium and water reabsorption from the distal tubule in the kidney, so increasing the circulating volume. The associated aldosterone release also stimulates the thirst response and the child drinks more. All these manoeuvres are ineffective as the original defect causing protein loss is still occurring. The resultant low plasma pressures in the blood cause the extra salt and water saved by the kidney or drunk by the child to leak out into the tissues – worsening the oedema.

Oedema settles in different places according to the age of the child. Water finds its own level and for a baby who spends most of its time lying down the oedema is predominantly periorbital. The skin around the baby's eyes is thin and loose and therefore has room for expansion. More mobile children have oedema around the feet and ankles. The oedema will reach legs, scrotum/labia, sacrum and eyes if it increases. All the internal tissues are oedematous, e.g. in the gut and bowel, giving rise to diarrhoea and vomiting.

Hyperlipidaemia is raised levels of circulating fat. It occurs because the liver is trying to respond to the lack of protein in the blood by increasing the protein synthesis to make up the deficit. The enzyme lipase which is responsible for limiting the lipid levels is only present in small quantities. The complete metabolic pathway of lipase is not yet certain but the presence of protein in the urine makes it frothy and smelly.

Diagnosis

- Confirm heavy proteinuria 3 or 4 +s
- Clinical examination
- Microscopic haematuria not macroscopic
- Low blood albumin
- High cholesterol and triglycerides
- Low calcium as 50% calcium bound to albumin
- C3 level is normal
- A renal biopsy is only carried out if the child is less than 3 months or older than 8 years at presentation or is resistant to steroid therapy

Nursing management of the fluid balance, hypovolaemia and blood pressure

The priority upon admitting a child with nephrotic syndrome is to assess the child's fluid status (see the ARF section above). The low plasma albumin can cause hypovolaemia. As nephrotic children are oedematous, fluid status is more difficult to assess. Skin turgor is less helpful, weight merely reflects the level of oedema and the oedema often masks the low Jugular Venous Pressure (JVP).

On recording the blood pressure, the oedema must be taken into account when choosing the appropriate cuff. Core-peripheral temperature gap in association with blood pressure are the most reliable indicators of fluid state. If a child has normal blood pressure for his or her age and a temperature gap of less than 2°C, the child is not hypovolaemic. Urinary sodium <10 mmol/L is an indicator of hypovolaemia; however, this investigation is only useful in the absence of furosemide.

Children often complain of abdominal pain when hypovolaemic. Severe, prolonged hypovolaemia can result in clotting of major blood vessels, so must be regarded as an emergency. If normal saline is given as in conventional treatment of hypovolaemia, the saline will quickly leak out of the circulation to become oedema. The circulation will therefore not be increased.

In severe hypovolaemia the child should be rehydrated with 4.5% plasma albumin which temporarily replaces both albumin and fluid in the circulation (10–20 mL/kg of 4.5% albumin). If hypovolaemia is less severe, 20% plasma albumin should be given slowly over at least 4 hours, with furosemide 1–2 mg/kg being given IV during the second half of the infusion. The dose is 1 g protein/kg body weight (up to 5 mL/kg 20% albumin) (Rees *et al.* 2007). This delivers concentrated albumin into the circulation, temporarily increasing the plasma albumin; this increases the oncotic pressure in the circulation, resulting in oedema fluid returning from the tissues to circulation.

Specifics for plasma infusion

There are a number of reports of intravascular volume overload with the development of pulmonary oedema associated with such therapy.

- The dose of albumin should not exceed 1 g/kg.
- The minimum infusion time is 4 hours to avoid this occurring.
- Strict monitoring of vital signs should take place.

- The infusion should be given during the day shift whenever possible as more staff are available.
- Record blood pressure and pulse respiratory rate quarter to half hourly, even if the child appears well and stable.
- If the child shows signs of fluid overload, commence oxygen saturations monitoring, suspend the infusion immediately and prepare intravenous furosemide as this may be required.

> **Top tip**
>
> It is important to nurse nephrotic children in the sitting position during plasma infusions to minimise the risk of pulmonary oedema.

Children with only mild peripheral oedema do not require fluid restriction, though where significant oedema is present, mild fluid restriction (70% of maintenance requirements) will help prevent further oedema formation. A low salt diet will control thirst. Where this measure alone is unsuccessful, the subsequent addition of diuretics (furosemide and spironolactone) will help resolve oedema.

It must be stressed that the child with overt nephrotic syndrome who is being fluid restricted with or without additional diuretic therapy should be kept under very close review to ensure that hypovolaemia (intravascular volume depletion) is avoided. The oedematous nephrotic child is at significant risk of hypovolaemia. This increases the risk of pre-renal failure, thrombosis and other complications. The child should undergo regular clinical assessment of peripheral temperature and capillary refill time, BP, pulse and weight during the presenting illness.

BP may be temporarily elevated in the acute phase, particularly if there is an element of hypovolaemia (low urinary sodium is a good objective clue to this): persistent hypertension is an unusual feature of minimal change disease and should prompt discussion with a nephrologist as alternative diagnoses should be considered.

Diet
A no added salt diet is a sensible measure in view of generalised oedema (salt and water overload) and the use of steroids.

Mobility
There is no evidence to support bed rest, which may increase the risk of venous thrombosis.

Infection
Children are at risk of bacterial infection because of urinary losses of immunoglobulins and complement proteins. Prophylactic penicillin V 12.5 mg/kg bd (against *Streptococcus pneumoniae*) should be given whilst oedematous and there should be a low threshold for investigating for, and adequately treating, infection should this be suspected.

Steroids
Administer prednisolone 60 mg/m^2 (maximum dose 80 mg) once daily for 28 days, followed by 40 mg/m^2 (maximum dose 60 mg) given on alternate days for a further 28 days (Rees *et al.* 2007). A response to steroid therapy is indicated by the resolution of proteinuria, urinary remission being defined as three consecutive days of zero or trace protein on Albustix®. Conversely those who fail to respond to steroid treatment require a renal biopsy to obtain a histological diagnosis to guide further therapy and have a poorer long-term prognosis.

Family information
Family members need to be taught urinalysis to allow home urine testing and the early detection of relapses prior to the development of oedema. Verbal information should be supported by written information on nephrotic syndrome. The prognosis for idiopathic minimal change nephrotic syndrome is good. If the disease presents classically and responds to treatment then it will follow a pattern of relapse and remission, with the gaps between gradually lengthening.

Haemolytic uraemic syndrome

The most common cause of ARF is haemolytic uraemia syndrome (HUS) (Taylor *et al.* 2004). At the height of the summer the regional paediatric renal centres may have up to six children at any one time. The most common form of HUS is typically preceded by *Escherichia coli* (type 0157 or VTEC) gastroenteritis with several days of bloody diarrhoea. Often members of the same family will have the same diarrhoeal illness which does not progress to renal failure, though it is uncommon for siblings to present with HUS together.

Signs and symptoms

Children presenting with HUS will typically have the following signs and symptoms:

- They will be pale and anaemic.
- They will have experienced recent weight loss from several days of diarrhoea.
- They will be irritable and lethargic.
- They may be either dehydrated from the diarrhoeal illness or fluid overloaded as a result of oliguria or anuria, depending on the stage of illness.
- Any urine is usually blood stained.
- Blood chemistry will reveal renal failure, raised creatinine uraemia and deranged electrolytes.
- Haematology will show low haemoglobin, fragmented cells and a low platelet count.
- Low platelet count impairs clotting.

Investigations

- FBC, blood film
- Chemistry including renal and liver function
- Clotting screen
- Group and save blood
- Urine dip stick for blood and protein
- Urine for M, C and S
- Urine albumin to creatinine ratio
- Verotoxin
- Stool microscopy and culture.

Treatment

The main treatment for HUS is early diagnosis and supportive care. The following are of major importance:

- Blood transfusion is indicated if Hb <6 or if 7 g/dL but symptomatic (e.g. shortness of breath, shock). It may worsen hyperkalaemia and volume overload. Platelet transfusion is rarely indicated unless invasive surgery is planned, or there is intracranial haemorrhage
- Dialysis
- Dietary/ total parenteral nutrition
- Fluid balance
- Electrolyte monitoring
(Siegler *et al.* 2005).

See the section above on specific nursing care of children with ARF for further details.

> **Stop and think**
>
> It is generally accepted that antibiotics are not part of the routine management of diarrhoea positive HUS. Some suggest that antibiotics may make HUS worse, although this remains controversial (Rees *et al.* 2007).

The most severe cases of HUS may require plasma exchange. Most children given good nursing and medical care will make a rapid recovery. Usually the first sign of recovery is the child looking better, then the haematology improves and finally the renal function recovers. Typically this takes 2–3 weeks.

Drug prescribing in renal failure

Basic principles

Varying degrees of renal failure will result in reduced clearance of drugs and their metabolites which are excreted primarily by the kidney.

Great care needs to be taken when prescribing in renal failure. Details of necessary dose adjustments are available in the British National Formulary for Children. Where uncertainty exists, consultation with an expert paediatric renal pharmacist should take place. Wherever possible, drug levels should be measured in renal failure.

Antibiotics and other anti-infective agents

Gentamicin and other amino glycerides (tobramycin and amikacin) need to be used with great care in renal failure as they are significantly nephrotoxic. Pre- and post-dose levels must be monitored. The risk of nephrotoxicity is increased by the presence of volume depletion, pre-existing renal impairment, hypokalaemia, hypomagnesaemia, and the concomitant administration of other nephrotoxic drugs such as diuretics etc. The penicillins and third generation cephalosporins require dose reduction in severe renal failure.

Family support

A variety of written and online information is available in a number of languages. Most units have family support workers, counsellors and specialist support nurses.

Chapter 9

CHILDREN WHO NEED MANAGEMENT OF PAIN AND SEDATION

Doreen Crawford and Sarah Roberts

Introduction

This chapter focuses on the needs of infants, children and adolescents who need management of their pain and who may be sedated. British nurses are reminded of the need to practise within the code of professional conduct (NMC 2008) and adhere to both local frameworks and the standards for medicines administration (NMC 2007), although it must be stated that these standards are generic and not paediatric specific. The care of infants and children needs to be holistic; they may be patients in hospital for the duration of their illness or they may have shared care packages involving community specialists and come into hospital for varying periods, for specific interventions or during crisis points in their lives. They may have intricate treatment protocols or infusions of complex pharmacology running as part of their care requirements but they are first and foremost children and require all the extra, special, psycho-social considerations for these age groups.

The neurophysiological framework by which infants and children feel pain will be considered; this may be anatomically similar to adults, but the interpretation and the meaning of the event are unique to the child. There are many definitions of pain. An acceptance that pain is what the person says it is (McCaffrey 1980) is a useful definition for the children's nurse when dealing with communicative children as it makes allowance for the fact that the pain experience need not be proportional to the degree of observable injury or disease to cause distress. This definition has limitations with younger less expressive individuals and infants; however, there are also the more biological definitions and there is increasing understanding of how pain is processed. Pain as a perceptive experience differs between children and adolescents and there are further difficulties in managing the pain of the preverbal and questionably cognitive patient.

Perhaps pain, distress and discomfort should always be assumed in the neonatal unit (NNU), high dependency unit (HDU) and children's intensive care unit (ITU) patient unless indicated otherwise. Certainly until evidenced otherwise, it might be safer to assume that any admission to a strange, noisy environment such as the NNU/HDU/CICU is likely to amplify the pain and distress experience. This said, severe, unremitting and unbearable pain in a highly dependent child is *not* exclusive to these areas and can affect these children in a variety of areas and at home.

Pain can be regarded as a special sensory sense. It could be regarded as a normal function and a normal reaction to wholly abnormal circumstances. Pain has a role in body protection, maintenance and defence. Response and reaction to pain has to be learned and there are socio-cultural factors which can influence this. Unfortunately pain is not a sophisticated sense and in health care its deployment can often be counter productive to the comfort and wellbeing of the individual. Pain can impede recovery. At its most primitive, the response to pain is reflexive; finer interpretation of the stimuli, its localisation and identification requires the functioning of a remarkable and imperfectly understood structure – the human nervous system.

Development of the nervous system

Potentially the most complex system, development of the nervous system is summarised in Table 9.1.

The biology behind the nervous system

The human nervous system is amazing and is responsible for the individual's ability to react with the environment as well as respond to internal triggers. It is a network of complex structures which can receive, emit and transmit electrochemical signals between tissues, organs and systems. The human nervous system functions as a unified whole but for convenience is divided into the central nervous system (CNS) and peripheral nervous system (PNS).

Table 9.1 Embryological and fetal development of the central nervous system and spinal cord.

Gestational age	Tissue and structure development
Embryonic period Gastrulation days 15–17	Gastrulation is the term used for the trilaminar period. The formation of the primitive streak is one of the signs of gastrulation. Cells along this streak migrate towards the interior (ingression) which results in the formation of three layers, the endoderm, mesoderm and ectoderm A thickening of the ectoderm forms the neural plate
Neurulation days 18–26	A cluster of cells central to the neural plate become columnar, giving the appearance of a groove and linear crests, rather like guttering. These crests progressively fold towards each other and, when the edges come into contact with each other, they fuse to form the neural tube. This eventually becomes the brain and the spinal cord Complete closure of the neural tube takes about 4–6 days. During the early part of the neurulation stage the neural tube is fused except for a small posterior neuropore and a larger anterior neuropore. The anterior neuropore will eventually subdivide into three vesicles representing the forebrain, midbrain and hindbrain. The anterior neuropore closes by day 24. The posterior neuropore is closed by day 26 Ectodermal cells from the margins of the neural tube detach to form dorsal clusters of cells called neural crest cells. These migrate peripherally to become sensory ganglia cranial and spinal nerves and so on
Early brain development weeks 4–6	The complex nature and shape of the human brain is determined during embryogenesis by flexures that result from bursts of rapid cell proliferation within the confines of the cranial vault During the three vesicle stage, representing the forebrain (prosencephalon) midbrain (mesencephalon) and hindbrain (rhombencephalon) the three part brain resembles a 'C' shape By week 5 the forebrain gives rise to the paired telencephalic vesicles which will eventually become the cerebral hemispheres and the diencephalon from which develop the optic vesicles. The midbrain remains tubular and undivided. The rhombencephalon (hindbrain) subdivides into the metencephalon and a more caudal myelencephalon By week 6, the cellular growth in a restricted area has resulted in the formation of the cephalic flexure, the pontine flexure and the cervical flexure. The metencephalon will form the pons and the myelencephalon will eventually form the medulla oblongata By week 5 and 6 all the cranial nerves are recognisable in the embryo except the optic and the olfactory

(Continued)

Table 9.1 Continued.

Gestational age	Tissue and structure development
Week 8	A period of rapid differentiation and neuroblast multiplication of the brain and spinal cord. By week 8 a cross section of the cord would reveal the characteristic butterfly shape of grey matter. Primitive spinal reflex arc is present The lateral walls of the spinal cord thicken, leaving a longitudinal groove which extends the full length of the spinal cord and into the midbrain. The divided grey matter forms dorsal and ventral plates. These plates signal the location of sensory and motor neurones and will eventually result in the sophisticated network of afferent and efferent neurones which will receive, transmit and respond to stimuli The ventricular system is established early from the division of the telencephalon
Weeks 12–20	Rapid vascularisation occurs The ventricles are well-defined C-shaped structures. A rich capillary network develops on the roof of the midbrain and hindbrain and this will become the choroid plexus which will secrete the cerebral spinal fluid which will bathe the CNS Rapid growth in restricted space forces the developing cerebral hemispheres to shroud and cover the midbrain. Initially the cerebral cortex is smooth Neurones start to myelinate. After week 18 neurones no longer divide. Surface area landmarks of the brain are increasingly identifiable. Neurones for nociception are located in dorsal root ganglion
Weeks 21–24	The density of cortical plate synapses increases Rapid growth of cerebral hemispheres causes convolution of the cortex and forms sulci and gyri, resulting in increased surface area A rapid increase in neurone cytoplasm gives rise to an increase in cell size
Borderline viability to term	As gestation progresses the cortical plate matures into the six layers of cerebral cortex. Pain experience elicits typical facial expression Rapid myelination occurs, and this will continue into the postnatal period

The CNS comprises the brain and spinal cord encased and protected by the skull and the spine. The PNS consists of nerve tissue outside the brain and spinal cord. These are nerve bodies/ganglia not entirely encased in the skull and spine and include the 12 pairs of cranial nerves and the 31 pairs of spinal nerves. Some of the cranial nerves are highly specialised and critical to the function of the 'senses' of taste, sight, hearing and smell. The PNS is differentiated into afferent and efferent pathways.

Neural transduction and transmission is complex, but to explain this simply it means that ascending nerves carry information impulses to the brain and descending nerves carry information and impulses from the brain to muscle tissue and glands and so effect the nervous systems' response. Affecters and effecters are specialist neurones and readers are advised to refer to an anatomy and physiology text such as those listed in the 'References, further reading and resources' section to further enhance their understanding.

Figure 9.1 shows the divisions of the nervous system. Complementary to the CNS and PNS is the autonomic nervous system (ANS) which is also subdivided into sections; the nerves of the sympathetic and parasympathetic have a primary role in regulating the individual's internal homeostasis.

The diagram depicts the ANS and the division into the sympathetic and parasympathetic

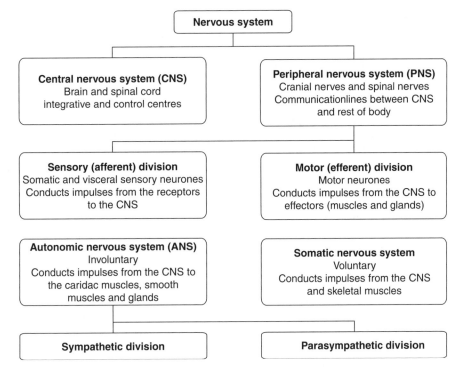

Figure 9.1 The divisions of the nervous system.

nervous system. The ANS exerts control mainly by involuntary action which in health does not impact on the conscious awareness of the individual. Although it is possible, with training in some circumstances, for the individual to exert control using biofeedback techniques, this will be considered in greater detail below and can be utilised to complement other therapies.

Components of the nervous system

The nervous system comprises two basic types of cell – the neurones and the supporting cells such as the neuroglia cells. Neurones vary in size from micrometers to meters and their shape and complexity differs with function and location. Generally speaking the neurones do not have direct access to good capillary networks and receive nutrients such as glucose more indirectly.

Neurone axons may be covered in a fatty sheath which acts as an insulator. Gaps in this covering allow for the flowing of ions at these intermittent junctions rather than along its full length. This is thought to increase velocity.

The covering of the axons takes place according to a developmental timetable and can be incomplete at birth. The interpretation of this knowledge lead to some 'experts' postulating that infants could not feel pain as their nervous system was immature. It is now accepted that the absence of a myelin sheath does not impede the transmission of stimuli which will then be perceived and experienced as pain. Fetuses and preterm infants from 24 weeks' gestation have a perfectly functional nociceptor system (Wolf 1999; Lee *et al.* 2005).

Neurones are categorised according to the number of branches they have. Unipolar have one process, bipolar two and multipolar several. Generally sensory neurones transmitting information to the CNS are unipolar and motor neurones transmitting information away from the CNS are multipolar.

Developmental aspects of the CNS

Neurones in the CNS do not regenerate. More neurones than are required are initially formed and some continue to divide following birth, with clear implications for early oxygenation and nutrition. If these neurones are not used and become part of a functional system they will die and this has possible implications for neonatal and infant experiences. Axons have limited capacity to repair, but successful function, following injury, depends on the type of injury and location of the lesion; the formation of scar tissue, which is an end product of repair, could impede transmission function. The olfactory neurones in the nose are unique in that they continue to divide and replace themselves throughout life.

How nervous tissue works

Neurones are not passive; they generate and respond to electro-chemical impulses by selectively changing the electrical charge over their membranes. All body cells are polarised, with the inside of the cell more negatively charged than the outside. This difference is due to the composition of the intracellular fluid compared to the composition of the extracellular fluid. There is more potassium inside the cells than outside and more sodium outside the cells; this difference is maintained by active transport on the surface of the cell membrane. Understanding this at its most basic level means that when this status of equilibrium is disturbed above a threshold, the neurone depolarises the signal transmitted along the axon. Most sensory nerve fibres are unimodal in that they respond to one type of stimuli, e.g. sound waves or light intensity. The afferent nerve fibres of the PNS are different in several respects;

they are polymodal and have the ability to trigger to the stimuli of mechanical, chemical or thermal reception. Once this information is transported to the CNS at the level of the spinal cord it means a variety of stimuli can be responded to and there is some ability to discern between the degrees of intensity. They do this as they have complex multi-transduction channels that can distinguish between different forms of stimulation and between intensities (McCance and Huether 2006).

Refer to a diagram of the cross section of the spine. Δ (delta) and C fibres are regarded as first order neurones. The transmission of stimuli from these fibres can be transmitted up the spinothalamic tract for interpretation by the third order and higher order neurones in the cerebral cortex, reticular and limbic areas of the brain. It is a little like a hierarchy of people passing on important messages to the management team. Understanding the essentials of this puts into perspective the value of the gate theory of pain first proposed by Melzack and Wall in 1965.

Once neurones have fired there is then a period of readjustment called the refractory period during which the neurone cannot fire. In some cases such as following an inflammatory response, cells can be regarded as hypopolarised and be more excitable than normal, as it takes less to trigger a signal. This state of hyperalgesia would have direct implications for the transmission of signals which went on to be perceived as pain and for the management of pain, as this state can prove to be very resistant to treatment.

Refer to a diagram of a synapse. Neurones do not physically connect, although they exist in close proximity. The gaps are called synapses, with impulses being transmitted across the gaps by electro-chemical messengers. Transmission occurs by chemical neurotransmitters, which are synthesised and stored by the neurones and released on instruction into the synaptic cleft. These chemicals pass over the synapse to reach a post-synaptic membrane and, depending on the level of excitation, have the potential to transmit the signal onwards.

Neurotransmitters

New substances that function as neurotransmitters continue to be identified; some are chains of amino acids, some are recognised as hormones and it is apparent that some have several roles which vary according to location. For example, norepinephrine can be both excitatory and inhibitory. Some have direct 'pain' implications, such as the neuropeptides, the endorphins and the enkephalins which are widely distributed throughout the CNS and the PNS. The increasing understanding of what happens in the synapse will potentially result in an increasing range of selective analgesics which will be capable of targeting and blocking the passage of stimuli. This will result in suppressing unwelcome sensations without impeding function; e.g. in a limb, pain will be removed, but the reception of other information such as the position and temperature of the limb remains available.

The importance of the biochemistry of the synapse is apparent every day in theatre and in ITU as this is the site of action that allows neuromuscular blockade; this permits a state of relaxation to allow intubation and ventilation, overcoming the normal body defence mechanism of cough and gag. Many of the children that the high dependency nurse cares for will have had experience of neuromuscular relaxation and the principles have implication for the understanding of the action of opioids, so, for the sake of completeness, this will be considered below briefly.

Chemically induced paralysis takes place at the neuromuscular junction which is the point where the motor neurones extending from the spinal cord make contact with the muscle fibres. Present, at that point, are the potential transmitters which if triggered will result in a muscle contraction. Neuromuscular blocking drugs target this action and prevent the transmission of electrical impulses in a number of ways. They can bind with the receptor sites of the neurotransmitters, so blocking the normal pathway, or they can compete with the neurotransmitters and bind with the site while not causing a muscle contraction.

Stop and think

It is important to remember while caring for an infant or child who has an infusion of muscle relaxant running is that these agents contain no analgesic or sedative properties. A child who is still and unresponsive may still be in pain and frightened.

As these children literally cannot move a muscle they can be considered trapped within themselves – they cannot communicate their fear and experiences to the outside.

Safety alert!

Before setting up, changing or increasing a muscle relaxant always check the respiratory support and the airway of the patient.

The biology of pain and sedation

The understanding of pain is as yet incomplete and ongoing research will continue to build on current knowledge. At present there is a consensus that there are two types of pain: fast and slow. The perception of fast pain occurs almost instantly and this is generally regarded as acute. It is precisely located, unique in character and identified by sudden sharp, pricking sensations. In contrast, slow pain is of later onset, perhaps a second or so after the initial stimulus. The unpleasant situation builds and escalates in intensity, becoming burning, aching and/or throbbing. It is less easy to localise and in some cases may be referred (Jenkins Kemitz and Tortora 2006, pp. 550–551). Relating the biology to the perception of pain is called nociception and depends on the intact functioning of the nervous system. The biology may be clearcut but the individual's experience of pain is less so. To counter pain experience and manage the clinical situation, pharmacological, cognitive strategies and holistic management can impede, mask or reduce the pain experience.

The stimulus of pain is transmitted in two pathways via a three neurone system to the cerebral hemisphere on the opposite side of brain from the pain location and by a two neurone system transmitting the stimulus to the cerebral hemisphere on the same side of the brain to the sensation (Waugh and Grant 2006, pp. 158–159). For pain to be experienced by the individual the following sequence has to take place:

- There has to be an event – a stimulus and a trigger strong enough to fire a receptor neurone. This stimulus will travel by neurone 1 to the spinal cord by the posterior route.
- Once in the spinal cord decussation takes place; this can be compared to a circuit with some messages being transported via one route and other messages by another. At this level it can be seen why some impulses generate a crude reflex withdrawal and others are conveyed for more precise interpretation.
- These impulses are transmitted via the anteriorolateral spinothalamic tract to the thalamus and neurone 3, where processing at the perceptual level can begin (Marieb 2004).

Pain processing

This section briefly considers the process from electrochemical transmitted stimulus to awareness and perception of pain. Neurone 3 conducts stimulus to the higher brain centres of the limbic system and the cerebral cortex. Areas of the cerebral cortex are representative of parts of the body and these areas are probably responsible for the interpretation of what we perceive as pain. In an instant this is matched up with previous experiences – the stored memories of pain. The pain stimulus is, in essence, made sense of and placed in context. There is also an understanding of what the individual's pain experience might mean to an outside observer, and further lightning-quick networking influences decision making about how the individual should react. This is conscious processing, it is complex and

for greater understanding the reader is advised to refer to text in anatomy and physiology. For children, there are fewer memories and less experience on which to draw, resulting in fewer learned clues on how to react. These factors account for the wide variety of pain responses and behaviours seen in children.

For the preterm and young infant there may be no previous experience and stored data on which to draw. There is significant debate as to the reception and perception of pain in the fetus (Fitzgerald 1995; Glover and Fisk 1996; Harrison 1996; James 1998; Lee *et al.* 2005). This debate could be extrapolated to include the extremely preterm infant (Slater *et al.* 2006). What can be accepted is that preterm and neonatal pain is physiologically disruptive and impacts on the physiological stability of the patient as it occurs at a time when the infant is developmentally unprepared for the stimulus. Exposure to stimulus, resulting in pain, may promote a heightened peripheral sensitivity or dampen down the normal expected behavioural responses to pain – indicative of altered development (Anand and Hall 2006). Neonatal nursing textbooks cover the topic extensively, but it is astounding that, in some textbooks of neonatal medicine, pain is not considered in the index. From a children's nurse perspective, an additional worry is the fact that children vary in their ability to develop the concept of time and infants have no concept of time; accordingly they do not have the ability to understand that the experience they are suffering is usually temporary and time limited. Infants do not yet understand that pain can come to an end and will not last for their eternity. Table 9.2 demonstrates the links between biology and practice.

Pain classifications

Nociceptive pain or non-nociceptive pain
The terms nociceptive (pronounced "no see cept ive") pain and non-nociceptive pain are an attempt to classify pain using biology as a basis and to

Table 9.2 Linking biology to the clinical interpretation of a child's pain.

Pain terminology	Definition
Pain threshold	The level at which the stimulus will exceed sensory tolerance and be perceived as pain. This seems not to vary much between individuals or in the same person if measured over time
Perceptual dominance	The phenomenon seeks to explain why an individual with several sites of pain focuses on the most extreme pain experience
Pain tolerance	The duration of time in which an individual will tolerate pain until prompted to seek relief. This varies considerably between individuals and within an individual over time
Radicular pain	The pain that arises from a major nerve and is felt along the distribution of the nerve
Referred pain	The pain perceived in an area removed from its point of origin. The point of origin is mainly visceral and is thought to occur as a result of the internal organs having so few sensory nerves
Incidence pain	Occurs when pain is provoked or intensified by movement or activity

create a taxonomy aimed at understanding the condition usually from a mechanical perspective.

Nociceptive pain originates from cell damage resulting in the release of inflammatory mediators; these bathe and sensitise the nociceptors which activate the pain cascade (Butcher 2004). Nociceptive pain can be superficial, from the skin, subcutaneous tissue or mucous membranes and can be characterised by well-localised sharp, pricking and throbbing experience (Butcher 2004) or may be somatic, from the deeper tissues such as muscle tendon and joints. This is less well localised and is characterised by aching, gnawing and constant pain. Visceral pain results from affected organs, causing sensations of deep, dull, dragging spasm or squeezing colicky pain and is frequently associated with vomiting and alterations in vital signs (Butcher 2004).

Non-nociceptive pain such as neuropathic pain can vary in nature and severity. This pain is often caused by oversensitisation of the nerves and is frequently associated with numbness or paraesthesia (Butcher 2004). The symptoms of which the patient complains reflect the nerve fibre affected. Burning and itching indicate that the C fibres are the causative nerves whereas colour and temperature changes are a result of activity of the B fibres (Butcher 2004).

Acute or chronic

Pain is further divided into chronic and acute pain in an attempt to define pain according to a time frame. Chronic pain is usually defined as 'pain which persists a month beyond the usual course of an acute disease or reasonable time for an injury to heal or is associated with a chronological pathological process which causes continuous pain – or pain which recurs at intervals for months or years'. Prolonged pain is disabling and can interfere with physical functioning (Shaw 2006).

From a clinical perspective there can be problems with all the information summarised above. Nurses seek to interpret what information is elicited from the assessment of an individual, but this is complicated when the child is cognitively impaired (Dowling 2004) or when dealing with a pre-verbal infant. Signs, symptoms and history of the event will assist, but the most effective pain assessment requires qualitative as well as quantitative analysis.

Signs and symptoms of pain

- Pain behaviour (may be socioculturally variable)
- Anxiety, vocal distress and facial expression
- Tachycardia – elevated heart rate/pulse above developmental norm
- Tachypnoea – elevated respiratory rate above developmental norm

- Fixed body posture and muscle tension
- Potential for alternation in blood gas
- Hypertension
- Diaphoresis – evidence of sweating, e.g. beads of perspiration on top lip
- Elevated temperature
- Elevated metabolic rate
- Hyperglycaemia
- Gastrointestinal disturbance

Because of the clinical complexity of pain, particularly chronic pain, the administration of an analgesic may not be sufficient to control the sensation or bring the experience into manageable proportions. In cases such as this there may be a requirement to use a joint approach with careful use of sedation.

Stop and think

Children in pain should rarely be sedated alone since this may mask signs of pain. You may need to challenge medical staff who have routinely adopted this strategy and insist on both pain relief and sedation.

Assessing a child's need for sedation

There are many validated tools for assessing an infant's or child's pain. There are fewer to assess the level of sedation (Bennett 2003). Sedation may be understood as a substance that works by producing a depression of the CNS; the greater the degree of depression the deeper the sedation. Sedation may be needed in HDU as well as in ITU as part of a strategy to prevent ITU syndrome (Baker 2004). Arguably the distress caused by childhood exposure to 'healthcare' can adversely affect an individual for the remainder of his or her life (Young 2000). There is some overlap between distress and pain and this has led to the development of joint sedation and pain tools such as the Nottingham score (Bennett 2003).

The distress of crying and the facial expression is one of the universal indicators of pain in infants and very young children and some pain tools have utilised these very effectively; e.g. the neonatal facial coding system (NFCS), initially developed by Grunau and Craig (1990), uses a range of facial expressions based on recognised responses to pain (the open mouth, lip stretch, taut tongue, eye squeeze and brow furrow). However, in some clinical conditions the facial expression is impaired. This is also the case if the child is effectively sedated and would complicate assessment if a muscle relaxant had been used. Extrapolating from this, facial expression is not always a reliable indicator of comfort in the care of HD children as facial expression could be absent. The appearance of a sleep state may give the possibly erroneous assumption of comfort. In these circumstances the multi-disciplinary team has little alternative but to focus on the physiological indications of pain and distress.

Sedation and analgesics are provided according to unit protocols and emerging clinical standards and the child should be continually monitored for any indication of breakthrough distress or pain. There is some evidence that there is scope for improvement in the way sedation is practised in children's hospitals (Babl *et al.* 2006). This has been recognised by DH, and NICE expect to have clinical guidelines for procedural sedation developed for use by 2010. Sedatives are powerful drugs and they can be an extremely useful mechanism for ensuring a child's co-operation. Sedatives are used in many areas of a hospital if a temporary quiet state is required for the duration of a procedure (Ruddle 2003).

However, the use of sedation is not without risk. It should be remembered that when these agents are employed children need continuous monitoring and supervision and should be regarded as HD children while under the effect of these drugs. Vital signs can be used to monitor physiological stability and may provide an indication of improvement or recovery. Continual monitoring can provide the nurse with information on the health status of the child, but a further less quantifiable indicator is developed through experience and involves a level of informed intuition.

This is what Benner (1984) alluded to and it does not sound very scientific, but the multidisciplinary care team can take some confidence in their combined years of clinical experience and an awareness that they are all bringing different assessment skills to the fore for the comfort of the child. At the same time the team needs to be mindful that the physiological indicators such as heart rate and blood pressure can vary for a myriad of reasons and also that a child experiencing unrelieved distress and pain cannot stay in the heightened state of arousal indefinitely, as his or her body systems will seek to achieve a balance and compensate. This biologically compensated status might result in the impression that the child is distress and pain free.

The child on CPAP, long term or minimal ventilation, who does not have infusions of muscle relaxation agents may still have infusions of sedation and analgesics. There is significant interest in the development and validation of a sedation scoring system (see Table 9.3) to be used in combination with or adjacent to a pain tool. The pharmacy of sedation is considered further below; however, sedation assessments like pain tools seek to measure a patient's status, but, like pain tools, measurement is not without difficulty as the data harvested cannot be quantified as interval or ratio. Assessment and measurement is complicated by the fact that there is significant subjectivity between assessors and this can be influenced by a nurse's and doctor's attitude to pain and distress and what they are inclined to do about it (de Lima et al. 1996; Melhuish and Payne 2006).

The higher the score the less well sedated the child is, but low scores are not necessarily indicative of good sedation. Children must be assessed against their entire clinical picture and every other detriment to their comfort taken into account, such as the risk of urine retention through immobility and pain (Steggal 2007) or a full postoperative bladder (Cropper 2003) and the need to facilitate optimum positioning (Griffiths 2005).

Pharmacological means of managing a child's distress

As a general principle, medicines should only be given when necessary and, in all cases, the benefits should be calculated against the possible risks and side effects (BNF for Children 2007). It is good practice to discuss treatment options carefully with children and their carers and in particular they should be educated to distinguish between the unpleasant consequences of the illness and injury and the potential side effects of the medication (BNF for Children 2007).

In all cases, prescriptions and instructions must be clear and guidelines followed. The children's nurse can help with compliance and concordance by observing and reporting if the child has difficulty in taking the medication and ensuring that the regime is as simple as possible. By working with the child and family the children's nurse can ensure that expectations are realistic. If medications are going to be required over an extended period, such as in chronic pain, ascertain that facilities and contingency plans are in place to make sure that treatment regimes are not interrupted while the child is at school etc. (www.dh.gov.uk).

Many of the more powerful medications prescribed to children in pain and requiring sedation

Table 9.3 Example of a simple sedation scoring chart.

Situation	Score
Unresponsive/hypotonic on handling	1
Moving or reacting to suctioning or major handling procedures	2
Moving and reacting to handling but poorly co-ordinated	3
Moving spontaneously with some co-ordination, can be roused by voice	4
Moving spontaneously with good co-ordination, will respond to directions	5
Awake but settled and relaxed	6
Irritable	7
Unmanageable	8

are subject to the Misuse of Drugs Regulations (2001), particularly preparations that are classified under schedules 2 and 3. In hospital, special principles apply to the administration of these medications. Safe storage and rigorous guidelines protect both staff and patient; in addition the supply and continuity of the agents are ensured. In the community, the situation has to be more flexible to allow for travel and holidays and the parents may need to be reminded about safe storage, protocols for keeping adequate supplies and the legal requirements, particularly if travelling abroad.

Sedation – the pharmacology

Chloral hydrate and triclofos

These remain popular hypnotics for use in hospital. They induce sedation and can be used for procedures or to maintain quiescent equilibrium for a short period. The effects of these drugs are cumulative and should be avoided in conditions complicated by renal and hepatic impairment. Children may build up tolerance and dependence and abrupt withdrawal ought to be avoided. They have an unpleasant taste and are gastric irritants. This gastric irritant effect can result in vomiting which leaves the quantity of drug available to sedate the child open to speculation, and an alternative plan may need to be in place for vital investigations to take place and avoid the need to cancel scheduled CT and MRI scans (Gray 2002).

In neonates, chloral hydrate is used where sedation is required without analgesia, e.g. to facilitate a 12-lead ECG or cardiac echo. It should be used with caution in ex-preterm infants as there have been a high number of adverse cardio-respiratory side effects (Anand and Hall 2006).

Trimeprazine, chlorphenamine and promethazine

These are sedating antihistamines and they have a relatively short action (promethazine may be active for up to 12 hours). They are useful for occasional use, such as for insomnia in hospital or to promote a drowsy sedated state, but should be used with caution in conditions complicated by renal or hepatic impairment. They have a range of side effects and in some cases have a paradoxical reaction. Older children may complain of the 'hangover' effect during the next day.

The benzodiazepines – examples diazepam, lorazepam and midazolam

These are indicated for short-term use (2–4 weeks) as there is a risk of habituation (BNF for Children 2006). Like the other sedatives they need to be used with caution in conditions complicated with renal and hepatic impairment. They can cause respiratory depression and drowsiness which can persist several hours after the initial administration. They are useful in that they can induce amnesia which is helpful in getting children to readjust from their stay in HD areas. Lorazepam has a prolonged sedative action of 8–12 hours and has potent anticonvulsant action where first-line medications fail. Midazolam has been subjected to frequent studies and as a result is not recommended for sedation in neonates. Its use is associated with changes in the cerebral blood flow and haemodynamic instability (Anand and Hall 2006).

Barbituates – for example phenolbarbitol

These have no analgesic properties. They are useful either in isolation or in conjunction with other therapies for conditions where there is excess sensitivity and excitability, such as the abstinence syndromes. They have a long history of use in neonates and there is some prescribing confidence, but, because of the potential serious side effects such as hypotension and respiratory depression, infants need close supervision (Anand and Hall 2006).

Nitrous oxide (Entonox)

This is a sweet-smelling colourless gas associated with anaesthetics but can be used in 50% combination with oxygen to induce procedural analgesic and co-operation without loss of consciousness (Bruce and Franck 2000). It must not be used if a pneumothorax is suspected as it expands in a closed space and would further compromise ventilation (BNF for Children 2007). It is increasingly popular for instant and short duration use and is becoming popular for children who need frequent interventions (Williams *et al.* 2006). Examples of where children would benefit from the use of Entonox include drain removal, clip/suture removal, urethral catheterisation, application of traction, complex dressings and packing of wounds.

Ketamine

In older children this has been extensively studied and provides analgesia, sedation and amnesia (Anand and Hall 2006). Ketamine is still occasionally used to induce sub-anaesthetic sedation. The main disadvantage is the risk of hallucinations and nightmares; although children under 16 are regarded as less at risk, recovery is relatively slow (BNF for Children 2007). In neonates ketamine causes slight increase in blood pressure, slight tachycardia and bronchodilation. Further studies are required. Anand and Hall (2006) recommend its use mainly when under approved research protocols.

Pain management

Use of tools for assessment

Because pain is private and subjective, it can only be measured indirectly, either by self report or by observing behaviours that are regarded as universal indicators of pain (Mathews and McGrath Pigeon 1993). Although it must be stated that the latter are learned behaviours, they can be culturally associated and socially influenced. There are now a range of pain tools that can be used to observe infants and children and identify those in pain. These use a variety of assessment methods which are designed to be applied to the different ages and cognitive abilities. These range from the preverbal tool FLACC (face, legs, activity, cry, consolability; Merkel *et al.* 1997) and neonatal

infant pain scale (NIPs) to the well-known Wong and Barker-type faces scale, and the idea has now been adapted and refined following a number of studies (Bayer and Wells 1989; Beiri *et al.* 1990; Hicks *et al.* 2001; Lyon *et al.* 2005). A useful resource for the nurse studying infants' and children's pain assessment tools can be found on the RCN website (www.rcn.org.uk/publications/pdf/guidelines/cpg_pain).

More sophisticated tests require co-operation. The poker chip tool (Hestor *et al.* 1990) can be used with negotiation and agreement; once a pain baseline can be defined chips are issued according to levels of hurt (Twycross and Smith 2006). Children need to be able to assess their own level of discomfort and quantify that in order to seek relief. Significant trust is invested in the assessing members of staff in order to allow children to be equally honest. In verbal children who can be reached and can respond sufficiently well to process information the visual analogue scale (VAS) can be used. This is a simple descriptive tool linking language to levels of pain – no pain to worst pain possible. The child needs to be able and willing to translate experience to analogue and to comprehend proportionality (Twycross and Smith 2006).

The ITU scales are more focused on a combination of vital sign recordings and subjective assessment of comfort. They are only as good as the nurses who use them and there are frequently discrepancies between individual assessors. Each patient should be independently assessed at various points during the day and, although there is some evidence to suggest that nurses with different experiences assesses children differently (Twycross 1997; Hall 2002), there is little point in taking an assessment and not doing anything about it. There needs to be a plan of action individually designed to manage the child and this should be discussed from a multidisciplinary perspective in consultation with the parents and implemented (Garland and Kenny 2006).

Despite the plethora of 'pain tools' and the management of a child's pain having a high profile in the National Service Framework (NSF, Standard 7, 4.28–4.33), there is evidence that children's pain is still not well addressed in today's health care. Coles *et al.* (2007) measured compliance in one strategic health authority and if these results are indicative of other Trusts the national picture might not be good. Although all Trusts audited claimed to have and use pain tools, there remained too few paediatric-specific pain teams in practice and the Healthcare Commission Report (2007) confirmed that children's pain is still being ignored in many Trusts.

Managing pain – the use of pharmacology

It should be remembered that analgesics are more effective in preventing pain than relieving established pain. Situations that are likely to cause pain and distress to children can often be anticipated and therapy planned and implemented in advance.

Analgesics – first level therapy

The non-opioid analgesics such as paracetamol and some non-steroidal anti-inflammatory drugs (NSAID) if used regularly and prescribed to therapeutic levels can be quite effective in the control of pain and discomfort. Individually tailored use of these can often avoid the need for stronger preparations. Paracetamol (acetaminophen) is a most useful therapeutic agent and can be administered in a range of ways, avoiding the use of the enteral route where necessary. Paracetamol has rapid action once absorbed, an anti-pyretic effect and it does not depress the respiratory drive. Paracetamol has relatively few side effects and reported adverse effects are rare, but the drug is extremely dangerous in over-dosage and strict adherence to the recommended dose needs to be strongly recommended. A disadvantage is that it has no discernable anti-inflammatory action so is often used in combination with other agents where this is thought to be beneficial. Many NSAID have analgesic action but can also be helpful in other ways as they can reduce inflammation. The

pain-relieving properties of these drugs should take effect soon after administration, but the anti-inflammatory mode of action may take time to build up to its most effective level. Ibuprofen also has an anti-pyretic action which, when given for this, may also improve the overall comfort of the child.

Stop and think

Ibuprofen is contra-indicated in children with asthma – check the medical history.

Drugs classified as NSAID have a similar mode of action – they reduce the metabolism of arachidonic acid to prostaglandins. Arachidonic acid is normally present in cell membranes; it is released when tissues are disturbed by disease process, trauma or irritation. Although prostaglandins do not cause pain in themselves, they sensitise the nerve endings to such an extent that ordinary, non-pain-producing stimulation can result in the perception of pain. NSAID are particularly useful in skeletal conditions, bone, joint and muscle pain. They form the cornerstone of management for rheumatic and arthritic conditions but may also be used for headache, dysmenorrhoea and dental pain.

Stop and think

Aspirin should be avoided in children under 16 because of its association with Reye's syndrome (BNF for Children 2007). Reye's syndrome is a devastating condition of young children characterised by encephalitis and hepatic failure. The condition carries a high mortality (Meadow and Newell 2002).

Side effects of NSAID are numerous and include gastro-intestinal disturbances, hypersensitivity and bronchospasm. In general children seem to tolerate these drugs better than adults and as there is a range of NSAID, if one is not tolerated, another can be tried. Children vary in their individual ability to tolerate and metabolise these agents. If NSAID were employed with the therapeutic aim of reducing the pressure caused by swelling or the discomfort from the inflammatory process and seem to be non-effective, a short course of steroids might be tried. The decision to use corticosteroids in children is not taken lightly as there are many serious side effects and it should be remembered that these agents do not have direct analgesic action, so if NSAID were being used in part for this purpose the child's entire pain-killing strategy might have to be revised.

Second and third level therapy

Moderate and strong analgesic agent such as codeine and morphine are opioid agonists and these are drugs that can build up dependence as an unfortunate side effect, but this is not a reason to withhold them from children if they are required. There was a general reluctance to prescribe opioids to infants because of these risks, but MacGregor *et al.* (1998) indicated that there were no differences between children who received morphine and a group who did not. Other studies have suggested that not providing analgesia affects later behaviour and responses to pain (Johnson and Stevens 1996).

Opioids have other side effects such as respiratory depression, impaired cognitive function, hypotension and gastro-intestinal disturbance. Often these side effects necessitate the use of other agents to treat and manage them and this can result in a whole host of further potential interactions. When this occurs, child medication becomes a complicated regime.

Good practice

Multidisciplinary review of a child's medication should occur frequently and agents that are no longer beneficial to the child should be removed from the prescription.

Opioids have been the subject of extensive research work and there is much more to be uncovered. The effect of 'poppy juice' has been known for centuries. For therapeutic and legal reasons the drugs synthesised from the plant have been classified and reclassified as greater understanding occurs. When the biology of pain was considered in the section above, the action of neurotransmitters in the synapse was reviewed. Different synthesised analogues of opium have different actions and this depends on the extent to which they mimic agonists or antagonist action. Fundamental to the understanding of pharmacology is the appreciation of the difference between agonists and antagonists:

- A neurotransmitter is considered to have agonist activity and initiates a pharmacological effect.
- An agent that is capable of blocking the action of a neurotransmitter is an antagonist.

Both have pharmaceutical roles. Sadly it is not as simple to state that opioid agents are all agonists; for example the antidote naloxone hydrochloride is an antagonist. The biochemistry is more complex and there are many receptor types and subtypes. As a consequence many of the narcotic agents are both receptor agonists and antagonists. This accounts for the varying degrees of action and the differing side effects of the natural opioids and the synthetic morphine substances. A mixed agonist/antagonist can offer the child analgesic effects without depressing the respiratory drive and are thought to have less potential for creating a dependency.

As opioid-type substances have relatively short-lasting action they are best administered either frequently in HD children or continuously. There are a few preparations that are considered to be long acting such as MST, the sustained release version of morphine salts. These modified release preparations are most used in palliative care. Essentially the total morphine requirements for 24 hours are given in two divided doses 12 hours apart, but plans must be in place for the management of breakthrough pain (BNF for Children 2007). Patient-controlled analgesia is considered below.

Occasionally analgesics alone are insufficient to manage a child's pain. Gabapentin is being increasingly tried to relieve pain (especially neuropathic pain). Gabapentin was originally developed for the management of epilepsy. It changes the way that the body "sees" pain. It is well tolerated and has relatively few side effects. It can be used in conjunction with existing analgesics.

In general the more common and minor analgesics should be tried first and their impact assessed before moving on to the stronger drugs which are more likely to have serious side effects. Analgesic drugs can be used singularly, in combination with each other or in combination with anti-inflammatory agents or sedation to keep a child comfortable.

This progression through the levels of potency can be considered almost as a stepladder, with the common and minor drugs situated on the lower rungs of the ladder and the stronger opioids appearing at the top. In all cases the nurse should utilise the most appropriate means of administration.

Stop and think

All prescriptions should be based on the child's weight and individually calculated. The strength of the preparation needs to be considered to make administration easier. Large volumes of dilute preparation might be more difficult for some children to swallow; others may prefer this to a stronger preparation which they perceive as less pleasant.

Many children hate needles and the intramuscular route is usually the last resort; needle phobia can develop but can be effectively managed (Thurgate and Heppell 2005). Arguably part of the phobia is the exposure to strangers who have less time to prepare the child or may be perceived as less sympathetic; this makes a good case for nurses to extend their role safely and learn to cannulate (Collins 2006). The rectal route can be a useful means to administrating medication but can be embarrassing for the child who needs

careful preparation in advance. This mode of administration is more common in Europe. The principles are the same as any other administration method and this route can be extremely useful where oral administration is not possible, there is no IV access or where the airway is compromised. Generally parents are a great help in reassuring their children. Where possible their wishes need to be respected. Whenever possible the consent of the child or the family needs to be obtained and real choices offered (Watt 2003).

One area where medical technology has really moved forward to the great benefit of the patient is in the way medication can be delivered. Intravenous access and infusions have become so common that their use has almost been taken for granted. However, the insertion of these can be a source of pain in itself. A topical application of local anaesthetic cream is recommended (Arrowsmith and Campbell 2000), but there are side effects to some of these mixtures; the location of application ought to be considered with care and the directions for use should be closely followed (Proudfoot and Gamble 2006). In addition there are potentially serious side effects to such access devices (Hamilton 2006a; 2006b) and so nurses need to be vigilant and observe the sites closely. It would be ironic that a cannula sited to give pain relief ended up causing pain and distress.

Stop and think

Before setting up, changing or adding a new infusion to an established line check cannula site, pump pressures and infusion compatibility.

Patient-controlled analgesia (PCA)

Children in control of their own pain management developed from an interest in self-administered analgesia as opposed to nurse-administered analgesia in the 1970s and represented a paradigm shift in the way a patient's pain was managed. As technology became more reliable and solutions more stable, this means of managing pain became popular and safe. PCA is fundamentally different from other means of administration in that patients can exercise their own control. PCA can be administered intravenously, subcutaneously or by epidural routes (Llewellyn and Moriarty 2007). The devices are sufficiently portable with battery back up to enable mobilisation and play for those having subcutaneous or intravenous therapy. Patients from the age of 5 and above can use the devices safely, but all children will need individual assessment and preparation and ideally this would be done by a 'specialist pain nurse'. The preparation of the child is all important and the technique is best used with an agreed pain assessment tool. Such co-operation is indicative of the unique blend of trust and sensitivity which can be established between children and their carers.

The technique can be used to augment background analgesia and the child is in control of the bolus on demand as part of post-operative management or anticipated painful procedures. Alternatively PCA may be used as a means of weaning the child down from stronger continuous infusions, e.g. in step-down care from ITU. As the analgesic requirement reduces, the device can be used when working the child towards oral maintenance. Weaning is not usually problematic, and local experience suggests that children naturally wean themselves off and frequently request removal of the devices as they become more mobile. The technique is sufficiently flexible to be of considerable value and an asset to community care management.

In palliative care the technique of continuous subcutaneous infusion can also be used to provide anti-emetic for the effective management of nausea and vomiting (Thompson 2004) or sedation. This can be particularly useful as a short-term procedure when the number of venous sites is limited or inaccessible. The technique – known as hypodermoclysis – was first described in the early 1900s but fell out of favour during the 1960s principally owing to the technique's misuse and the increasing safety of intravenous fluid and drug administration (Baura and Bhowmick

2005; Khan and Younger 2007). However, in selected cases for specific substances and with proper preparation the technique could emerge once again to the benefit and ease of management of children and adolescents who need additional flexibility in the administration of therapy.

The use of epidural analgesia has revolutionised post-operative management. It is highly effective in controlling acute pain in the lower limbs, pelvis, abdomen and chest (Weetman and Allison 2006). Most epidurals are administered without incident, but there is a risk of life-threatening complications and safe administration requires an informed, skilled, multi-disciplinary approach (Royal College of Anaesthetists 2004; Medical Devices Alert 2006). The general surgical children's wards sometimes do not have adequate staff levels to observe epidural infusions and this has led to otherwise conscious and stable children being cared for in HDU/ITC environments. This will have unfortunate results in the way these children can rest and recover. Sleep and rest are complex phenomena and there is increasing evidence to implicate deprivation in altered healing (Bennett 2003). The HDU is not the most tranquil of areas to spend post-operative time and may contribute to a child's emotional distress.

Neuro-surgical techniques

These are more common in the USA and in adults and are only just beginning to make an impact in the management of chronic intractable paediatric pain. The aim is to block or interrupt the sensory pathway of the peripheral nervous system or to provide counter stimulation. It is a highly specialised technique but increasingly used. A brief summary is provided below. In some cases it can be used to palliatively decompress areas where disease states, such as overgrowth of a tumour, have resulted in intractable and unmanageable pain.

Cordotomy

This is when the dorsal root supplying 'information' to the spinal cord for transmission to the brain is divided either by open surgery or by a percutaneous route. It is usually a short-term procedure for patients with malignant disease. Although good effect is obtained in the majority of patients this tends to wear off over time and is indicative of the plasticity of neural tissue.

Sympathectomy

This is division of the nerves of the sympathetic nervous system. Again it is of greatest use as a short-term measure for intractable pain from cancer and in patients who could have greater quality of life where they not requiring such enormous quantities of drugs to keep them comfortable. The likelihood of success can be gauged by temporary pharmacological blocking. These techniques are not without risks and side effects as total anaesthesia of an area is difficult to live with and there can be ischaemic changes to distal parts even with highly selective sympathectomy.

Electrical nerve stimulation

Although transcutaneous electrical nerve stimulation devices have now reached the high street and are available without prescription, implanted devices directly to the dorsal column are rarely used. These are expensive and controversial, but they can at least be removed if ineffective.

Non-pharmacological means of supporting a child and promoting coping

This is where the art of nursing can be fully appreciated and where children's nurses and doctors get to be most creative. The child can benefit from a number of strategies which range from watching television (Bellieni *et al.* 2006) to looking through virtual reality glasses (Sandler *et al.* 2002).

Relaxation

Tension will make pain worse; muscle tension is uncomfortable in itself so muscle relaxation methods may make a significant contribution to pain management. These can be taught and practised as a strategy pre-operatively or may be used as part of a chronic pain management strategy. These relaxation techniques can work surprisingly well for children (Payne 2000):

- The child is invited to contract and hold a major muscle mass for a specific time. When performing the muscle contraction the child is distracted and focused away from the seat of the pain, then the child is told to relax. This muscle work may be beneficial in itself as the contraction and relaxation will improve blood flow and may relieve ischaemic states.
- Complying with instruction and the attention and investment of another individual may improve perception of self worth and this boost may alter brain chemistry such as serotonin states.
- During the relaxation stage the child is invited to remember the 'good, calm, warm' feeling of the relaxed muscle and there may be a facet of suggestion.
- These sequential and rhythmic tension/relaxation exercises may be accompanied by controlled breathing exercises and the child instructed to slowly blow the pain away.
- In some children these techniques are particularly beneficial to aid sleep and therapists who use guided imagery may utilise relaxation states to instil the positive and pleasant thought processes.

Relaxation has no direct analgesic effect and can never replace analgesics but may enhance their action. Some children cannot facilitate this technique on their own. They can become dependent on their carers or their therapists to induce such states, although audio recordings might help.

In older children, with good attention spans and commitment to the therapy, a biofeedback technique might be helpful. In this the child is taught to monitor an inner state such as pulse, muscle tension, breathing or temperature and work to control it and reduce it. This requires significant concentration and distracts the child away from the pain.

Massage

Massage under appropriate circumstances is enjoyable, safe and popular with patients but often not one of the first therapies considered by clinicians, possibly because of its portrayal by the media and its links to adult entertainment (Vickers and Zollman 1999; Kemper 2001). However, the therapy is increasing in popularity within the neonatal unit where it can be employed as part of a developmental care package. In HDU, its use could be considered as part of a counter-irritation strategy or distraction.

Hypnosis

Hypnosis is essentially an altered state of consciousness which is incompletely understood. Mantle (2001) defined it as a state of daydreaming where external stimuli are tuned out and the focus of concentration is narrowed and the attention is selective. In pain it can be used to relocate the child from a passive helpless enduring state to one of control. Hypnotherapy is a flexible tool and the child's own imagination can be creatively used. The therapist needs to be sufficiently skilled to use the child's own language and sufficiently familiar with the child to realise just what that language means to the child. Because of the way the therapist uses language to suggest alternative experiences to the child the therapy has restricted use in children with uncertain cognitive abilities and there are also age limitations in using the therapy with infants.

The value of play

This can never be overemphasised and the support of a trained play therapist can be invaluable. This strategy can be used with the very young child as well as older children and can be used for short procedures such as dressing change or cannula insertions as well as for longer-term pain management strategy. Artwork can be surprisingly revealing of how children see life, can reveal their hopes and fears and can indicate how they feel about their illness and circumstances. In particular, drawings can be a vital enhancement to communication, but nurses and art workers need to be appropriately prepared to cope with the very sensitive material that can be revealed (Wellings 2001). Therapeutic play work with puppets can help children with chronic conditions and pain to express and act out the difficulties they face in their daily lives and this is a valuable addition to the long-term management of a child (Savins 2002).

> ### Think point
>
> To assess how the child sees scale and proportion ask him or her to draw a child having an injection.

Play therapy can be used in many ways, e.g. role playing and behavioural rehearsal. During this (in safety and without risk of judgement) children can trial and model possible reactions to procedures and situations. Coping states can be promoted and although anxiety and worries may still be manifest, the model would be to work towards overcoming the anxiety.

Family therapy

This is a 'catch all' term that encompasses many strategies and techniques. Essentially, as the child in long-term pain does not exist in isolation, the entire family needs to support the child and in turn be supported. This is especially important in palliative care but also where the child has psychosomatic pain and maladapted behaviour. Family therapies have many aims but among them are the improvement of communication, the resolution of past conflicts, the enhancement of family decision making and the promotion of the independence and autonomy of the child.

Alternative therapies

There is considerable scepticism from mainstream medicine as to the efficiency and validity of some alternative therapies. As there is considerable competition for clients, funding and recognition, this is perhaps not an unexpected reaction. However, the use of complementary and alternative medicine is common (Kemper 2000) and can play an important supporting role in relieving symptoms and improving the quality of life of children (Scrace 2003). For parents, it allows them to feel that they are in some control over attempts to relieve some of their child's distress (see Table 9.4). There is some emerging evidence

Table 9.4 Alternative therapies.

Therapy	Description
Acupuncture	Acupuncture is part of a traditional Chinese medicine system, developed over millennia and becoming increasingly common in the West over the past 40 years. It may have particular relevance to the management of difficult-to-treat pain as traditional Chinese medicine (TCM) does not distinguish between physical and psychological components of health states. The theoretical basis of TCM focuses on 'opposing forces' and requires some understanding of Chinese metaphysics to appreciate the therapies fully. However, the treatment aims are to establish a balance and harmony within the individual
	There is considerable evidence that the therapies work, whether by belief placebo, liberation of the body's own endorphins or by masking or interfering with the transmission of pain stimulus
	Acupuncture is used extensively in some enlightened clinics to good effect (Currie 2006). In the author's experience young children are less than enamoured at the prospect of repeated sessions involving needles, however fine. Considerable effort may be required to get them to engage with the concept. Perseverance may be worth it as there is some evidence that the investment in the experience is perceived as pleasant and helpful (Kemper *et al.* 2000). The therapy might be more applicable to the young person who may be able to grapple with the philosophy behind the process and fully engage with the therapist
	Therapists ought to come well recommended and there is a specialist licencing body. Acupuncturists differ in how many children they treat per week (Lee *et al.* 1999) and this might have an effect on their confidence. There could be considerable risk in using this therapy in isolation. There is a risk of contamination and infection so sterile needles must be used and the insertion sites well mapped
Aromatherapy and reflexology	Aromatherapy is based on the positive effects of stimulation of areas of the brain by the smell produced by volatile agents, usually plant esters and oils, and is most usefully used in conjunction with massage. There is probably a considerable 'feel good factor' at work during the use of these substances and this has to be a positive factor in the management of patients in desperate states. The patient should not have unrealistic expectations of the therapy or be promised that this is a viable substitute to conventional management. In the author's experience some aromas have the capacity to induce feelings of nausea as well as feelings of wellbeing. There are attendant risks with the use of burners and vaporisers. Oils inserted into hot water to inhale must be used with caution with young children. Some oils are toxic in concentration and can cause skin rashes and irritation. Some such as ergot should not be handled by pregnant women
	Reflexology can be used in conjunction with aromatherapy or used in isolation, the massage being facilitated by use of light unscented oil. It is based on the principle that the hands and the feet are dense with nerve networks and plexus and that some areas correspond to major organs. Stimulation of these areas can work beneficially remotely
Therapeutic touch	The research base for this is small but it is gaining popularity, particularly in neonatal units. Despite the name, the body is not touched and the therapy is said to work by rebalancing the body's natural energy pattern. There are also therapeutic touches and massage strategies which do involve contact and it is recommended that nurses refer families to the relevant experts or undergo proper training before deployment (Hallett 2004)

that children with chronic conditions are more likely to use alternative therapy than 'healthy children' and worryingly this was often without the knowledge of their paediatricians (McCann Newell 2006).

> **Stop and think**
>
> The NMC standards for management of medicine (2007) include a reminder that nurses who practise alternative therapy need proper training and preparation in order to protect their patients.

Neonatal considerations

Non-nutritive sucking has long been used to distract and settle infants and many parents choose to use this technique to good effect at home. It can be used with equal effect in hospitals. Some infants self settle and take comfort from their thumb. Some of the more interesting and applicable distraction techniques for infants in hospital include the administration of glucose or sucrose (Haouari *et al.* 1995). This was popular during the 1980s and is gaining popularity again. It is a simple strategy to implement and can be administered with or without the additional distraction of sucking; the evidence is very supportive of the intervention (Stevens *et al.* 2003). The analgesic effects of allowing infants access to the breast is a contentious issue and worthy of further significant study (Carbajal *et al.* 2006); certainly access to the breast and breast feeding is increasingly indicated as having a range of benefits to the individual, some of which have long-reaching implications for a lifetime of health, adjustment and wellbeing (Montgomery *et al.* 2006).

Long-term implications of pain

There is some controversy over the possible or likely long-term effects of pain and distress on survivors of the NNU and the CICU/PICU/HDU.

Table 9.5 Psychological components to pain.

Psychological component	Result
Sensory-discriminative	Allows injuries to be identified in time and place
Motivational-affective	Produces autonomic responses such as movement away from the source of the injury
Cognitive-evaluative	Pain stimuli are influenced by anxiety and culture

Adapted from Butcher (2004).

The long-term sequels of pain events are not fully understood (Taddio and Katz 2005), so complementary to analgesics and pain management is the need to be aware that some counselling, behavioural follow up or some psychodynamic therapy may be useful in chronic or unresolved problems which may follow from the original pain state or as a result of the child's management.

Psychosomatic pain

Children usually have a lot more to do in their lives than fake pain, so the child, first and foremost, ought to be believed. There are psychological components to pain (see Table 9.5). These are all normal responses and are not part of the psychosomatic picture, although they may have been a feature in the development of it.

This is not to say that children do not play-act to avoid the unpleasant or the dreaded, just as some adults can do. This is in order to take time out and give them space to mentally rebalance or recharge their energies. Some children model their behaviour on adults and may display a learned behaviour to get attention and it can be regarded as a coping mechanism of sorts. However, there are a few psychiatric disorders in which the perception and reporting of pain plays a prominent role.

Somatoform pain disorder is a condition where no organic source for the pain can be located or the pain is significantly out of proportion to the source. The question has to be asked what 'pain' means to this patient. Some patients, in an attempt to displace abhorrent situations and experiences such as sexual abuse, may present with abdominal or other unexplained pain. Other children may be at risk as their parents, following psychiatrically driven desires of their own, fabricate illness in their child and prepare the child to collude with them. The child is subjected to a battery of tests and investigations, some of which will have attendant risks.

Spiritual aspects and holism

There is a lack of literature informing nurses on the spiritual perspective of pain and suffering. From a Jewish-Christian religious perspective suffering can have a complex dimension which goes far beyond the human understanding. For some, an ability to accept one's fate may lead the sufferer into a state of grace. For those who believe in this, offering sedation and analgesia might be unacceptable, particularly the concept of terminal sedation. Naturally there are related cognitive and developmental issues of the child's level of understanding to consider. For nurses caring for children there is the concern that although the families might be devout and fervent in their beliefs the child might be denied the choice to be allowed to choose this option of comfort. There is also the possibility that although a child's physical pain is controlled, the fear and uncertainty is not being addressed and what the nurse needs to address are the spiritually holistic needs of the patient.

Appendix

Table A1 demonstrates common drugs and their effects.

Table A1 Common drugs.

Drug	Dose	Mode of administration	Physiological effects	Side effects	Contraindication/caution
Paracetamol	Consult BNF Example dose: 1–5 years: 20–90 mg/kg in divided doses 6–12 years: As above but not to exceed 4 g daily or for longer than 48 hours	Oral – tablets, melts or suspensions Intravenous Rectal	Inhibits cyclo-oxygenase in CNS but not in the periphery Analgesic but not anti-inflammatory effect	Rare occasional rashes Hepatic failure in very high doses	Hepatic failure
Ibuprofen	Consult BNF Example dose: Infant up to 3 months 5 mg/kg 3–4 times daily after feed	Oral – tablets or suspensions	Inhibits cyclo-oxygenase in the periphery Analgesic and anti-inflammatory effects	Gastro-intestinal upset nausea hypersensitivity reaction	Cardiac failure Liver disease Renal impairment Peptic ulceration *Caution:* risk of bronchospasm
Diclofenac	Consult BNF Example dose: Child 6–18 years rectal 0.5–1 mg/kg (max 75 mg) 2 times daily up to 4 days	Oral – tablets or dispersible tablets Rectal	Inhibits cyclo-oxygenase in the periphery Analgesic and anti-inflammatory effects	Gastro-intestinal upset nausea hypersensitivity reaction	Cardiac failure Liver disease Renal impairment Peptic ulceration *Caution:* risk of bronchospasm
Codeine	Refer to BNF Example dose: Child 1 month–12 years 0.5–1 mg/kg every 4–6 h (max 240 mg) daily	Oral – tablets or syrup Rectal Injection – SC, IM or IV	Acts on opioid receptors in the CNS and the periphery to block pain transmission	Respiratory depression Constipation Drowsiness Nausea	Hepatic impairment Renal impairment Respiratory conditions and impairment
Morphine	Consult BNF Example dose: Infant 1–6 months bolus IV 100–200 μg/kg Infusion 20–30 μg/kg/h	Oral – tablets or liquid Injection – SC, IM or IV	Acts on opioid receptors in the CNS and the periphery to block pain transmission	Respiratory depression Constipation Drowsiness Difficulty in micturition Nausea and vomiting Flushes and rash	Raised intracranial pressure Hepatic impairment Renal impairment Respiratory conditions and impairment

Chapter 10

CARE OF THE CHILD WITH A BURN INJURY

Jane Leaver and Clare Thomas

Introduction

A burn is arguably one of the worst injuries a child can suffer, often causing disfigurement, disability and psychological trauma which necessitates the involvement of a multidisciplinary team to meet the needs of the burnt child and his or her family. This chapter focuses on the care of a child who has suffered a burn injury. It will discuss the common causes of burn injuries, and look briefly at the anatomy and physiology of the skin, burn physiology, assessment of size and depth of burn, emergency management, wound and pain management, nutrition, toxic shock and psychological management.

Overview of anatomy and physiology of the skin

The skin is the largest organ of the body and consists of two layers, the epidermis and dermis. The epidermis is the outer layer of the skin and is constantly shed and regenerated. The dermis layer lies under the epidermis and within this layer nerve endings, hair follicles, blood vessels, sebaceous and sweat glands are situated.

The skin has several major functions including:

- Temperature control
- First line of protection against infection
- Protection of internal organs

- Sensory activity
- Production of vitamin D
- Waterproofing
- Excretion of waste products

If the skin is damaged, these functions will be impaired and the treatment of burn injuries need to take this into consideration

Causes of burn injury

A burn occurs when the skin is damaged by heat in the form of flames, scalds, chemicals, radiation, electricity or by contact with a hot surface. Most injuries in children are accidental although there are cases where non-accidental injury may occur; therefore obtaining an accurate history is essential in trying to establish the cause of the injury. This will also help with education on accident prevention prior to discharge.

National statistics are not currently readily available due to the ongoing restructuring of burns service provision and the development of a national database. General statistics for the UK include:

- 26 000 under 5 years are burnt or scalded in the home each year.
- Every 2 hours a child less than 18 years of age with burns or scalds is admitted to emergency departments or specialist burns units.
- Every day 10 children under 5 years of age are admitted with burns and scalds.

Table 10.1 Causes and incidents of paediatric burns from a regional burn centre for children (2006).

Cause	Incidence (%)
Scald	70
Contact	13.5
Flame	10.5
Flash	3
Chemical	1.5
Electrical	1
Friction	0.5

- Forty five percent of all severe burns and scald accidents occur in the under 5 age group (http://www.childrensfireandburntrust.org.uk).
- Around 450 children under 5 are admitted to UK hospitals each year with severe scalds caused by bath water, and a further 2000 suffer less severe scald injuries. There are over 20 deaths a year as the result of scald injuries from hot baths (www.kernoweb.myby.co.uk/salamanders).

Table 10.1 provides some more specific data for 2006 from one of the regional burns centres in the UK, reflecting the percentage of children seen within each broad category of burn injury.

Scalds

Scalds are the most common type of injury in children, particularly in the pre-school age group, with a higher percentage of males to females (Hankins *et al.* 2006). The main reasons for so many scalds occurring in this age group are linked to the immaturity of cognitive and motor skills development which means a lack of danger awareness and poor coordination (Settle 1996). On occasions the accident happens in unfamiliar environment or when the child is momentarily unobserved and manages to perform a motor activity such as a crawl or roll not previously achieved.

Contact burns

These burns are being seen more frequently. The most common culprits being irons and hair straighteners, which have been left on the floor to cool down, and also unguarded domestic heating appliances.

Flame burns

As children get older, flame burns become more common as they, particularly adolescents, are more prone to experimenting with the use of matches and flammable substances.

Chemical, radiation and electrical burns

Chemical burns may cause injury to the outer skin or injury to internal organs through ingestion of chemical products such as bleach or a combination of both. If a child is admitted to hospital having ingested a chemical it is essential to ensure that any other child at the same address is not exposed to the same danger.

Causes of electrical burns include coming into contact with faulty electrical equipment, insertion of products into electric sockets and in the young person coming into contact with outside electric equipment, e.g. pylons or electrified railway lines.

Radiation burns are extremely rare, particularly in children, although occasionally cases of severe sunburn necessitating hospital care have been reported. Burn injury may occur as a consequence of intensive radiotherapy, and while most incidences of this are relatively mild, the pain and possible long-term damage caused should never be underestimated.

Burn physiology

Damage to the skin by a burn injury produces both localised and systemic effects on the body. Local tissue is destroyed which sets off an inflammatory response releasing cytokines and other chemical mediators.

The release of these substances in a burn of greater than 30% of total body surface area

Table 10.2 Zones of a burn wound.

Burn zone	Tissue damage
Coagulation zone	This is the point of contact of the burn and there is tissue death
Stasis zone	This is the area surrounding the coagulation zone. It has less damage but the circulation is compromised. It has the potential to recover, but any further damage which could be caused by infection, hypovolaemia or oedema could cause necrosis, causing the wound to deepen and enlarge
Hyperaemia zone	This is the outermost layer of the burn. It has an increased tissue perfusion due to inflammatory mediator and will usually recover. In a large burn this can involve the rest of the body

Adapted from Herndon (2007).

(TBSA) will have a systemic effect on the whole of the body (Hettiaratchy and Dziewulski 2004), causing cardiovascular, respiratory, renal, metabolic and immunological changes.

Jackson (1953) described the burn wound as having three zones (Table 10.2) – coagulation, stasis and hyperaemia (cited by Herndon 2007).

Electrical burns have some differences in their pathophysiology. Initially, an electrical burn may appear visually quite small. However, if the electricity was of a high voltage (>1000 V) the electrical current will enter at the point of contact and travel a path to the exit point at earth. As the current passes through the tissues, damage will occur from the heat generated (Australia and New Zealand Burn Association 2006). This causes more damage than initially seen and makes it harder to assess the size of the burn. There may also be other injuries present such as torn muscles/ligaments due to muscle tetany and fractures due to falls. Cardiac arrhythmias may also be present due to the impact the electrical current may have on the conduction pathways within the heart.

Assessment of burn size and depth

Burns are described in two ways:

- The size of the burn
- The depth of the burn

Calculation of size

Calculation of burn size is an estimation of the total burn surface area (TBSA). One of the most common methods employed is the Lund and Browder chart (Figure 10.1). Areas of burn injury on the body are transcribed onto the chart with as much accuracy as possible and then the percentage is calculated for each area and added up to give a total. This is the most accurate method in use.

The Wallace rule of nines (Figure 10.2) can also be used, which, although not as accurate, is easier to remember if a Lund and Browder chart is not available. However, for use in children some modification is required, as shown, to account for the fact that children have larger heads compared to the rest of their body surface area than adults. It should also be remembered that for a quick estimation of small areas the child's hand equates to 1% of his/her body surface area.

For children, the rule of nines needs to be adjusted as follows:

For a child up to one year, the head equals 18% and each leg equals 14%. For each year after the first, the head decreases by 1% and each leg gains 1/2%. Therefore, adult proportions are attained by the age of ten years.

Calculation of depth

Appearance
The depth of the burn is defined by the amount of skin loss that occurs. This can be divided into partial thickness and full thickness skin loss (Hettiaratchy and Papini 2004).

CHART FOR ESTIMATING SEVERITY OF BURN WOUND

Name _____ Ward _____ Number _____ Date _____

Age _____ Admission weight _____

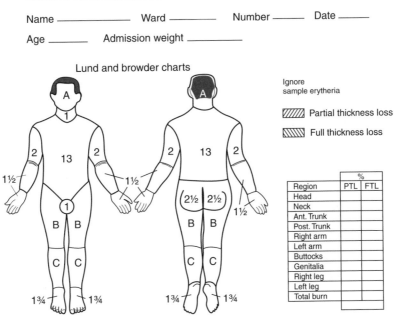

Lund and browder charts

Ignore
sample erytheria

▨ Partial thickness loss

▧ Full thickness loss

Region	%	
	PTL	FTL
Head		
Neck		
Ant. Trunk		
Post. Trunk		
Right arm		
Left arm		
Buttocks		
Genitalia		
Right leg		
Left leg		
Total burn		

Relative percentage of body surface area affected by growth

Area	Age 0	1	5	10	15	Adult
A = ½ of Head	9½	8½	6½	5½	4½	3½
B = ½ of One thigh	2¾	3¼	4	4½	4½	4¾
C = ½ of One leg	2½	2½	2¾	3	3¼	3½

Figure 10.1 The Lund and Browder chart for accurate assessment of the % BSA.

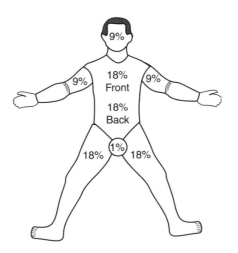

Figure 10.2 Wallace Rule of Nines chart.

Partial thickness burns may be further subdivided into:

- A superficial burn – where only part of the epidermis is destroyed. The area looks red and is very painful as in sunburn
- A dermal burn – where all the epidermis and part of the dermis is destroyed. This can be further divided into superficial dermal, which looks red and blistering can be seen, and deep dermal, which looks drier and is paler in colour

In contrast, a full thickness burn is where both the epidermis and dermis have been destroyed. The area will be charred looking or waxy white in colour and can sometimes be mistaken for unburned skin.

Sensation, bleeding and blanching

Other methods of estimating the depth of the burn apart from appearance are sensation, bleeding and blanching.

The deeper the burn the less sensation is present as the nerve endings have been destroyed. A superficial burn is very painful whereas a full thickness burn has no sensation. Similarly, bleeding on a pin prick is brisk in a superficial burn but becomes delayed in a deep dermal burn and non-existent in a full thickness burn.

However, both of these can be difficult to assess and a more accurate non-invasive method is to assess the capillary return on blanching of the burn wound with pressure. With a superficial burn the capillary return is brisk. This then becomes slower as the burn becomes deeper, until there is no blanching in deep dermal and full thickness burns.

Some burn services also have the facility and the expertise to use laser imaging doppler technology to aid burn depth assessment. This process uses a red laser to scan the burn wound and then produce a diagrammatic colour image of the blood flow in the wound. This can be helpful in determining borderline full thickness depths and establishing whether surgery is indicated. For the scan to be accurate the child needs to remain still for the duration of the procedure, which can be problematic especially in the younger age groups.

Consequently this may need to be performed under sedation or general anaesthetic.

Emergency management

The National Burn Care Review Committee (2001) suggests that all paediatric burns greater than 5% should be referred to a specialist burns service and those greater than 10% require formal fluid resuscitation which would then require high dependency care (along with any patients who potentially have an airway problem due to swelling or smoke inhalation). Advice and support should always be sought from the regional/national specialist burns service for children in any of the following categories:

- Under 5 years of age
- All 5% TBSA and over or >2% if full thickness
- If the face, hands, perineum, feet, neck and/or axillae are involved
- Circumferential burns
- Chemical burns
- Electrical burns
- Burns with associated inhalation injuries
- Burns with additional trauma
- Children with pre-existing medical conditions
- Child protection issues
- Sepsis or other complications of burn care
- Delayed wound healing

Immediate actions

The primary action for the treatment of a burn injury, after ensuring personal safety, should be removal of the heat source to reduce tissue damage, e.g. smothering of flames or removal of clothing with scalds.

Following this the burn wound needs to be cooled with copious amounts of cool water at a temperature of 15°C to reduce the release of chemical mediators and to prevent the burn becoming deeper (Australia and New Zealand Burn Association 2006). Cold tap water should be adequate for this purpose.

Following cooling, the burn wound should be covered. This not only keeps the wound clean but also helps to reduce pain as the nerve endings are not left exposed. Cling film is an ideal covering as it keeps the wound moist and does not stick to the wound on removal, reducing any further injury. The burn can also be viewed through the cling film without removing it if necessary. Application of any topical creams should be avoided until the child has been formally assessed by the burns team, as they could cause changes to the burn wound which would impede the assessment.

Initial assessment and management

A primary survey is required using the advocated ABCDE approach as for any child following trauma (Table 10.3). For the child with a burn injury, additional consideration needs to be given to these areas as there may be life-threatening complications arising even as the assessment is being carried out.

Fluid resuscitation

Once the size of the burn has been assessed then fluid resuscitation can be calculated. Children with burns of less than 10% can usually compensate for the fluids that they will lose with the administration of additional oral fluids.

Those with burns larger than 10% will need fluid resuscitation to ensure adequate tissue perfusion due to the amount of fluid that is lost through capillary permeability from the circulation, particularly in the first 8 hours following burn injury. There are many fluid resuscitation formulae

in use; however, one of the most commonly used formulae in the UK is the Parkland formula as it is relatively simple and easy to use (Table 10.4).

Some burn services, although using crystalloids initially, will introduce albumin after about 8 hours when the capillary permeability leak begins to reduce. This is more to replace the oncotic protein loss than increase the circulatory volume (Hettiaratchy and Papini 2006).

Patient monitoring

Replacement of fluid is not a precise procedure and the formulae are only a guide; therefore it is important for children to be carefully monitored to ensure that they are neither under- nor overloaded with fluid. Although the pulse, respiratory rate, BP and capillary refill time give an indication of the child's condition, urine output

Table 10.3 Specific considerations of primary assessment and management of the burn-injured infant/child.

Assessment	Notes/considerations
Airway	The history of the accident will give vital clues as to the risk of airway involvement, with the following key factors being causes for concern: • Enclosed environment • Presence of smoke • Evidence of facial burns, singeing of nasal hair and/or eyebrows • Hoarseness of voice (consider the child who is whispering in response to questions) • Breathing difficulties • Altered level of consciousness Anaesthetic assessment is required for any burns to the face/neck or if there is a possibility of smoke inhalation injury It is recommended that if there is a risk to the airway, intubation occurs sooner rather than later, especially if transfer to another hospital is required (Australia and New Zealand Burn Association 2006) Ensure that the cervical spine is protected if there is history or suspicion of associated trauma
Breathing	Full respiratory assessment should be undertaken as soon as possible Oxygen should be given to maximise tissue oxygenation and perfusion and to combat any carbon monoxide intoxication Circumferential burns to the chest may require escharotomies to facilitate ventilation. This is an excision through the burnt eschar to viable tissue in order to relieve constriction pressure, allowing for chest expansion
Circulation	Assessment of peripheral and central circulation Any bleeding should be stopped and this is especially important if there has been a delay in treatment as hypovolaemia will also be present due to fluid loss from the burn Assessment of peripheral circulation is essential to detect any circumferential deep burns causing compartment syndrome. If this is present then the child will require escharotomies (as above) Any jewellery should be removed as swelling may occur which will make it harder to remove at a later time
Disability	Assessment of the child's neurological status using first the AVPU (alert verbal painful unresponsive) score and then age-appropriate tools is essential Reduced level of consciousness may result if there has been a head injury in addition to burn injury Level of consciousness will be reduced if there is hypoxia from smoke inhalation and/or carbon monoxide intoxication
Exposure	It is vital that the child is kept warm due to risk of hypothermia In addition to this risk the body will have a hypermetabolic response resulting in the hypothalamus setting a higher temperature threshold and the body will aim for a core temperature of 38.5°C The environment consequently needs to be warmed to between 28 and 33°C to reduce the hypermetabolic state (Barrow and Herndon 2007)

will give a more accurate guide to the child's fluid resuscitation status.

A child in HDU may need to be catheterised in order to keep an accurate hourly fluid balance. Approximately 1 mL/kg/hour of urine is required in order to excrete waste products and maintain homeostasis. If the urine output is less than 0.5 mL/kg/h then consideration should be given to increasing the amount of resuscitation fluid and conversely

if it is greater than 2 mL/kg/hour consideration should be given to decreasing the amount of resuscitation fluid. The main exception to this final point is in the presence of rhabdomyolysis (the destruction/breakdown of skeletal muscle cells). Myoglobin is found inside muscle cells where it acts as a storage depot for oxygen. As the muscle membranes break down during rhabdomyolysis, myoglobin leaks out along with potassium and is carried to the kidneys.

Table 10.4 Parkland formula for calculation of fluid requirements following burn injury.

	Requirement
Resuscitation fluid The amount of fluid to be given in the first 24 hours from the time of injury	4 mL Hartmann solution $\times$ Wt (kg) $\times$ TBSA Half of the calculated volume is given in the first 8 hour post injury and the remaining half of the volume given over the following 16 hour
Maintenance fluid Maintenance fluid should take into account any oral or enteral feeds. This maintenance fluid should not be hypotonic as this increases the risk of hyponatraemia (National Patient Safety Agency 2005)	100 mL/kg/24 hour up to 10 kg of body weight plus 50 mL/kg/24 hour between 10–20 kg of body weight plus 20 mL/kg/24 hour for each kg over 20 kg of body weight

Adapted from Australia and New Zealand Burn Association (2006).

In the kidneys, myoglobin can break down into a toxic chemical called ferrihaemate which damages kidney cells. In this scenario, urine output needs to be increased to maintain filtration through the renal tubules, preventing the accumulation of ferrihaemate and subsequent renal impairment. The child may also have a central venous line (CVL) inserted and the central venous pressure (CVP) measurement can be a useful indication of the fluid status of the child. As with any clinical information this reading should not be taken in isolation but used in conjunction with other clinical indices.

Blood gas analysis may also be of use at this time (see Chapter 2).

Initial pain management

Burns are excruciatingly painful. The trauma of the injury will add to the distress of the child and family along with being in unfamiliar surroundings. It is important to provide adequate analgesia from the onset, which may necessitate intravenous opioid administration titrated to the needs of the patient.

Ongoing management considerations

Pain management

Children with thermal injury may require larger doses of analgesia/opiates than expected as they build up increased tolerance over a period of time (Meyer *et al.* 2007).

The use of regular paracetamol and a non-steroidal anti-inflammatory drug in conjunction with the opiate can be very effective for controlling background pain.

Gabapentin has also been shown to be effective in combating neuropathic pain from burn injuries in children (Mendham 2004) and should be considered along with amitriptyline, depending on the child's clinical status. The use of an age-appropriate pain scale to score the amount of pain is extremely useful in assessing the child's pain management and aiding the adjustment of analgesia (see Chapter 9).

Further analgesia will be required for dressing changes. For some children anxiety is also a problem and can increase their perception of pain, in which case it may be advantageous for oral sedation to be considered for dressing changes. A general anaesthetic or intravenous analgesia and sedation may be appropriate for some children.

Practitioners must always check prescribed medication against recognised national formulary (e.g. the British National Formulary for Children 2007) and administer in accordance with the local policy and their Code of Professional Conduct. Distraction therapy can be an effective way to reduce distress and pain levels (see Chapter 13). Other non-pharmacological interventions have also been shown to be effective in reducing anxiety and pain, e.g. music therapy, massage and hypnotherapy.

Wound management

Dressings are an important part of burn care; however, they should not be the first thing considered. There is a risk that the hugely visible impact of a burn on the child and family may lead practitioners to want to dress the wounds quickly, but more life-threatening problems need to be the priority of treatment.

There are many dressings and products on the market that could be appropriately used such as:

- Urgotulle and Urgotulle SSD® (or other low adherent antimicrobial dressings containing silver
- Acticoat® – silver-coated primary wound dressing, which is used as an antimicrobial barrier layer for partial and full-thickness wounds such as burns, donor sites and graft recipient sites that are judged to be at risk from infection
- Duoderm® – a hydrocolloid dressing
- Flamazine® – silver-sulphadiazine cream which is used for the prophylaxis and treatment of soft-tissue infections
- Mepitel® – a porous, semi-transparent, low-adherent wound contact layer, consisting of a flexible polyamide net coated with soft silicone

- Aquacel Ag® – primary wound dressing containing silver which absorbs and interacts with wound exudate to form a soft, hydrophilic, gas-permeable gel that traps bacteria and conforms to the contours of the wound. It is thought to provide a micro-environment that facilitates healing
- Polyfax® – a topical antibacterial ointment which contains two antibiotic agents – polymyxin B and bacitracin zinc

The ideal dressing for a burn is one that protects against infection, promotes moist wound healing, absorbs the large amount of wound exudate produced and is comfortable for the child.

The wound appearance and the primary aim of treatment would need to be taken into consideration when deciding on a dressing, i.e. protection, debridement or treating infection. This would also influence the frequency of the dressing changes. Other factors to consider when determining the frequency of changes are the condition of the child, the burn wound and the type of dressings being used.

Any dressing that is applied needs to be secured well but without pressure as children can be prone to excessive movement and will fiddle with the dressings.

Cleaning the burn wounds is an important aspect of wound management; however, there is controversy regarding the cleaning of wounds (Watret and Armatige 2002). Some literature advocates not cleansing wounds as it will interfere with the healing process and this is an appropriate course of action with clean healthy granulating wounds. A burn wound with more exudate, however, requires more attention and showering or bathing the child is a good option or irrigating with a sterile solution of chlorhexidine and cetrimide.

is that blister fluid contains growth factors and that by leaving blisters intact you are maintaining a moist sterile wound environment, aiding epithelisation. The other opinion held by many burn specialists is that the blister fluid may contain potentially harmful inflammatory mediators, that the blister may impede assessment and is likely to rupture, creating an environment favourable to bacteria (Hanumadass and Ramakrishnan 2005).

The authors would advocate the debriding of burn wound blisters and other dead tissue from the burn wound to create a clean wound bed that can easily be assessed. It is also often easier to debride the blisters initially soon after injury than a few days later when the blister fluid has jellified. Advice should always be sought from the regional/national specialist service.

In addition to dressings there are skin substitutes that are available to apply to partial thickness burn wounds (e.g. Biobrane®, a biosynthetic wound covering which provides a scaffold on which new skin cells can grow) and allografts. These skin substitutes are temporary dressings and although they initially cause closure of the burn wound, reducing pain and fluid loss and encouraging migration of epithelial cells, they will lift off after a week or so when epithelisation has occurred. However, caution needs to be used if devitalised tissue or colonisation is present due to risk of infection. These skin substitutes are expensive and should be applied to a clean wound bed, by experienced staff, usually in theatre.

Most full thickness burn wounds will need to be grafted to minimise scarring. Early excision and grafting is advocated to minimise blood loss (Papini 2006), to remove potentially harmful bacteria, reduce pain, quicken recovery and reduce hospital stay (Janzekovic 1977). The gold standard for wound coverage is the patient's own skin (autograft), but there are times when there is insufficient autograft to cover the wound and a bioengineered product may be used to act as a dermal matrix so that grafting may occur at a later stage, e.g. Integra®. Certain areas of the body require specific consideration with regards to wound management (see Table 10.5).

Scarring

Once the burn wound has healed, scarring is likely if it has been grafted or has taken several weeks to heal. Although it is not possible to avoid scarring, some scar management techniques can improve the appearance of the scar. The most common are moisturising, pressure and silicone. Regularly massaging the scar with a simple non-perfumed moisturiser helps to replace moisture in the skin that is deficient due to lack of sebaceous glands; this can also help to temporarily reduce itching, a common problem. Pressure garments have been shown to reduce hypertrophic scarring. The mechanism for this is not really clearly understood, but it is thought that the pressure helps the collagen fibres to realign and thus aids the scar maturation process (Gollop 2002). Topical silicone either in the form of a sheet or gel has also been shown to soften scars. It should not be used on open wounds.

Splinting and physiotherapy is another vital aspect of wound management and rehabilitation, helping to maintain function and movement and to reduce or prevent wound contractures. This should be considered at the beginning of treatment as incorrect positioning can lead to complications.

Nutrition

Nutrition is a vital aspect of burn care for several reasons. First, because a large wound is created there is an increased requirement for proteins, carbohydrates, vitamins and minerals to facilitate good wound healing. Second, albumin is lost through the burn wound exudate and extra protein is required to compensate for this. Third, there is an increased hypermetabolic response due to stress from the trauma and the nature of the burn wound.

Table 10.5 Specific considerations for body areas.

Body area	Notes/considerations
Face and head	The face is very vascular with good healing potential but it is not easy to dress well The treatment of choice for facial is often regular cleaning to remove exudate, followed by the application of white paraffin or Polyfax® to keep the wound moist but prevent bacterial contamination If the wound extends under the hairline the hair may need to be shaved to facilitate accurate assessment, wound care and to prevent hair becoming matted and creating an environment that encourages bacterial growth Facial burns are also prone to swelling which is often at its greatest 24–48 hours post injury. This has possible implications for the safety of the child's airway
Ears	If the ears are burnt care needs to be taken that any exposed cartilage does not dry out and die
Eyes	Any child with burns around the eye area should have an ophthalmic assessment as corneal damage may have occurred.
Hands/arms/feet	The hands are another challenging area to dress especially in a small child If it is possible to dress the hand to facilitate movement then this should be done, otherwise the use of a boxing glove dressing is advocated, taking care to maintain a functional position. Splints may be required to achieve this If there is a circumferential full thickness burn to the arm then the hand may need to be placed in a clear plastic bag, which acts as a dressing but enables observation of the circulation. If the circulation becomes impaired then an escharotomy may be indicated The same principles of care apply to the feet
Perineal and buttock area	This can present difficulties especially in the non-toilet-trained child due to risk of infection The use of Flammazine® in the nappy which is frequently changed can be effective. Sometimes in the older child it is feasible to use a bowel management system to keep the area free from faecal contamination

It is important that a proper nutritional assessment is carried out by a dietician and the appropriate nutritional requirements calculated on a regular basis. In addition it is important to monitor the adequacy of nutrition through blood protein and glucose results, the estimation of the body's nitrogen balance from 24-hour urine collections and a weekly weight check.

It is recommended that the serum level of trace elements is monitored, as trace elements, in particular zinc, copper and selenium, have an important role to play in growth and repair, metabolism, immunity and as antioxidants (Voruganti 2005). It has been shown that these trace elements are reduced in burns and it is advocated that high doses of trace elements are given IV to patients with major burns (Berger et al. 1998; see Chapter 5).

Often children will not take enough of their nutritional requirements orally. It is recommended that for these children and in particular those who have a percentage burn greater than 20%, supplementary feeding should be instigated by enteral feeding. Ideally a fine-bore nasogastric tube should be put in place in the first 24 hours to facilitate feeding as soon as possible and to help maintain the integrity of the gut, reduce bacterial translocation and help prevent paralytic ileus (Norman et al. 2002). Sometimes a nasojejunal tube is preferred in children with larger burns so that their feeding regime is not interrupted as much from frequent theatre visits. There is evidence to suggest that jejunal feeding can safely continue during surgery (Jenkins et al. 1994).

Because of the stress response to the burn injury and the physiological compromise, the burn patient may also be prone to a Curling (stress) ulcer and appropriate medications will be required such as H$_2$ receptor blockers.

Toxic shock

Toxic shock syndrome is a systemic illness which occurs mainly when *Staphylococcus aureus* endotoxins or less commonly *Streptococcus* and *Pseudomonas* endotoxins enter the blood stream. It has a reported incidence in children with burns and is thought to be due to the fact that the child has not yet developed the appropriate antibodies (White *et al.* 2005). If a child with a burn injury becomes very unwell with fever in conjunction with any of the other signs noted in Table 10.6 then toxic shock should be considered. Toxic shock syndrome can proceed very rapidly from observation of the first signs and symptoms to multi-organ failure and death. Early recognition and prompt treatment are essential to effect a good recovery. Treatment includes the administration of fresh frozen plasma or IV immunoglobulin concentrate which contain the antibodies required. Intravenous antibiotics such as flucloxacillin should also be given to prevent further growth of *Staphylococcus aureus*. Other supportive measures should be initiated as required by the child's condition.

Table 10.6 Clinical indicators of toxic shock syndrome.

Early signs and symptoms	Late signs and symptoms
Pyrexia	Lethargy/drowsiness
Rash/erythroderma	Decreased urine output
Vomiting	Tachycardia
Diarrhoea	Tachypnoea
Cool peripheries	Reduced saturations
Restlessness/irritability	Shock/collapse/hypotension
Low white blood cell count	

These can occur at any time but mostly between 48 and 72 hours after the burn injury and may occur in small burns.

Environmental and continuing care considerations

The environment in which these children are nursed is an important component of their care. As they have sustained skin loss they require an environment that can help keep them free from infection, keep them warm and prevent the loss of body fluids due to evaporation. A cubicle in which the ambient temperature may be constantly monitored and adjusted is the ideal environment where this is possible. The attention to hygiene of both staff and visitors is very important; consequently hand washing and wearing of protective clothing is encouraged by all.

Top tip

It is worth noting that is also important to keep visitors and nursing staff well hydrated as they are also in a room with a high ambient temperature.

In addition to the specific considerations discussed within this section it is important to remember that these children require the same fundamental nursing care as for all unwell children, including oral care, normal hygiene needs and play activities. Consideration needs to be given to pressure area management and specialised pressure-relieving equipment may be required. The position that these patients are nursed in is also important, as this may affect their long-term outcome. Children with neck burns should be nursed without a pillow to encourage neck extension. Depending on where the burns are, their head or limbs may need to be elevated. Splints to stop contractures of some areas, e.g. hands and feet, will need to be made and fitted. Physiotherapists and occupational therapists have an important role to play in the care of these children.

Psychosocial needs

As with all children and adolescents admitted to hospital for treatment, their and their families' needs should to be taken into account. In some circumstances due to the nature of the injury and incident there is more than one family member injured, which has an increased impact on the family. Burns are a traumatic occurrence and therefore the admission is rarely planned. The family may have had to travel to the treatment centre and may need accommodation. They will need explanation about treatment and may share in the care of their child; many will require help in order to cope with the appearance of their child.

The psychological trauma is not just at the time of the accident and the patient and family may require the involvement of the psychologist over a long period of time, especially after discharge in order to come to terms with an altered body image. This may include help in returning to school and reintegrating with peers. There are various support groups available nationwide that can be of benefit. It is also worth remembering that the staff involved in caring for these patients may also need support.

Useful resources

www.nationalburncaregroup.nhs.uk – provides information and policy guidance for healthcare professionals involved in the care of people with burns in the UK.

www.childrensfireandburntrust.org.uk – provides support and advice for children and their families after a burn or scald injury.

www.kernoweb.myby.co.uk/salamanders – provides a contact site for children following burn injury.

www.burnsupportgroupsdatabase.com – provides a database of burns support clubs and activity camps organised by various burns associations.

www.changingfaces.org.uk/home – This is a UK charity that supports and represents people who have disfigurements of the face or body.

www.capt.org.uk – Provides information and researches the number of children and adolescents killed, disabled or seriously injured in accidents.

The editors hold no responsibility for the identified websites above and would encourage individuals to access them prior to offering them to parents and the child.

Conclusion

The successful outcome for the patient who sustains a burn relies on a large multidisciplinary team working together planning the care of the patient from admission to discharge and beyond, as even though the patient will be discharged from hospital he or she will need ongoing treatment as an out-patient and help getting back to his or her pre-accident life.

Chapter 11
INFECTION AND INFECTION CONTROL

Katie Anderson, Felix Hay and Doreen Crawford

Introduction

The aim of this chapter is to introduce the children's nurse to infectious disease and infection control. The chapter does not intend to be a 'prescriptive dictionary' of pathogens; it is more a helpful and practical guide for the nurse working with highly dependent children. It is worthy of note that the immune response to infectious disease is very complex; therefore not all areas are discussed extensively. However, this chapter will cover the challenges that nurses face as a result of infection and will consider:

- The normal physiological response of a child to infection
- What makes the highly dependent child more susceptible to infection
- Some fundamental measures that may be used to strengthen a child's immune system
- What the nurse caring for highly dependent children can do to aid diagnosis and treatment, and prevent the transmission of infection

Background information

The world is a rich microbiological 'soup'. Diverse micro-organisms exist in the air that is inhaled and in the food that is consumed. As far as the human environment is concerned, both internally and externally, micro-organisms are everywhere. Some micro-organisms cause disease but most do not. Many play a critical role in processes that make life possible, some even prevent disease, and new therapies are being developed to use micro-organisms to cure disease. Some pathogens have challenged civilisation and arguably changed human history, such as those that caused plague, cholera, smallpox and the childhood diseases, still exist. However, eradication, understanding and management have made them less dangerous, at least in the Western world. Some micro-organisms thought to have been almost eliminated such as tuberculosis and gonorrhoea have returned and malaria continues to kill millions worldwide. With global warming and modern travel there are many opportunities for microbial spread as national boundaries are no barrier (Campbell 2007). In response, governments have implemented some seemingly successful strategies and recommendations designed to prevent outbreaks, such as in the case of threatened severe acute respiratory syndrome (SARS), H5N1 avian influenza (bird flu) and HIV pandemics.

Equally as important as threatened pandemics are those pathogens that cause nosocomial (hospital-acquired) infections. Methicillin/multiple resistant *Staphylococcus aureus* (MRSA) and *Clostridium difficile* (C-Diff) are examples of these and they have affected many patients, some with tragic outcomes. These, often avoidable, infections have hindered clinical activity and have shaken public confidence. Arguably these microbes have also changed the National

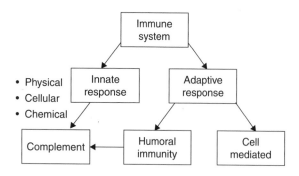

Figure 11.1 Two-pronged immunological response.

Health Service (NHS). The NHS has faced many challenges since its inception and has undergone many changes; although most are politically driven others make sound biological sense. Caring for patients, whenever safely feasible, in their own homes or in smaller units with fewer caregivers is one such example. It is logical to expose vulnerable patients to as little variety of micro-organisms as possible. At times, exposure to health care cannot be avoided and it is important that staff caring for children in hospital have an appropriate knowledge of infection and its implications.

Normal physiological response

Having an understanding of the basic principles of the immunological response is vital if nurses are to effectively contribute to the diagnosis, treatment and prevention of transmission of infection. The immunological response is primarily a 'two-pronged' approach: the innate response (non-specific) and the adaptive (specific) response (see Figure 11.1).

Innate response

This response is present from birth and includes chemical, physical and cellular defences. It is designed to identify and destroy the 'non-self',

but is restricted to a limited number of basic disposal methods and reacts in the same way to all 'non-self' matter.

Physical barriers to infection

Skin

Provided it is unbroken and fully keratinised skin is an effective form of protection. It forms the barrier between the internal workings of the human body and that of the environment. The skin also harbours Langerhan cells that engulf pathogens and take part in antigen presentation, therefore initiating the adaptive immune response. Langerhan cells are also found in the mucous lining of the nose, stomach, lungs and intestine. Lactic and fatty acids in sweat and sebaceous secretions lower the pH of the skin environment and have a direct inhibitory effect on pathogens.

Respiratory tract

The respiratory tract has a complex defence mechanism; pathogens rarely find their way into the lower regions unaided. Ciliated epithelial cells aid in the prevention of pathogen invasion by producing mucus. This traps pathogens and transports the mucus upwards in its path to excretion, either by coughing or sneezing.

Gastrointestinal tract

Ingested material is a common means of pathogen invasion. However, the majority of potential disease-causing pathogens are halted by the actions of bodily functions. Hydrochloric acid and bile salts provide extremes in the environmental pH, in which many pathogens cannot reproduce or survive. Enzymes are designed to split proteins and the larger microbes can be damaged in this way. Powerful peristalsis is also a potent means of preventing pathogens from taking hold in the intestines.

Chemical

Cytokines are the chemical messaging service for cells and are released to bring cells involved in the immune response to an infected site. The complement system is also utilised, but is complex and not fully understood. Essentially it is a collection of proteins that interfere with a pathogen cell membrane using a biochemical cascade which kills the invader. It is involved in the innate response, but is also utilised by the adaptive response.

Cellular

Many cells take part in the innate immune response. The majority have phagocytic properties, in that they engulf an invading pathogen and destroy it. Mast cells can be found in connective tissue and mucous membranes. They release histamine and cytokines in response to pathogen invasion; this dilates the blood vessels and generates a greater flow of neutrophils to the infected area. The neutrophils are attracted to the toxins produced by the pathogen and pass through spaces in the blood vessel walls to arrive at damaged tissues. The neutrophils then ingest the pathogen and destroy it. This is seen as inflammation. Finally, natural killer (NK) cells are responsible for destroying the host's cells that have already become infected by a pathogen, thereby limiting the spread of infection.

Adaptive response

This response to infection is ordinarily limited at birth because of the sterile environment of the amniotic sac. This, of course, may not be the case if a fetus has come into contact with pathogens from the mother. Although a new-born will be able to produce an innate response, and have some immunity from the mother, this defence alone is not substantial enough for childhood and adulthood. It is the development of the child's adaptive immunity that will prevent the majority of pathogen invasions from doing damage to the body, as it is a more explicit response.

Cell-mediated response

This response utilises the T-lymphocytes, which are derived from the thymus. There are three types:

- *T-cytotoxic cells (CD8)*: these cells seek out pathogen-infected cells and mediate an influx of water and ions. The infected cell cannot manage this influx and its cell membrane fractures (lysis).
- *T-helper cells (CD4)*: these cells release interleukins that increase T-cytotoxic and B-lymphocyte production.
- *T-suppressor cells*: these cells stop T- and B-lymphocytes from acting when the antigen presenting macrophage has been deactivated.

Humoral immunity – the primary response

In order to understand the humoral response, it is vital to have a basic understanding of some key terms (see Table 11.1).

The process by which humoral immunity is gained can be split into five stages:

- Antigen presentation
- Clonal selection
- Clonal proliferation
- B-lymphocyte differentiation and antibody production
- Antibody activity

Antigen presentation

Macrophages engulf the 'non-self' and present the 'non-self' antigen on its own cell surface.

Table 11.1 Key terms.

Term	Description
Antigen	A molecule that initiates an immune response. They are like codes found on cell surfaces and aid recognition. The 'self antigens' identify cells that do not display the same code, e.g. bacteria, mismatched blood, organs
Antibody	A plasma protein, often termed immunoglobulin. Produced by B-lymphocytes and having a unique binding site for every individual antigen. The 'lock and key' analogy is often useful here to understand the specific nature of these molecules
Macrophage	A large cell which develops from monocytes, originating from red bone marrow (myeloid cell). They engulf 'non-self' material by phagocytosis

Clonal selection

Within the lymph nodes, T-helper cells and B-lymphocytes that have the corresponding shape to the antigen presenting macrophage are selected.

Clonal proliferation

T-helper cells secrete cytokines that induce B-lymphocytes to divide, producing large numbers of clones. This allows the body to keep up with the large numbers of bacteria as they divide rapidly.

B-lymphocyte differentiation and antibody production

Some of these clones will become memory cells and some plasma cells. The plasma cells go on to produce equally specific antibodies, at a phenomenal speed. Memory cells are stored and can be triggered in the future to produce antibodies, if the body were to be re-infected by the same pathogen. This is known as a secondary response and is much swifter than a primary response.

Antibody activity

Antibodies work in many ways to destroy/hinder pathogen activity. Some bind to numerous pathogens, clumping them together. This is known as agglutination. Other antibodies release antitoxins that neutralise toxins produced by pathogens. Lysis digests the pathogen membrane in order that the pathogen explodes and therefore dies, whilst opsonisation coats the pathogen in a protein that identifies it as the 'non-self' and subsequently induces phagocytosis of the pathogenic cell.

Immunoglobulin development

Immunoglobulin G (IgG)

Term infants are born with high levels of maternal IgG as it readily crosses the placenta and will offer a range of protection for approximately 3 months against pathogens to which the mother has been exposed. This is known as passive immunity. IgG is the most versatile as it is capable of functioning like all immunoglobulins and can be found in both blood and interstitial spaces. Levels are 40% of that of an adult by the age of 12 months (Hockenberry and Wong 2003).

Immunoglobulin M (IgM)

IgM is responsible for clumping micro-organisms together ready for elimination from the body and for combating Gram-negative infections. It is the first to be produced by the fetus *in utero*; however, levels at birth are still comparatively low. Adult levels are not reached until 9–12 months (Hockenberry and Wong 2003), therefore newborn infants are at increased risk of contracting Gram-negative infections. IgM does not cross the placenta due to its large molecular size.

Immunoglobulin A (IgA)

IgA levels are low at birth, but breastfeeding improves its concentration. IgA is predominantly found in the respiratory and gastrointestinal tracts (MacGregor 2000).

Immunoglobulin E (IgE)

IgE is predominantly associated with the allergic responses of the body.

Immunoglobulin D (IgD)

The function of IgD is not yet recognised.

The concentration of all immunoglobulins increases as children grow. At what age they achieve their full quota varies between immunoglobulin groups.

Environmentally acquired defences

There are some aspects of infection prevention that should be actively encouraged by both hospital and community staff, as part of their role in good health promotion. Two examples are breastfeeding and immunisations, as prevention is better than cure. Also effective and very simple to implement is teaching good parent-craft. This can be a useful tool in the fight against infection. Teaching the correct methods of sterilisation and informing parents about selective contact and hand washing would prevent common infections, such as the invasion of gastrointestinal pathogens which cause diarrhoea and vomiting.

Breastfeeding

Breastfeeding is one particularly good way of supporting the immune system. It is thought to reduce mortality from common infections (especially gastrointestinal) in infants and children who are, or were, breastfed (World Health Organisation (WHO) 2003). Breastfeeding is also thought to aid recovery from such infections, and should be encouraged exclusively for the first 6 months of life (WHO 2003). Colostrum and breast milk contain IgA and lactoferrin, which are useful components in fighting gastrointestinal infection, particularly *Escherichia coli*. *E. coli* has a high metabolic requirement for iron, needed for growth and replication. However, lactoferrin has a high affinity for iron, and so deprives the *E. coli* of its vital iron source. This makes the *E. coli* susceptible to attack by IgA. This immunoglobulin does not cross the placenta so it can only be obtained via breast milk in newborn infants.

The document 'Ten Steps to Successful Breastfeeding' can be found on the WHO website, as a useful aid to supporting mothers. It is of note that for a highly dependent infant, if breastfeeding is not temporarily possible, mothers should be encouraged to express milk, so that the infant may continue to have the benefits of breast milk. Kangaroo care/cuddles should be encouraged during this time to continue the vitally important bond and close contact between mother and child that is partially responsible for lactation.

Immunisations

Immunisations are an important aspect of infection prevention. As a result of immunisation programmes, alongside improvements in sanitation and public health awareness, infection and death rates have plummeted and some diseases have been completely eradicated. Immunisation has the ability to confer herd immunity and this may alter disease patterns in whole communities. If a community has herd immunity, the vulnerable, i.e. those not yet vaccinated and those who are not able to tolerate vaccination, are protected.

The process of primary response to a pathogen can last several weeks, which in severe disease could prove too lengthy. Immunisations act by inducing the body to generate a primary response to a given pathogen, in a safe manner. If the disease pathogen were then to invade the body at a later date, there is a quicker secondary response. The memory cells produce plasma cells, which results in a high concentration of antibodies (higher than in a primary response). This high concentration of antibodies results in the pathogen being destroyed before symptoms occur.

It is the healthcare workers' responsibility to give parents up-to-date, evidence-based information regarding immunisations so that they may make an informed decision.

Increased vulnerability of the highly dependent child

Some infants are born highly dependent as a result of their prematurity. Some children are highly dependent because of a long-term or life-limiting condition. Others are highly dependent for short periods while they are treated for accidents or serious conditions in high dependency/intensive care units. However children have become highly dependent, they are at greater risk of contracting infections because of his/her need to have multiple invasive interventions, while possibly having a compromised immune response. If nursed in hospital, the risks are greater still as a result of the hospital environment – i.e. multiple carers, shared equipment and being in close proximity to other patients.

Indwelling equipment/invasive procedures

Highly dependent children, whether nursed in the community or in hospital, often have indwelling apparatus in order to help them survive or to remain comfortable – e.g. a tracheostomy, gastrostomy/nasogastric tube, central venous access or urinary catheter. These devices, though vital, can be vectors for infection as they break the protective layer of the skin or bypass the protective mucous membranes of entry to the body. Although these pathogens can be environmentally acquired, many are normal flora of the body that have found a means by which to enter the body. For example, *Staphylococcus epidermidis* found on the skin has a high affinity for attaching to plastic prostheses such as IV and urinary catheters (Engleberg *et al.* 2007). It is with this knowledge that it becomes clear that carers, whether health professionals or family members, should be made aware of the importance of maintaining good standards of hand hygiene and care of the indwelling equipment. They must also be aware of the signs of infection in order that treatment can be administered and the equipment be swiftly removed. Specific guidelines regarding the safe care of a patient with a urinary catheter, central venous catheter or patient requiring enteral feeding can be found in the NICE guideline on infection control (2003).

Invasive procedures range from the placement of indwelling equipment to the undertaking of major surgery. Many hospital procedures are conducted if not under aseptic conditions, with a non-touch clean technique to reduce the risk of contracting infection (Hart 2007). However, by the very nature of these procedures being invasive, it is clear that the body's normal defence mechanisms may not prevent colonisation by pathogens.

Hospital environment

In addition to indwelling equipment, the hospitalised highly dependent child has many additional risk factors for infection. The first and arguably most significant is that of multiple carers. The use of good hand hygiene, alcohol rubs and universal precautions is fundamental yet vital in the prevention of infection transmission between patients and carers. Effective occupational sickness and uniform laundering policies are also of great importance. It could be speculated that a return to the system of 'in-house' uniform laundering could reduce rates of infection, by reducing the risk of staff bringing in community pathogens and in making sure that uniforms are washed to the most up-to-date and regularly assessed standards. Uniforms laundered at home should be washed separately, and need to be able to tolerate a temperature of 60° (DH 2007). Uniforms can now be coated with microbe-resistant material.

The communal nature of many hospital environments is clearly another issue to be discussed. A good deal of the equipment and toys used in neonatal and paediatric services is communal. Flemming and Randle (2006) found that 85% of toys sampled from an intensive care unit (ITU) harboured viable bacteria that could have been detrimental to a child's health. Equipment used that can be sterilised should be sent to the sterilisation department within individual hospitals. If this is not possible due to the size or nature of the equipment/toys, local infection control policies should be met regarding cleaning. Obviously this is not an ideal situation, but equipment is vital to the care of the patient and toys are a fundamental part of family-centred, development-friendly units and wards. Bringing a child's own toys for sole use may be an option, particularly if the child is found to be colonised by an infectious pathogen. If this is the case, then isolation is necessary in a cubicle or incubator, thereby removing some risk of the communal nature of hospitalisation. Additional precautions would also need to be undertaken, as discussed later in this chapter. It is worth remembering that such isolation can also prove to be a risk for infection, particularly in neonates who spend their first weeks or months inside a warm, often moist, environment. This environment is a perfect incubation area for pathogens; therefore risks must be minimised by changing incubators regularly as per local policy.

Recognition and diagnosis of infection

The swift recognition of infection or risk of infection in highly dependent infants and children is vital if its effect on the body is to be minimised and its spread contained. The diagnosis of specific pathogens is not immediately obtained, though screening is important for sensitivity testing and therefore ultimately appropriate antimicrobial therapies. The list of infection signs below is in no way exhaustive, but gives an indication of the huge range of infection markers and the response the body has to invasion by pathogens. This is particularly true of young children or those who are very sick, who have little or no verbal communication skills. Parents and nursing staff can often pick up when patients do not seem to be themselves. This allows nursing and medical care to be optimised, preventing further harm to the patient and further distress to the family.

It is important to note that these signs and symptoms are not always triggered by toxins secreted by pathogens, but rather as a result of the body's response to pathogen invasion.

Signs of infection

- Pyrexia
- Pain
- Lethargy
- Irritability
- Altered skin colour – pallor/flushed/cyanosed
- Increase in secretions
- Change in consistency/colour of secretions (thick/green, etc.)
- Core – toe temperature gap
- Altered vital signs
- Increased incidence of apnoea/desaturation/ bradycardia
- Reduced feed tolerance (vomiting/bile aspirates/ abdominal distension or discomfort)
- Elimination changes (diarrhoea/lack of bowel motion/offensive odour/colour/ward urinalysis changes/pain)
- Rashes (N.B. few rashes are indicative of serious infection)
- Inflammation and erythema

- Visible exudates
- Development/increased need of oxygen or ventilator support

Infection screen

In some patients the source of infection may be more obvious than in others. If an obvious source can be identified then the process of specimen sampling may be swift and reasonably simple. However, some sampling methods are more painful or more laborious than others. Below are some infection screening procedures:

- Lumbar puncture
- Supra-pubic aspiration or mid-stream urine
- Blood tests (include culture, CRP, FBC, U&Es and gas)
- Radiography (X-rays/ultrasound)
- Swabs – eyes/throat/nose/skin lesion/entry sites to body (catheter/central line/gastrostomy/ tracheostomy)
- Stool culture
- Naso-pharyngeal aspirate
- Sputum culture
- Tips of lines/tubes (e.g. endo-tracheal tube, longline)

However, if the source of the infection is not clear then a general infection screen may be undertaken. Infection screens often have many elements of the procedures listed above, though not all of them have to be utilised if medical and nursing staff feel they are not necessary or if it is clear that the patient is too sick to tolerate the procedures involved.

Specimen collection and laboratory techniques

Nurses spend a great deal of their time collecting specimens. To ensure this is not time wasted and to increase the likelihood of disease detection there needs to be some awareness and compliance with laboratory requirements. The type of specimen container used will determine the acceptable delay

allowed before processing the specimen in the laboratory. An example is the common use of sterile universal containers for urine, instead of a urine container with boric acid. A boric acid container places the urine sample into 'stasis', affording the time needed to get the specimen to the laboratory. However, these bottles require a minimum urine sample of 10 mL. This is not always possible if collecting from preterm infants or highly dependent children who may be suffering from oliguria. If a sample must be placed in a universal container for insufficiency reasons, it should be taken to the laboratory promptly; otherwise there is an increased risk of false results. Urine bag samples are also liable to give false results if a sterile sample is needed for microscopy, culture and sensitivity (mc&s). A urethral catheter sample is often useful as it should be a sterile sample. Supra-pubic aspiration (SPA) sample is a gold standard for urine sampling, but is very invasive. A mid-stream urine (MSU) sample into a sterile field is the least invasive method, but is often unsuccessful in younger children.

In general, swabs, secretions, endo-tracheal tube tips and intravenous line tips should arrive at the laboratory within 4 hours of being taken. If this is not possible, certain specimens may be placed in a refrigerator without significant detriment to the culture results. Notable exceptions to this are specimens looking for delicate organisms such as *Neisseria gonorrhoeae*, blood culture bottles and certain virological studies such as *Chlamydia trachomatis* isolation. In these cases the transport of the specimen direct to the laboratory specimen reception should be arranged and, if outside normal working hours, consideration must be given to contacting the laboratory to arrange for processing urgently or appropriate storage upon receipt.

The details provided by medical and nursing staff on request forms is of great importance in determining the extent of investigation undertaken and the significance placed on any findings in the laboratory. Date of onset of symptoms, duration of illness, other predisposing medical conditions, all recent and current

Table 11.2 Examples of Gram stain reaction and bacterial morphology of bacterial pathogens.

Gram reaction and morphology	Common pathogens
Gram positive cocci	*Staphylococcus aureus* β-haemolytic streptococci
Gram positive bacilli	*Listeria monocytogenes* Clostridia group such as *Clostridium difficile*
Gram negative bacilli	*Escherichia coli* *Pseudomonas aeruginosa*
Gram negative cocci	*Neisseria gonorrhoeae*
Gram negative cocco-bacilli	*Haemophilus influenzae*

antimicrobial therapy, as well as a full description of specimen site and the patient's details will all influence the final laboratory report and should therefore be included, wherever possible.

The Gram stain

The Gram stain is a laboratory technique that allows visualisation of certain micro-organisms and human cells. When performed directly on specimens, this stain can give an indication of the cellular response to infection (i.e. presence of leucocytes) as well as the type of bacteria/fungi present. The Gram stain also has a use in the preliminary identification of bacteria according to their Gram reaction. Examples of Gram stain reactions for commonly encountered pathogens are given in Table 11.2. The morphology of bacteria is also included in a Gram stain result to aid any presumptive diagnosis of infection.

Pathogens and disease

Pathogens that invade the body are usually categorised into four groups:

- Bacteria
- Viruses
- Protozoa
- Fungi

Bacteria

Bacteria are single-celled micro-organisms with no nucleus. They contain a capsule within their cell wall, which protects them from human granulocytes.

Viruses

Viruses are parasitic micro-organisms that can only reproduce within living cells. Unlike bacteria, viruses have a centre of genetic material of either DNA (deoxyribonucleic acid) or RNA (ribonucleic acid) (see Table 11.3).

Protozoa

Protozoa are primitive single-celled animals which are parasitic and disease causing. Malaria is a protozoan.

Fungi

Fungi are eukaryotic cells and are made up of a number of hyphae (thread-like structures). They reproduce by means of spores.

Pathogens

Methicillin/multiple resistant *Staphylococcus aureus* (MRSA)

This can be found in skin folds, perineum, axillae and anterior nares. It commonly survives in these places without causing infection. A patient becomes clinically infected with MRSA when the organism breaks the skin barrier and proliferates to cause a systemic response. Children with indwelling equipment are at particular risk of contracting MRSA and if signs of infection are suspected at these sites, MRSA must

Table 11.3 Classification of virus.

Family	Type	Examples of virus/disease
Adenoviruses	DNA	Tonsillitis, respiratory tract infections, conjunctivitis
Papovaviruses	DNA	Benign tumours (e.g. warts), some cancers
Herpesviruses	DNA	CMV, chickenpox, glandular fever
Picornaviruses	RNA	Myocarditis, meningitis, common cold
Retroviruses	RNA	AIDS, leukaemia. Can convert RNA into DNA
Orthomyxoviruses	RNA	Influenza (fever, cough, sore throat)
Paramyxoviruses	RNA	Mumps, measles, croup, respiratory synctial virus (RSV)

Adapted from Dorling Kindersley Human Body (2001).

be considered. If, after formal diagnosis, treatment is indicated then the antibiotic of choice is often vancomycin. This antibiotic must be given intravenously and needs levels monitoring as it is excreted by the kidneys and absorption can be variable.

Clostridium difficile (C-Diff)

This bacterium tends to proliferate in individuals who have undergone antimicrobial therapy, particularly with cephalosporins and clindamycin (McConnell 2002). This occurs because the bacterium has less competition from the normal flora of the gut, which has been suppressed by such anti-microbial therapies. It is an anaerobic, Gram-positive bacterium and it produces spores that can remain in the environment for long periods of time. The pathogen commonly exists in infants without causing symptoms as the toxins it produces do not affect their immature intestinal cells (DH 2007).

It is also found in some individual's guts alongside the natural micro-flora. However, in vulnerable children and young adults, the toxins produced by the microbe can cause profuse diarrhoea, sometimes with associated colitis and even peritonitis. It is transmitted from patient to patient by direct contact, via staff or an infected environment. Diligent infection control measures will control the spread (for example, hand washing, patient isolation, and use of chlor-clean for

the environment, gloves and aprons). Alcohol, common disinfectants, acids, drying and heating do not kill the spores of *C. difficile* (Hall and Horsley 2007). The use of anti-diarrhoeal therapy is not indicated as it may predispose patients to mega-colon and delay clearance of the toxins (McConnell 2002).

Human immuno-deficiency virus (HIV)

This virus destroys CD_4 'helper' lymphocytes and as cell numbers are reduced the immune system struggles to fight opportunistic pathogens. The virus also interferes with humoral immunity by making B-cells and macrophages dysfunctional. Congenital infection with HIV is now relatively rare owing to an effective prophylaxis management regime with antiretroviral agents for mothers and newborn infants. However, as a result of undiagnosed pregnancy, non-compliance with medication, breastfeeding, modern migration patterns and the improved health of women with HIV, the children's nurse is at some point likely to care for a child with HIV. If hospital treatment is required for these children, it is important that staff be aware of the child's increased susceptibility to infection, and provide care appropriately. Any specimens sent to the laboratory from an HIV positive patient/patient at high risk of developing HIV from the mother should have 'high risk' status made clear upon them.

Hepatitis B virus (HBV)

Congenital HBV infection is predominantly a perinatal infection since intra-uterine infection accounts for less than 5% of cases. The HBV can be acute or chronic. With acute infection, the virus is spontaneously cleared by the body's immune system within weeks to months. However, neonates and children are much less likely than adults to clear the infection. Almost 100% of newborns and 50% of children that contract the HBV will develop chronic hepatitis (NICE 2006). The main clinical significance of chronic HBV infection is the long-term sequelae of cirrhosis and hepato-cellular carcinoma. Studies have shown that, unlike HIV, breastfeeding by HBV-positive mothers is not contra-indicated and should therefore not be discouraged.

Staphylococcus aureus

Staphylococcus aureus is a Gram-positive coccus responsible for a wide range of infections. Since the organism is ubiquitously distributed in the environment, colonisation of the nose and skin occurs readily. The most common manifestations of Staphylococcus infection are conjunctivitis and skin infections, although abscesses, osteomyelitis, septicaemia and respiratory infections can also occur. Infections usually respond to flucloxacillin, but certain MRSA strains must be treated differently.

Pseudomonas aeruginosa

Pseudomonas is a Gram-negative bacillus. Favourable conditions for the growth of this bacillus include warm, humidified environments. Therefore, those children with a tracheostomy or those requiring respiratory support via a humidified circuit are at increased risk. Humidified circuits should be changed weekly at a minimum and weekly tube changes especially for tracheostomy patients should be adhered to.

Planned endo-tracheal tube changes may alter in length depending upon individual units and patient status. One characteristic of P. aeruginosa is the production of green pigments, which when visible in infected secretions and discharges and accompanied by the rancid smell of heavy Pseudomonas infection, may assist diagnosis before laboratory reports are available.

Respiratory synctial virus (RSV)

This virus is particularly common in infants and young children, especially during the winter months. In mild infection, rhinorrhoea and coughing are the most common symptoms. In severe infection, bronchiolitis is seen and fluid and/or respiratory support may be required. Severe RSV infection can render a child highly dependent. It is worthy of note though that RSV infection can occur in an already highly dependent child as a nosocomial infection, and this is particularly true in neonates and those who are immune suppressed. Infants with suspected or proven RSV infection should be nursed in isolation; older children can be cluster nursed and appropriate infection control measures put in place. Vaccination of vulnerable infants and young children should be considered.

Examples of infectious diseases

Bacterial meningitis is categorised by the inflammation of the meninges covering the spinal cord and brain. The most common infective agents are Neisseria meningitidis and Streptococcus pneumoniae. Haemophilus influenza type b (Hib) was once a common causative agent, but since the introduction of the Hib vaccine numbers of cases have been significantly reduced. Neisseria meningitidis (meningococcal) has 13 known subgroups, with group B being the most common, for which there is no vaccine. Meningococcal meningitis is particularly serious as there can be rapid progression to septicaemia and shock (refer to Chapter 2). *Streptococcus pneumoniae* is less common owing to the introduction of a pneumococcal vaccine into the childhood immunisation programme. In newborns, group B *Streptococcus* and *E. coli* are the most common infective agents causing meningitis. Antenatal screening for group B *Streptococcus* is increasingly common and successful.

Pneumonia is a reasonably common condition in children and infants, but does not have a universally accepted definition, largely because microbiological identification of bacterial pathogens in the lower respiratory tract is very difficult without invasive procedures (Haque 2007). Consequentially, diagnosis is primarily based upon clinical and radiological signs. These are often difficult to interpret as bronchiolitis can often give a similar clinical picture (Haque 2007).

Urinary tract infection (UTI) is a very common condition in children, and is the second most common association in children presenting with febrile convulsions (Haque 2007). To diagnose a UTI, laboratory/dipstick testing must be accompanied by clinical symptoms. Highly dependent children requiring catheterisation are at an increased risk of UTI, so close observation of the site should be employed and catheters passed with an aseptic technique. Daily dipsticks may be done whilst the catheterised child is hospitalised in order to monitor for any pathological signs of infection, such as leucocytes, nitrites, blood and protein. It is worthy of note that these signs individually may not be indicative of infection (especially in neonates) but when found in conjunction with one another, and other symptoms, may be significant.

Severe combined immunodeficiency disease (SCID) is characterised by a lack of humoral and cell-mediated immunity. These children are very susceptible to infection. It is usually suspected if a child has repeated infections, infections from rare pathogens, or after failure to recover from an infection (Hockenberry and Wong 2003). The only treatments are supportive, such as the administration of IV immunoglobulins and preventing the child from particularly risky activities in terms of pathogen colonisation. This of course is difficult the older the child becomes, from a social and developmental aspect. If admitted to hospital very strict isolation rules must be put in place to protect the child from serious infection.

Treatment of infection

The mainstay treatment for infection remains antimicrobial therapy. However, many serious systemic infections often require complex supportive care in addition to appropriate antimicrobial therapy because of the multiple destructive effects a pathogen invasion can have on the human body.

If infection has been suspected sufficient to warrant screening, it would be poor practice to then not prescribe and deliver antibiotics immediately. Antibiotics should be prescribed based upon clinical symptoms and individual hospital policy. Once cultures and results of tests have been completed, discussions with microbiologists may prove vital in treating any infection found. Antibiotic therapy may need altering to cover certain pathogens and some antibiotics need microbiology approval to be used for any length of time. It is of note that microbiology results will not usually be available until 24–48 hours after the sample has reached the laboratory, and specific sensitivity testing often takes a further 24 hours.

Antibiotics are used not only to treat current infection, but also often on patients for prophylactic purposes, e.g. after major or invasive surgery. Prophylaxis is used in neonates in whom there is an inherent risk from the mother, e.g. with group B *Streptococcus* presence or a premature rupture of membranes (particularly if more than 48 hours). It is also used when infants are born prematurely or with low birth weight.

Oral versus intravenous antibiotic therapy

Oral antibiotic therapy is not commonly used in sick neonates due to the risk of poor absorption, complications of altering gut pH and increasing the risk of necrotising enterocolitis. In paediatrics, oral antibiotics are used frequently, though their use in the acute highly dependent child is limited, as a great deal of serious infections often have a systemic element to their infective status and therefore require swift production of therapeutic levels of antibiotic.

Preventing transmission of infection

Standard principles

Hand hygiene

Meticulous hand washing by staff and visitors is a vital process in breaking the infection cycle and is regarded as the most successful and cost effective way of controlling nosocomial infection (Gould *et al.* 2007). Despite hand washing being a simple measure, it has compliance rates as low as 50% (Creedon 2005). Research suggests that staff members do not wash hands enough, at the right time or employ optimal technique. As a result many Trusts implement audits and campaigns to highlight the importance of effective and timely hand washing. A multifaceted, multidisciplinary approach to this education has been found moderately, but consistently, effective (Naikoba and Hayward 2001; Creedon 2005). These conclusions have been made in the literature both historically and currently and would suggest that interventions to increase compliance are not overly successful. The problem of effective hand washing is a continuing issue.

Staff members have reported certain issues that inhibit their ability to wash hands effectively, such as dermatitis and associated skin problems. Contributing factors to this occurrence include the frequency of washing, the products used, water temperature and inadequate drying (Pellowe 2007). Some of these factors can be improved upon by staff members themselves, such as the drying of hands and the use of adequate water temperature (Pellowe 2007). Other factors could be improved by hospitals such as the use of good soap and hand creams.

Hand washing is not the only aspect of hand hygiene that is very important in preventing the transmission of infection. Other notable aspects include the use of artificial nails, nail polish, fingernail length and the wearing of jewellery. The wearing of artificial nails and jewellery (particularly jewelled rings and wrist watches) is not recommended as part of good practice in infection control. They inhibit good hand washing, they can tear gloves and they harbour high percentages of micro-organisms. Infection control policies also recommend that fingernails be short and clean, as higher proportions of microbes are found in those with longer nails. The evidence regarding the wearing of nail polish is limited. Ward (2007) suggests that wearing nail polish *per se* is not an issue as no more microbes were found on nail polish than on natural nails. The problem develops with chipped nail varnish in which microbes can collect and multiply in the uneven surface (Ward 2007).

Protective equipment

Gloves should be worn whenever a healthcare professional's risk assessment suggests possible contact with the mucous membranes, bodily fluids, blood, secretions/excretions or non-intact skin of a patient. They should also be worn when handling sharp/contaminated equipment or sterile sites and during invasive procedures. This precaution should be undertaken regardless of whether a patient is infected with a known pathogen or not. It is suggested that it is the unknown patient who poses the greatest risk to staff and other patients in terms of infection transmission; therefore universal precautions must be adhered to. When gloves are removed, hands should be decontaminated as appropriate. Gloves do not negate the need for effective hand washing.

According to the most up-to-date NICE guideline (2003), plastic aprons should be worn when the risk of uniforms becoming soiled with blood, bodily fluids or secretions/excretions is present. Some intensive care settings are, in fact, taking this protocol one step further, utilising plastic aprons upon all close contact with patients, such as in moving and handling procedures. The need for face masks, eye protection, respiratory equipment and full body clothing should be assessed by healthcare professionals on an individual basis, founded upon their own risk assessment. This could be made in conjunction with appropriately trained staff, such as infection control nurses and microbiologists.

Use and disposal of sharps

Intravenous medication administration now allows for the use of a 'needle-less' system. This reduces the risk and occurrence of sharps injuries (particularly from 'dirty' sharps) significantly. Despite this, accidents still occur and all sharps injuries should be appropriately reported regardless of circumstance, even if the needle is clean, as it is important for occupational health services to log the rates of injury in order that new standards may be implemented to reduce these. NICE (2003) recommendations for safe needle handling include: never re-sheath a needle, never pass sharps from hand to hand and dispose of sharps in appropriate containers which are not overfilled. Sharps should also be disposed of quickly and by the health professional having used them, as only he/she will know that all have been accounted for and disposed of appropriately. Between use, sharps containers should be closed and they should be secured out of the reach of mobile children.

Source isolation

If a patient is suspected of or formally diagnosed with an infectious illness, as outlined by local hospital policies and national guidelines, then strict isolation measures must be put in place to protect patients and staff from transmission. Children in high dependency areas must be placed in cubicles, as appropriate. Aprons and gloves should be placed outside the door of the cubicle and designated linen and clinical waste bins should be made available inside the cubicle itself. All linen and clinical waste bags must then be 'double-bagged' immediately outside the cubicle so that they may be safely moved through the ward and around the hospital. An infection control alert should also be placed upon the entrance to the cubicle so that staff and visitors have an understanding of the requirements upon them to prevent transmission. An infection control team referral should also be made at this time for monitoring purposes.

The 'cubicle crises' of the winter months are often stressful periods for those staff involved in the admission process, and the infection control team are often called upon to facilitate decisions regarding the appropriate transfer of children out of cubicles.

Recent moves to reduce hospital acquired infection (HAI) rates

The introduction of 'modern matron' posts within the NHS was designed to improve the patient experience, one example of which was the hope that they would implement and oversee measures to reduce HAI rates. The Healthcare Commission and the Health Act were established in 2006 to implement a code of practice for the prevention and control of HAIs. The commission is currently embarking on a programme of unannounced hospital visits. Trusts found to be failing from an infection control perspective will be issued with 'improvement notices'.

Conclusion

The diagnosis, treatment and care of highly dependent children with infection are complex subjects that have been given an overview in this chapter, but due to their magnitude this should not be considered exhaustive. In cases of infection caused by pathogens that are not detailed here or where further knowledge is required, the bibliography may be of some use. Drawing on these resources will allow the children's nurse to not only deliver care in a more informed way, but also support families who will need reassurance if their child is to be protected from or is ill due to infection.

Glossary

Term	Definition
Agranulocytes	White blood cells with no granules in their cytoplasm. There are two types: monocytes and lymphocytes
Bacillus	Rod-shaped bacterial cell
Coccus	Bacterium that is almost spherical in shape. It divides and arranges itself into specific patterns, allowing for specific identification
Complement	Series of enzymes present in serum that, when activated by antibodies, produce widespread inflammatory effects as well as lysis of bacteria
Congenital infection	Infection present at birth
Cytokines	A group of proteins and peptides that act as a chemical signalling service for cells
Dendritic cells	Function as antigen-presenting cells. When activated by pathogens they transfer to lymphoid tissues where they aid in the adaptive immune response
Gram positive	Have thick cell walls
Gram negative	Have thin cell walls that have a toxic element within them that stimulates the innate response and cytokine release
Granulocytes	A type of leucocyte (white blood cell) that has a lobed nucleus and a granulated cytoplasm. Produced in the bone marrow. Examples: neutrophils, basophils and eosinophils
Herd immunity	The proportion of a community that has to be immunised for those who have not been immunised to be protected
Interleukins	A group of cytokines
Langerhan cells	Dendritic cells that act as antigen-presenting cells in certain tissues
Lymphocyte	Small cell in the blood, tissues and lymph that 'polices' the body for non-self material. It can recognise individual antigens and divide into numerous cells of identical specificity. They also have a long lifespan
B-lymphocytes	Secrete antibodies
T-lymphocytes	Thymus derived. 'Help' B-lymphocyte cells kill infected cells and activate macrophages
Lysis	Cell membrane damage causing leakage of cell contents. In the case of bacteria, this is fatal
Mast cells	Basophils that inhabit tissues
Monocytes	Known as macrophages once they leave the blood stream and enter tissues
Natural killer cells	Lymphocytes found in the blood. Kill infected host cells
Pathogen	Disease-causing organism
Phagocytes	Cells that engulf particles/non-self cells into their cytoplasm where they are contained within a vacuole and digested by enzymes

Chapter 12

CARE OF THE CHILD WITH HAEMATOLOGICAL AND ONCOLOGICAL CONDITIONS

Karen Selwood, Michelle Wright and Doreen Crawford

Introduction

This chapter focuses on children who have haematological and oncological conditions and need high dependency support, care and monitoring. The chapter reviews the more common malignant conditions of childhood and considers the main treatment strategies and the many complications of these. The more common haematological conditions such as sickle cell anaemia and idiopathic thrombocytopenia are considered.

Background to the malignant conditions of childhood

Cancer occurs when cells within the body rapidly multiply and become out of control. These cells are no longer able to function effectively and as their numbers increase they form a lump or tumour. When cancer cells break away from their original site and spread to other parts of the body they may produce secondary tumours known as metastases (Children's Cancer and Leukaemia Group (CCLG) 2007). Cancer is the leading cause of death, by disease, in childhood (National Cancer Institute 2007), although it is rare and only 1 in 600 children under the age of 15 years develops the disease (CCLG 2007). There are approximately 1700 new cases of

paediatric cancer annually in the UK (CCLG 2007). These statistics are based on children from 0 to 15 years; however, many regional paediatric units also look after adolescents as their outcomes are more favourable with paediatric treatments as apposed to adult protocols.

Causes of cancer in children

There are no clear answers as to what causes cancer. There have been suggestions that there may be a link with electromagnetic fields or environmental pollutants. However, there is no clear evidence (Plon and Peterson 1997). Some children are more at risk than others. Children with Down's syndrome are more likely to suffer from leukaemia. Children who have Beckwith–Wiedemann syndrome have an increased risk of developing hepatoblastoma, Wilm's tumour and rhabdomyosarcomas and are followed up regularly (Shafford and Pritchard 2004). Some paediatric cancers are hereditary such as retinoblastoma and some medical conditions such as neurofibromatosis can increase a child's risk of developing certain tumours; however, both are rare.

Development of treatment strategies

Paediatric cancer treatments have progressed. In the 1960s the cure rate for children with cancer was only 3 in 10, compared with today's rate of 7 in 10 (CCLG 2007). The success of paediatric oncology treatments can be attributed to clinical trials. Treatments within oncology are advised by protocol, based on randomised and controlled trials. There are several current trials aimed at improving the survival of children with cancer and the focus of many of these has moved towards event-free survival with a reduction in long-term side effects (CCLG 2007).

Types of paediatric cancer

Wilm's tumour

Wilm's tumour is a malignant tumour of the kidney. The majority of children diagnosed are under the age of 7. Treatment includes a combination of surgery, chemotherapy and occasionally radiotherapy depending on the stage of the disease. Staging of the disease is done at the time of surgery and will depend on the histopathology of the resected kidney. Overall survival of a child with a Wilm's tumour is about 90% depending on the stage of the disease reached (Metzger and Dome 2005).

Non-Hodgkin's lymphoma (NHL)

The number of children suffering from NHL has increased over the years. It is a malignancy of the lymphoid cells and is classified into several categories (Lymphoma Information Network 2007):

- Burkitt's lymphoma – 40%
- Large B-cell lymphoma – 20%
- Anaplastic large cell lymphoma – 10%
- Lymphoblastic lymphoma – 30%

NHL has a peak incidence between the ages of 7 and 10. Staging (from 1 to 4) is dependent upon the site or sites of disease at diagnosis, but if the bone marrow or central nervous system are involved they are automatically at stage 4. The most common primary site is the abdomen (30–45%) followed by the mediastinum (25–35%). Until recent years NHL had a very poor prognosis, with many children dying following diagnosis; however, improvements in chemotherapy, surgery and occasionally radiotherapy have increased survival rates dramatically (Patte 2004). Chemotherapy is the treatment of choice often accompanied by surgery of the residual mass. Indications for radiotherapy are rare and often only used in emergency situations (Patte 2004).

Hodgkin's disease

Hodgkin's disease is a malignancy of the lymphatic system and usually affects children over the age of 5. Sixty to seventy percent of children present with enlarged cervical nodes; other areas are the axilla (10–15%) and the groin (6–12%), with the inguinal nodes being affected (Hoffbrand and Pettit 1997). Staging of the disease is dependent on the extent of the disease at presentation and whether there is dissemination. Treatment depends on staging and mainly consists of chemotherapy and radiotherapy. The prognosis for Hodgkin's disease is excellent, with a 95–100% cure rate at 5 years (McDowell et al. 2004).

Leukaemia

Leukaemia is the most common form of paediatric cancer, representing around 30% of all childhood cancers (Smith and Hann 2004). The word leukaemia refers to cancer of the blood-forming or haematopoietic tissues (Colby-Graham and Chordas 2003). Leukaemia is classified in terms of the prominent cell line affected and whether it is chronic or acute.

Acute lymphoblastic leukaemia (ALL) accounts for approximately 75% of all childhood leukaemia and myeloblastic/myeloid leukaemia (AML) accounts for 15–20%. Chronic leukaemia is a less rapidly progressing disease, with chronic myeloid leukaemia accounting for 5% of paediatric leukaemias (Altman and Fu 2006). The prognosis for children with ALL has increased dramatically over recent years, with event-free survival being approximately 80%. AML has approximately a 60% disease-free survival rate. Chemotherapy is the main type of treatment for leukaemia; however, the regimes are very different depending on the type of leukaemia. Radiotherapy has a role in the treatment of central nervous system disease, but this is not common. Clinical features of childhood leukaemia relate to the inhibition of normal cell production owing to leukaemia cell replacement within the bone marrow (Smith and Hann 2004).

Neuroblastoma

Neuroblastoma represents approximately 10% of all solid malignancies in children, however it is the most common malignant tumour seen in early childhood (Pearson and Pinkerton 2004). Neuroblastoma is derived from nerve cells, initially developing in the adrenal glands and commonly spreading throughout the abdomen and throughout the body. This is a malignant condition with a high mortality rate. Poor prognostic factors include diagnosis over the age of 18 months, tumour stage and biological features, including the amplification of the MYCN myelocyto matosis viral-related oncogene proto-oncogene (Kushner and Cheung 2005). Sixty per cent of patients present stage 4 disease including bone metastases and bone marrow disease and have only a 20% survival rate. Treatment includes chemotherapy, radiotherapy, surgery and stem cell rescue.

Bone tumours

Ewing's sarcoma and osteosarcoma represent over 90% of all childhood and adolescent primary bone tumours (Whelan and Morland 2004). Treatment is a challenge for the child, family and carers, involving intensive chemotherapy, reconstructive limb-salvage surgery or amputation and radiotherapy (Whelan and Morland 2004). The most common site to develop a Ewing's sarcoma in childhood is the pelvic area, followed by the femur. The most common sites for osteosarcomas are the femur, tibia or humerus. Prognosis depends on the presence of metastasis, the size of the tumour and the histological findings following removal of the tumour (Whelan and Morland 2004).

Central nervous system tumours

Tumours of the central nervous system represent 20% of paediatric cancers, with the highest percentage of cancer-related death and significant associated morbidity (Hargrave et al. 2004). There are around 100 different types of brain tumour, which are generally named after the type of cell they developed from or the area that they have grown in. Examples of common paediatric brain tumours are astrocytoma/glioma, ependymoma and primitive neuroectodermal tumour (PNET) and the most common of these is medulloblastoma. Treatment can include surgery, radiotherapy or chemotherapy or a combination of all three depending on the type of tumour.

Retinoblastoma

Retinoblastoma is a malignant tumour of the retina of the eye. It is a disease of infancy and is often picked up quickly by health visitors, midwives, GPs or from parental concerns, with a white reflex or white pupil being observed (Melamud et al. 2005). In 40% of children it is inherited. Non-inherited tumours tend to be unilateral but bilateral disease can occur. Treatment depends on the size and location of the tumour and the extent of disease progression at diagnosis, with the primary aim of saving the child's life and secondarily saving the eye. Commonly enucleation or removal of the eye is required with or without adjuvant treatment such as laser therapy, chemotherapy, cryotherapy, thermotherapy or radiotherapy. Prognosis for children with retinoblastoma is very good especially if detected early.

Soft-tissue sarcomas

Soft-tissue sarcomas consist of a group of malignancies that involve a variety of tissues within the body, including contractile, connective and supportive tissues (Carli *et al.* 2004).

Rhabdomyosarcoma

Rhabdomyosarcoma accounts for approximately half of all soft-tissue sarcomas in children and young adults and arises from primitive muscle cells and can develop anywhere within the body. There is a presumption that there are micrometastases at diagnosis and this influences treatment. Treatment is primarily chemotherapy with local control which may involve both surgery and radiotherapy (Breitfield and Mayer 2005). Prognosis depends on the site of original presentation and extent of disease but is between 50 and 70% (Flamant *et al.* 1998).

Non-rhabdomyosarcoma

Non-rhabdomyosarcoma is rarer and mainly consists of extraosseous Ewing's sarcomas, malignant peripheral nerve sheath tumours, fibrosarcoma and synovial sarcomas. Treatment depends on the type of disease but can include all modalities already mentioned. Prognosis varies depending on the type of tumour (Carli *et al.* 2004).

Hepatoblastoma

Hepatoblastoma is a malignant tumour, of embryological origin, affecting the liver and accounts for 2–5% of paediatric cancers (Shafford and Pritchard 2004). The majority of children who develop hepatoblastomas are under the age of five years, with the disease being more common in girls than boys. Treatment consists of a combination of surgery and chemotherapy and staging is related to the degree of metastases present at diagnosis and if complete resection was possible at surgery. Children with a complete resection at surgery have an 80% survival rate (Shafford and Pritchard 2004).

Chemotherapy and the cell cycle

This section briefly reviews cell replication and division. For further details of mitosis and diagrammatical representation of these cell phases readers are referred to the anatomy and physiology (A&P) textbook of their choice. Both malignant and normal healthy cells go through the same five steps in preparation for cell division – stages G0, G1, S, G2 and M.

G0 is often referred to as the resting phase, where cells lie dormant and are not actively involved in the reproductive cycle. Most normal cells spend the majority of their time in the resting phase and are only recruited back into the cell cycle in response to stimuli, e.g. hormones or growth factors.

G1 is the first active phase in the cell cycle and is characterised by the production of ribonucleic acid (RNA), enzymes and proteins, which are all required in the later stages of the cell cycle.

The S phase involves deoxyribonucleic acid (DNA) synthesis and the amount of DNA is doubled. In the G2 phase, cells are preparing for mitosis, with continual RNA synthesis and mitotic spindle construction; this phase is very much characterised by growth and the final preparations for cell division. The cell cycle is concluded with cell division and the production of two daughter cells – the M stage (Young 1999; Morgan 2003).

A basic understanding of the cell cycle is important to understand how chemotherapy works. Chemotherapy is a chemical agent which has anti-cancer or cytotoxic (cell killing) properties. It is used with the aim of eradicating or controlling the growth of cancer cells. Chemotherapy is given orally or intravenously, depending on the diagnosis and protocol. As a powerful agent it has a systemic effect on the whole body.

Cancer is a disease of uncontrolled or abnormal cell growth. The aim of treating a malignancy with chemotherapy is to find the drugs that the disease is sensitive to and then use them at appropriate intervals to treat the malignancy. This is usually done in the form of a clinical trial

Table 12.1 Chemotherapy agents.

Cytotoxic drug	Effect on the cell cycle	Common side effects
Alkylating drugs		
Cyclophosphamide	Cell cycle non-specific	Bone marrow suppression
Ifosfamide		Hair loss
Busulfan		Nausea and vomiting
Melphalan		Haemorrhagic cystitis
Cisplatin	Cell cycle non-specific	As above, plus hearing loss
Carboplatin		
Cytotoxic antibiotics		
Bleomycin	Cell cycle specific	Bone marrow suppression
Dactinomycin (actinomycin D)		Heart muscle toxicity
Daunorubicin		Nausea and vomiting
Doxorubicin		Hair loss
Epirubicin		
Mitoxantrone (mitozantrone)		
Antimetabolites		
Cytarabine (cytosine)	Cell cycle specific. Most active during the	Mucositis
Fludarabine	S phase of the cell cycle	Liver toxicity
Mercaptopurine		Renal toxicity (methotrexate)
Thioguanine (tioguanine)		Fever (cytosine and fludarabine)
Methotrexate		
Vinca alkaloids		
Vincristine	Cell cycle specific	Peripheral neuropathy
Vinblastine		(e.g. jaw pain, foot drop)
Vinorelbine		Constipation
		Paralytic ileus
		Seizures
Miscellaneous		
Asparaginase	Not a cytotoxic drug. It is an enzyme that deprives leukaemia cells of essential nutrients so that they die	Anaphylaxis
		Pancreatitis
		Coagulopathy
		Liver dysfunction
Etoposide	Inhibits DNA synthesis in S and G2 phases	Bone marrow suppression
Dexamethasone (steroid)	Pharmacological action uncertain	Gastrointestinal effects
		Musculoskeletal effects
		Diabetes
		Hypertension
		Avascular necrosis
		Cushing's syndrome
		Neuropsychiatric effects

where all drugs and treatment processes are then monitored in response to efficacy, side effects and outcomes. There are several different groups of cytotoxic drugs. They all have different actions and side effects (see Table 12.1).

Radiotherapy

Radiotherapy can be used individually as the sole mode of treatment for certain paediatric cancers, or with adjuncts such as surgery, chemotherapy or, in some cases, all three (Hopkins 1999). Radiotherapy is commonly used in the treatment of paediatric tumours such as rhabdomyosarcomas, Ewing's sarcomas, Hodgkin's disease, neuroblastoma, leukaemia with central nervous system involvement and Wilm's tumour.

Radiotherapy also has an important palliative role to play in controlling the symptoms of progressive disease (Hopkins 1999). Radiation is described as the transference of energy from one point to another (Hopkins 1999). Radiotherapy uses targeted high energy rays to kill cancer cells by damaging the cells' internal molecules. When radiotherapy rays hit a molecule, the bonds holding electrons together break up, forming free radicals. Free radicals are very unstable and attack the nearest molecule, causing cell damage (Cancer Research UK 2007).

Because of its action, radiation therapy has to be exact; it is applied directly to the tumour site or the metatastic area. With the use of computed tomography and magnetic resonance imaging the ability to define a target volume that tightly conforms to the tumour shape is increased. This accuracy means that high doses are given directly to the tumour and not to any healthy tissue. As treatment is more accurate there are fewer risks of complications (Symonds 2001). Total body irradiation is used in the preparation for bone marrow transplantation.

Side effects

These include both short-term and long-term effects. The effects depend on the organ receiving treatment and the type of radiotherapy. Although radiotherapy is applied to the treatment area, non-cancerous cells can also be damaged. For example, short-term side effects of abdominal radiotherapy include abdominal cramps, nausea, vomiting and diarrhoea; long-term effects include infertility (Hopkins 1999).

Surgery

Surgery is an effective method of removing a solid tumour. Paediatric malignancies such as neuroblastoma, osteosarcomas, Ewing's sarcoma, Wilm's tumour, hepatoblastomas and brain tumours require surgery in combination with chemotherapy and/or radiotherapy. Children with brain tumours often require surgery at diagnosis, whereas children with osteosarcoma will have chemotherapy to reduce the tumour followed by surgery. The effect that chemotherapy has on that removed tumour will dictate the degree of chemotherapy the child will receive.

Novel therapies

Traditional treatments of chemotherapy, surgery and radiotherapy for children with a malignancy are not always sufficient to successfully treat and cure some malignancies. A variety of 'newer' therapies is emerging and application of these may benefit children in the future.

Molecular-targeted therapies

These inhibit tumour growth and progression without harming healthy, rapidly dividing cells and include monoclonal antibodies and tyrosine kinase inhibitors.

Gene therapy

Gene therapy is the process of transferring selected genes into a host with the hope of halting or curing a disease (Robertson and Fritz 1996). It can be used to destroy cancer by correcting a genetic defect, manipulating genes or both (Reiger 2001).

Tumour vaccines

Vaccination involves administration of an agent that stimulates the immune system to react against the foreign substances (antigens) of the vaccine. The person will then develop immunity. Subsequent exposure to the antigen will then initiate an immune response to destroy the antigen (Muehlbauer and Schwartzentruber 2003). The development and deployment of a vaccine against the human papilloma virus that causes cervical cancer will make an impact on this disease.

Stem cell rescue/bone marrow transplantation

This is used for the treatment of high risk or relapsed leukaemia and certain haematological conditions. Bone marrow transplantation involves the administration of high dose chemotherapy with or without total body irradiation. Following treatment children are nursed in isolation until bone marrow recovery is achieved. Due to the high doses of treatment administered and a prolonged period of neutropenia, bone marrow transplantation is associated with a high risk of severe infection and even death. Children may receive bone marrow/stem cells from a related or unrelated donor, depending on the availability of a suitable match.

Stem cell rescue enables children with solid tumours to receive a higher dose of chemotherapy than they could receive without a rescue. Chemotherapy is given to the child, followed by the administration of a growth factor – granuloctye-colony stimulating factor (G-CSF) – to boost the production of stem cells. Stem cells are then harvested from the child. A high dose of chemotherapy is then given and the child's own stem cells are re-infused. As with bone marrow transplantation, stem cell rescue is associated with a prolonged period of neutropenia and a high risk of infection. Stem cell rescue is commonly used in children with stage 4 neuroblastoma, following initial chemotherapy, surgery and/or radiotherapy.

Access to the circulation

Most children and adolescents will have a central line inserted for ease of administering chemotherapy, use of blood products and antibiotics. They can be skin-tunnelled devices, e.g. a Hickman line, or completely implanted, e.g. a subcutaneous port. The totally implantable devices have no external catheter which may have a positive impact on body image and the patient's life style. Consideration needs to be given to the amount of treatment required and how the child copes with needles. Peripherally inserted lines can

also be used but generally have a shortened life expectancy, and where possible a more permanent central line needs to be inserted.

The placement and use of a central line is not without potential problems, the most common being infection. This can result from migration of skin organisms from the insertion site to the catheter tip (Parker 1999). Infection can be localised or systemic. Local infection can be treated with topical antibiotics and, depending on the type of organism cultured, may need systemic antibiotics.

A patient with systemic infection would be treated as a febrile neutropaenic patient (with sepsis) with broad-spectrum antibiotics. A persistent fever in a child with febrile neutropaenia which does not improve with antibiotics may be a result of a line infection which may require removal. IV antibiotics would then be administered through peripheral access lines (Campbell 2000).

The central line can become partially occluded. This should be suspected when sampling from a previously good line deteriorates and the blood return becomes sluggish or stops. This is usually related to fibrin deposits around the catheter tip or a blood or fibrin clot in the line. Complete occlusion can also be caused by malposition of the line or kinked or cracked tubing (McCloskey 2002). Treatment of a partial occlusion is usually by the administration of a thrombolytic agent, e.g. urokinase over a period of 2–4 hours but can be left *in situ* for up to 24 hours. If the catheter is completely obstructed then the line will need to be replaced.

Complications of the disease and the therapy

Spinal cord compression

Spinal cord compression is a medical emergency and a serious complication of a malignant process (Haas 2003). Spinal cord compression, although rare (5–30% of general oncology patients), may be seen on any high dependency unit and is associated with considerable morbidity and mortality (Osowski 2002; Joseph and Tayar 2005). In adults, cord compression is associated with carcinoma of the lungs, breast and prostate (Joseph and Tayar 2005). In children, it is associated with a variety of malignancies including lymphoma, neuroblastoma, osteosarcoma, leukaemia, posterior fossa brain tumours and metastatic disease (Haut 2005).

Spinal cord compression is described as a compression of the thecal sac by a mass in the epidural space (Quinn and DeAngelis 2000). The vertebral column consists of 26 vertebrae and a malignant invasion of the spinal cord can occur at several locations within the spinal cord (Flounders and Ott 2003). Spinal cord compression can be apparent at diagnosis. Accurate imaging is crucial to ensure the child commences the right treatment. An MRI is required for comprehensive imaging of the central nervous system (Kwok *et al.* 2006).

The signs and symptoms of spinal cord compression depend on the extent and the location of the spinal cord involvement. Back or neck pain is a common symptom, which may progress from a vague discomfort to weakness in limbs, a loss of sensation, autonomic dysfunction and occasionally paralysis (Osowski 2005). Symptoms may resolve with treatment; permanent neurological impairment may occur following a delay in treatment (Higdon 2006).

Spinal cord compression requires prompt intervention in order to prevent permanent loss of neurological function (Slocombe and Boynes 2005). Decompression surgery is one option; other strategies include radiotherapy and chemotherapy. Dexamethasone can be administered in an attempt to reduce swelling and inflammation and give temporary relief of pressure (Haas 2003). This is possibly one of the few situations where chemotherapy is administered as an emergency.

Nursing care of a child with spinal cord compression depends on the position and size of the mass in relation to the spinal cord. Adequate pain relief and ongoing neurological assessment are fundamental to ensure that the compression is not increasing (Flounders and Ott 2003). Preventing the complications associated with sensory-motor deficits and immobility are important factors to consider in the care of these children (Wilkes 1999). High standards of essential nursing care of pressure areas, bladder and bowel, mouth and eyes, infection control and wound care all play a part in the child's care management.

Psychological care of the child and family should not be forgotten when caring for a child with spinal cord compression. Families not only are dealing with an acutely ill child but also can be trying to cope with a diagnosis of cancer, as well as the prospect of ongoing neurological symptoms.

Superior vena cava syndrome

Superior vena cava syndrome is an obstruction of blood flow through the superior vena cava (SVC). The SVC is a major drainage vessel, draining venous blood from the upper extremities, upper thorax, head and neck (Kallab 2005). Superior vena cava syndrome in oncology patients is predominantly related to the disease process at diagnosis or a relapse.

The syndrome can also be associated with infection and central venous lines. Obstruction of the SVC in children is rare and can be a result of any malignant process causing a mediastinal mass, such as non-Hodgkin's lymphoma, Hodgkin's disease and chest tumours. The initial signs and symptoms may be few; however, they increase as the malignant disease progresses and invades the SVC. Symptoms include dyspnoea, oedema to the face and upper body (including extremities), engorgement of the face and veins, protruding eyes and subconjunctival haemorrhage. Patients may experience a cough, wheeze, tachycardia, headaches and dizziness/visual disturbances (Haut 2005). The onset can be insidious but can also happen very quickly, leading to major respiratory problems.

The diagnosis can be established by chest X-ray or CT scan, but is often established through an accurate history taking and clinical examination (Haut 2005; Kallab 2005). Management is related to the underlying aetiology of the tumour. An accurate prompt diagnosis is essential for this group of patients to ensure the correct, appropriate treatment is commenced. Adjunctive therapy is often required such as steroids and diuretics if oedema is present (Beeson 2007). Supportive management in an ITU with immediate intubation and ventilation may be appropriate when superior vena cava syndrome is suspected (Haut 2005).

Nursing care of a child with severe acute upper airway obstruction such as superior vena cava syndrome is a challenge (Hon *et al.* 2005). Children should be nursed in the position that is most comfortable for them in order to increase lung capacity (Hon *et al.* 2005). Psychological care is crucial as the child and family are dealing with an acute life-threatening episode, as well as the prospect of ongoing chemotherapy/radiotherapy.

Tumour lysis syndrome

Tumour lysis syndrome (TLS) consists of several metabolic abnormalities that result from the death of tumour cells. It can occur prior to treatment but more commonly occurs 12–72 hours after initiation of treatment (Rheingold and Lange 2006). Children who are most at risk usually present with a large tumour burden, e.g. lymphomas or high white cell count leukaemia, although tumour lysis can be seen with other solid tumours. The risks to the child are increased if renal function is compromised on diagnosis.

The metabolic abnormalities that can occur are hyperuricaemia from the rapid release and catabolism of intracellular nucleic acid which is normally cleared through the kidneys (Cairo and Bishop 2001), hyperphosphataemia from the rapid release of intracellular phosphorus from malignant cells, hyperkalaemia from the potassium released by the tumour cells, and hypocalcaemia which relates to the hyperphosphataemia.

Initially the kidneys can cope with all these events, but eventually problems will arise, leading to potential renal failure. The signs and symptoms of the metabolic abnormalities can include nausea, vomiting, lethargy, oedema, fluid overload, heart failure, cardiac arrhythmia, seizures, muscle cramps, tetany and possible death (Cairo and Bishop 2004).

Management, which includes the prevention and early recognition of potential problems, is vital. Prevention consists of having an awareness of the potential for patients to develop TLS. Aggressive hydration at a rate of 3 L/m^2 of body surface areas should be commenced before chemotherapy is administered and during treatment. Renal function needs to be observed closely (Jeha 2001; Cairo and Bishop 2004). There should be frequent weight measurements performed and the recording of the fluid balance needs to be diligent

Potassium should not be added to any fluids for a child with a newly diagnosed malignancy. Frequent electrolyte sampling should occur and early recognition and correction of abnormalities is important. The use of allopurinol or rasburicase is also necessary. Allopurinol prevents the formation of uric acid whereas rasburicase metabolises uric acid into a soluble form. Allopurinol does not produce an immediate effect so rasburicase should be administered to high risk patients. Often only one or two doses are required (Secola 2006). Any blood samples taken from a patient on rasburicase needs to put on ice immediately. If the samples are stored or transported at room temperature, uric acid will degrade and the result may indicate a false low level (Branyt 2002; Lim *et al.* 2003).

Management of specific metabolic abnormalities

Electrolytes are considered in Chapter 5; however, in malignant conditions specific metabolic abnormalities may be seen.

Hyperphosphataemia

Hyperphosphataemia may be corrected by the use of oral phosphate binders, e.g. aluminium hydroxide, which are not very palatable and may require a nasogastric tube for them to be administered. In severe cases renal dialysis may be required.

Hypocalcaemia

If the phosphate is corrected then hypocalcaemia should correct itself. However, if the patient is showing signs of low calcium then calcium gluconate should be administered intravenously, although this may increase the risk of calcium phosphate deposits and obstructive uropathy (Jones *et al.* 1995).

Hyperkalaemia

There are several ways to reduce a patient's potassium level and these may include oral or rectal sodium polystyrene sulphonate, insulin and glucose infusions and nebulised salbutamol (Cairo and Bishop 2004). Furosemide may also be useful in increasing urinary potassium excretion (Flombaum 2000).

Hyperuricaemia

The use of allopurinol or rasburicase should minimise this. However, if symptoms persist renal dialysis may be required.

General side effects of chemotherapy

Chemotherapeutic agents not only have an effect on the specific disease process but also have a systemic effect on the bone marrow, hence the associated significant side effects. The acute and often potentially life-threatening side effects are related to chemotherapy's effect on cells which have a rapid mitotic rate, such as gastrointestinal mucosa, hair follicles, gonads and critically the bone marrow. Some of the side effects that may happen are discussed here.

Anaemia

Anaemia is the deficiency of red blood cells or haemoglobin (Hb) leading to a reduction in the oxygen-carrying capacity of the blood (Hastings *et al.* 2006). There is no agreement regarding the definition of anaemia in oncology patients, but it may be considered if the Hb falls below 7–8 g/dL. Children with bone marrow disease may present with anaemia, but it can also occur as a complication of the treatment received.

The signs and symptoms of anaemia include:

- Pallor
- Breathlessness
- Headaches
- Loss of appetite
- Dizziness
- Fatigue
- Irritability

There is no consensus regarding the Hb level at which transfusion may be required to correct anaemia. Different hospitals have varying protocols; most will take into consideration the symptoms of the child as well as the Hb.

Adolescents are often less able to tolerate a reduced Hb and need to receive blood products sooner than younger patients. Treatment of anaemia can improve the child's quality of life. Children with normal Hbs have more energy, can concentrate better and enjoy life more.

Risks of administering blood and blood products

There are risks that need to be considered when administering blood products and these include adverse reactions and the potential for infections (also see Chapter 5). The risk of infections has been reduced since blood products are leukodepleted. This is especially seen in the reduction of cytomegalovirus (CMV) infections. If these occur in an immunocompromised patient there is a significant risk of morbidity and mortality. Many oncology units will administer CMV negative blood products as well to reduce the incidence of transmitted CMV.

The risks of blood transfusion have resulted in strategies designed to boost the child's own response to anaemia. Endogenous growth factors such as erythropoietin can support the body's response to anaemia by regulating the proliferation, maturation and differentiation of red blood cells. Administration of erythropoietin has been shown to be safe and is well tolerated for the treatment of anaemia in children, although the evidence is limited (Porter *et al.* 1996; Leon *et al.* 1998; Feusner and Hastings 2002).

Thrombocytopenia

A low platelet count can result in bruising or bleeding and this may lead to diagnosis of the primary condition; however, chemotherapy may also cause a low count. Signs and symptoms of thrombocytopenia include bleeding, purpura and petechiae.

The management of thrombocytopenia can be conservative; platelets are usually not transfused unless the child is severely affected. Platelets have a short life span and there are potential problems from using multiple blood products. If a child is to undergo a procedure, e.g. lumbar puncture or central line insertion, then prophylactic platelets could be given to bring the count to above 50×10^9 L (British Committee for Standards in Haematology 2003).

Some children who have had a haemorrhagic problem in the past, e.g. a cerebral bleed, may have a platelet count set by their consultants to try to prevent a reoccurrence of this problem. Children with a fever may have decreased platelet production and/or increased platelet destruction so may require platelets on this basis to avoid haemorrhage (Zimmerman 2004).

Neutropenia

The normal neutrophil count is $2.5–7.5 \times 10^9$/L. Neutropenia is a common complication of cytotoxic chemotherapy. It occurs about 10 days after treatment and usually recovers by 21 days depending on the treatment given. It puts patients at significant risk of morbidity and mortality from the risk of life-threatening infections. The definition of neutropenia differs within various hospitals but is commonly referred to as an absolute neutrophil count of $<0.5 \times 10^9$/L.

Gram-negative bacteria (e.g. *Escherichia coli*, *Pseudomonas aeruginosa* and *Klebsiella*) used to be the most common organisms seen in these children. Now Gram-positive bacteria (coagulase-negative staphylococci, *Staphylococcus aureus*, α-streptococci) are seen more often, possibly due to the use of indwelling central lines.

The signs and symptoms of infection are often subtle to start with; pyrexia may be the only indication that there is an infective process taking place as the inflammatory response is altered in the presence of neutropenia. Fever is usually defined as one temperature recording above 38.5°C or two recordings above 38°C (1 hour apart). The usual signs of infection may not be present. Some children, especially the very young, may be generally unwell but do not have an abnormal temperature. Where infection is suspected they should be treated as a febrile neutropaenic.

Investigations require a full assessment of the child and include inspection of the skin, mucous membranes, perianal area and the entry sites of any central venous lines. Blood cultures should be taken from the central line or peripherally if no line is *in situ*. Swabs should be taken from any potentially infective area, e.g. the central line and percutaneous endoscopic gastrostomy (PEG) tube. Blood tests (including a full blood count), urea and electrolytes and liver function tests are also needed.

Prompt treatment is essential, with broad-spectrum antibiotics ideally within 30–60 minutes (Pizzo 1999). Consensus varies in the choice of antibiotics that are used, but they usually consist of an aminoglycoside and either a piperacillin- or cephalosporin-based drug. Usually the antibiotics are continued until the child has been afebrile for 48 hours unless blood cultures show positive. If so, the child would continue on the appropriate antibiotics until a full course of appropriate treatment has been given.

Antifungal treatment is usually commenced after the child has been pyrexial for approximately 4 days. If there is a positive fungal result from the culture sampled or other signs of fungal infection, treatment would be started earlier.

The use of haematopoietic colony-stimulating factors can decrease the duration and severity of neutropenia in adults and children (Lehrnbecher and Welte 2002; Sung *et al.* 2002). Some protocols advocate the use of them electively to reduce the duration and severity of neutropaenia and to enable chemotherapy schedules to be maintained. Some patients will only receive them if they have a prolonged neutropaenia or are significantly unwell.

Management of cachexia

This is a progressive deterioration with muscle wasting that occurs when protein and/or calorie requirements are not met (Cunningham and Bell 2000). It is common in children and is mainly caused by reduced oral energy intake relative to energy expenditure (den Broeder 2000). It is often seen in children who have a large tumour burden, especially abdominal tumours.

Nutritional support can be given orally, intravenously or enterally. Methods can be used alone as well as in combination. Aggressive use of parenteral nutrition may be advocated, allowing the body to cope with the chemotherapy whilst also attempting to address the weight loss. Weight loss will have an impact on body image and this will also need to be addressed (see Table 12.2).

Management of nausea and vomiting

Nausea and vomiting is a distressing side effect of treatment and can be extremely debilitating.

Table 12.2 Reasons for poor nutritional intake and some tips to overcome them.

Symptom	Advice
Anorexia	Small frequent meals
	Variety of foods
	Add calories to food/drinks, e.g. butter, sugar
	Drink supplements/replacements
Taste changes	Try different foods to find out what they can taste/enjoy
	Small amounts often
	Often like strong tasting foods
Constipation	Encourage lots of fluids
	Use laxatives/stimulants as required
Diarrhoea	Check cause of diarrhoea is not infective – if not, drugs like loperamide may be used
	Encourage fluid intake
Nausea/vomiting	Administer antiemetics which control nausea/vomiting
	Offer food/fluids after antiemetic administered
	Small frequent meals
	Lots to drink when able
	Avoid strong cooking smells
Sore mouth	Ensure adequate analgesia – systemically and topically
	Ensure adequate fluids
	Encourage soft diet

Table 12.3 Management of nausea/vomiting.

Drug	Action	Potential problems/side effects
Dopamine blockers Metoclopromide Domperidone Haloperidol	Increase gastric emptying	Extrapyradimal effects Gastrointestinal disturbances
5-HT3 blockers Ondansetron Granisetron Tropisetron	5-HT3 antagonist	Headache Flushing Constipation
Antihistamine Cyclizine	Action unclear has mild sedating properties	Drowsiness Headache
Phenothiazine Levomeprazine Chlorpromazine	Antipsychotic effect Acts centrally on CTZ	Hypotension Drowsiness
Benzodiazipine Midazolam Lorazepam Nabilone	Anxiolytic, sedative and amnesia-inducing action	Drowsiness Vertigo Euphoria Sleep disturbances
Corticosteroids Dexamethasone	Action unsure but may reduce inflammatory damage to mucosal cells, reduce 5-HT3 release and affect the blood–brain barrier	Range of side effects, some very serious such as adrenal suppression and electrolyte imbalance

It can occur at any time and some patients may even experience anticipatory vomiting related to an association between something in the environment (may be physical, sight or smell) and chemotherapy. Some drugs used have a more emetic potential than others, but there may be other factors that lead the patient to vomit or feel nauseous, e.g. previous experiences or motion sickness. Chemotherapy agents induce vomiting by either stimulating the vomiting centre (located in the medulla lateral reticular formation) itself or direct or indirect stimulation of the chemotherapy trigger zone (CTZ, located in the floor of the fourth ventricle). This in turn activates the vomiting centre to produce nausea and vomiting (Berde *et al.* 2006).

Nausea, retching and vomiting are unpleasant symptoms and regular use of antiemetic drugs are essential and should be commenced prior to the administration of chemotherapy to attempt to block the receptors responsible for nausea and vomiting. There should be a plan in place to administer antiemetics depending on the emetic potential of the chemotherapy drugs and ensure that the medication is administered regularly and at the appropriate times. This usually considers a combination of antiemetics which will act in a variety of ways to prevent nausea and vomiting (see Table 12.3).

It is important also to consider non-pharmacological interventions to prevent nausea and vomiting and these can include acupuncture, relaxation, guided visual imagery, acupressure and sea bands (Dibble *et al.* 2007). There is limited evidence regarding their efficacy, but the child and family should be given the choice to use them if able.

Gastrointestinal problems

Mucositis

Chemotherapy targets rapidly dividing cells. The endothelial lining of the mouth and oropharynx can be badly affected and this will result in a sore, inflamed mouth and oral infections. It usually occurs 7–10 days after the commencement of chemotherapy. There is also a risk that any infection present in the mouth can migrate through the broken mucosa into the bloodstream, leading to a systemic infection (Brown and Wingard 2004). A sore mouth has an impact on a child's ability to maintain adequate nutrition and fluid intake.

Signs and symptoms of mucositis are pain, inflammation, swelling, ulceration, dry mouth, dry, cracked lips and bleeding. Management includes the education of the child and family towards the maintenance of good oral hygiene and ways to minimise the problem. Basic oral hygiene should involve cleaning the teeth with a soft toothbrush and fluoride toothpaste at least twice a day (Glenny 2006). If oral thrush is present then an absorbable antifungal such as fluconazole, itraconazole or ketoconazole is recommended (Glenny 2006).

A comprehensive assessment of the oral mucosa is important and a tool such as the Oral Assessment Guide developed by Eilers *et al.* (1988) may be beneficial. Gibson and Nelson (2000) have successfully adapted this tool for use in children and developed an algorithm of care that reflects the needs of the individual. Ideally a national tool and management algorithm should be developed.

Oral assessment needs to happen regularly; families need to be vigilant and taught to observe for problems and should be advised on what action should be taken. When a child presents with a sore mouth, pain relief should be a priority. This can by a combination of topical and systemic relief. Topical anaesthetic mouthwashes or sprays can be useful but should be used with caution especially in young children. Sensible advice should be given regarding the consumption of excessively hot or cold drinks following the administration of these. Systemic pain relief needs to be considered as well as intravenous analgesia. If there is pain from a sore mouth but it is controlled then children are more likely to perform oral hygiene and maintain adequate hydration and nutrition.

Nutritional issues

Weight loss is common in the child with cancer. This can be apparent on diagnosis or occur at any time during treatment. It may result directly from the effect of the tumour or as a result of treatment (Cunningham and Bell 2000). It can have a prognostic effect; children who are well-nourished are better able to resist infection and tolerate treatment (den Broeder 2000). It also has an impact on quality of life and the psychological wellbeing of the child.

There are many issues that can exacerbate nutritional problems – anorexia, taste changes, nausea and vomiting, constipation, diarrhoea and fatigue. Table 12.2 gives some hints on how to manage some of these problems.

Nutritional assessment is vital; however, there is not an established valid tool in use in paediatrics. Assessment should include dietetic history, any eating problems that the child has experienced and clinical examination. Weight and height measurements should be taken to establish a baseline. These assessments should be repeated several times throughout treatment and should pick up children with problems or who are at risk of developing problems (McMahon *et al.* 1998). It is vital to have a multidisciplinary approach to nutrition and dieticians are part of the team involved in offering support and advice.

Encouraging a child to eat and drink can be a difficult task and may turn into a battle between children and parents. Small frequent meals of a variety of foods may need to be offered, including foods with high calorific value. A variety of oral supplements are available to try which can be added to drinks or foods or may be taken on their own. Enteral feeding is an effective means to supporting nutrition in a child with a functioning gut and there is evidence to show it does maintain weight (den Broeder 2000).

Some children find a nasogastric tube difficult to come to terms with as it generates problems regarding body image and can be uncomfortable

(Brown 1999). This can be overcome and families taught to care for such tubes, which may facilitate earlier discharge home. However, there is increased use of PEG tubes which are now often inserted in children where weight loss is going to be a problem. Radiotherapy may affect their ability to eat normally.

Parenteral nutrition (PN) may be considered when the gut is not functioning or weight loss continues despite enteral nutrition (Lowis *et al.* 2004). A centrally placed catheter is required to administer PN, but most oncology children will already have some type of central access. PN is considered in Chapter 5 and will be calculated to meet the individual child's needs. PN does have risks associated with it and for the oncology child these include infections, hepatotoxicity, suppression of oral intake and metabolic abnormalities.

Typhlitis

Typhlitis or neutropaenic colitis is chemotherapy-induced damage to the intestinal mucosa primarily in the terminal ileum, ascending colon and caecum; this occurs when the patient is neutropaenic. Mucosal ulceration and possibly necrosis occur. The organisms mainly involved are anaerobes and Gram-negative bacilli, especially *Pseudomonas aeruginosa.Clostridium difficile* is also an important cause of typhlitis (Walsh *et al.* 2006).

The signs and symptoms may be non-specific. Initially abdominal pain may be localised to the right lower quadrant and there may be fever and diarrhoea (Gomez *et al.* 1998). Other symptoms may include nausea and vomiting. A CT scan is the most sensitive way to look for typhlitis and to assess caecal wall thickening (King 2002). Management tends to be conservative at first with intravenous fluids, broad-spectrum antibiotics which may also include an antibiotic against anaerobes, e.g. metronidazole, nutritional support, nil orally and analgesia (Otaibi 2002).

Surgery may be considered if there is evidence of impending perforation, persistent

gastrointestinal bleeding after correction of thrombocytopenia and general deterioration of the child, but is not routinely performed (Jain *et al.* 2000). G-CSF may be commenced to help stimulate recovery of the neutrophils to help aid recovery of the gut. Antifungal treatment may be added if the child remains febrile (McCullough and McDonald 2003).

Altered elimination – constipation

Constipation is defined as a decrease in the frequency of the passage of stool which then becomes hard. It is caused by the ineffective actions of the bowels and can occur in children undergoing treatment for cancer for a variety of reasons, including spinal cord compression, intestinal obstruction and some medications such as opioids or vinca alkaloids (Smith 2001).

Signs and symptoms include hard, infrequent stools, pain, discomfort, bloating, nausea, abdominal distension and poor appetite. Prophylactic management is preferred with the recognition of children who are at risk. Appropriate fluids and diet will help, but the child may not always feel like eating. Regular assessment of bowel actions is important and if the child has not had his or her bowels open, action should be taken to address this. Treatment may be needed with stool softeners or laxatives and monitored for efficacy as they may need to be changed, increased in dose or stopped once the child has maintained adequate bowel actions.

Suppositories and enemas are sometimes used. They may be well tolerated, but there is a potential risk of trauma to the anal area, leading to infection, bleeding and anal fissures.

Altered elimination – diarrhoea

Diarrhoea can be caused by several chemotherapy drugs and can cause many problems to the child. It can result in dehydration, electrolyte imbalances and general debility (Hogan 1998).

Chemotherapy is often the primary cause, but diarrhoea can also be caused by infection, antibiotics and the overuse of laxatives. There can also be damage to the gut from surgery or radiotherapy which may lead to malabsorption and diarrhoea.

Signs and symptoms are an increased frequency of bowel movements, abdominal pain, abdominal cramps, weight loss and dehydration. Management includes detection of the primary cause and, if possible, this is treated directly, e.g. stop laxatives, treat infection, change antibiotics. Some foods exacerbate the diarrhoea and these need to be avoided. If the child is dehydrated then fluids and electrolytes are required to correct this. Careful observation of the anal area is important to observe for any excoriation and inflammation that may need to be treated. If there is no infective cause for the diarrhoea then one of the opioids, e.g. loperamide, may be used to reduce peristalsis in the intestines (Wadler et al. 1998).

Other systemic complications of treatment

Cardiac problems are associated with the anthracycline drugs and can include acute arrhythmias, conduction abnormalities and decreased left ventricular function. Usually the more anthracyclines that have been given, the more the child is at risk; however, some children will develop problems after minimal treatment. Cumulative doses of anthracyclines should be recorded and regular echocardiograms performed to detect any problems with the ejection fraction. Symptoms of cardiac failure may occur many years after completion of treatment so long-term follow-up is required.

Some chemotherapy drugs can cause problems to the kidneys. Observation of renal function is vital and regular monitoring may be required to see if there is any deterioration. If this occurs, and it is often associated with cisplatinum,

methotrexate and ifosfamide, then doses of these drugs may need to be reduced or omitted.

Chemotherapy may affect the liver and cause transient elevations in the liver enzymes in the blood. Veno-occlusive disease (VOD) (sinusoidal obstructive syndrome) is a serious complication and is associated with significant mortality and morbidity. VOD involves injury to the sinusoidal endothelial cells in the liver. This leads to hepatocyte necrosis, with cellular debris causing small occlusions in the hepatic veins, leading to liver dysfunction. The children who get VOD include those who have had bone marrow transplants and those chemotherapeutic agents such as actinomycin, or long-term use of azathioprine or 6-thioguanine.

The signs and symptoms include jaundice, weight gain with fluid retention, ascites and hepatomegaly resulting in right upper quadrant pain, thrombocytopenia, impaired liver function and rarely renal failure (Rheingold and Lange 2006). The majority of cases of VOD can be diagnosed by clinical features, using elevated liver function tests, particularly high ALT, AST and bilirubin (Veys and Rao 2004). Doppler ultrasound is used if VOD is suspected and may show altered hepatic artery indices or reversal of hepatoportal blood flow, but the results may be inconsistent and clinical features are more important.

Prevention of VOD is the gold standard for children at high risk of developing this. Two drugs are commonly used – ursodeoxycholic acid is thought to protect hepatocytes from cholestasis, and defibrotide which is a fibrinolytic and antithrombotic agent. The treatment of VOD is also defibrotide, which is given intravenously and has been associated with increased survival (Rheingold and Lange 2006). Nursing management of children with VOD involves maintaining a strict fluid balance, weighing the child twice a day, undertaking girth measurements, monitoring the blood picture, full blood count (FBC), clotting, renal function and liver function tests.

Platelets may be administered. Other management strategies are supportive, including analgesia, good skin care, nutritional management and promotion of a positive body image.

Body image

The loss of body image during treatment for a malignancy can cause distress to children and their families. Often the child will lose weight and look different. Some may also gain weight, especially children who receive steroids as part of their treatment.

As some chemotherapy affects rapidly dividing epithelial cells, hair growth is reduced, leading to alopecia. This can be distressing to both the child and family and can have a severe effect on body image. This occurs usually 2 weeks after commencing chemotherapy and the hair usually will not grow again until chemotherapy has stopped. Many children will wear a wig, but some choose to wear scarves and hats.

Dealing with changes in their body image adds another problem for children to cope with and some may need help and support to deal with this.

Haematological disorders

Sickle cell disease

Sickle cell disease is the most common genetically inherited disorder in England (NHS 2006) affecting 1:2000 live births. It is the collective name given to a range of haemoglobin abnormalities which affect the structure and function of the haemoglobin contained in the erythrocyte. A single amino acid substitution of valine for glutamate in the beta chain of the haemoglobin molecule is responsible for the disease. This affects the shape and the flexibility of the erythrocyte particularly when oxygen tension is reduced, hence the name sickle cell. Abnormal erythrocytes have a shorter life span than the normal erythrocyte and there is a degree of co-existing anaemia. Generally speaking the greater the proportion of abnormal cells present the more likely the individual is to suffer crisis and complications.

The disease is prevalent in populations of African and African-Caribbean origin but can also be found in people who have a Mediterranean or Asian background; 'white' indigenous UK carriers have also been identified (Bennett 2005). It is an autosomal recessive trait which means that it can be carried by healthy 'unsuspecting' individuals who are unaware of their status until they have affected children by another carrier. The risks of two individuals who are both carriers having an affected child in each pregnancy are 1:4 (25%), with a 50% chance of passing on the carrier status (Ross and Wilson 2006). It is estimated that there are 240 000 carriers of sickle cell in England. With increased migration this number is likely to increase.

It is important to detect the condition early as effective management can reduce infant mortality, improve the quality of life and increase the life expectancy. Although the disease has a wide range of severity, it is anticipated that as many as 300 lives could be saved each year as a result of the new neonatal blood screening (NHS media release 2006).

Clinical features

Although symptoms of sickle cell disease can be present in infancy, most patients present after 6 months old. Sickle cell erythrocytes are more likely to deform than normal erythrocytes, leading to haemolysis and thrombosis within small-diameter blood vessels. This can result in ischaemia to the distal part which has the impaired blood supply and may result in end organ damage. There are four classic presentations of crisis.

Vaso-occlusive crisis

This can be triggered by infection, dehydration, hypoxia, stress and cold. This painful crisis typically involves the chest, abdomen, spine and limbs. In infants the digits may be involved and the hands or feet appear swollen. These children need to be taken seriously and an acute chest infection may present with a persistent cough, tachypnoea, dyspnoea and pain. Although the initial chest X ray may be unremarkable there are often changes 2–3 days later.

Splenic sequestration

This usually occurs in children younger than 5 years old following an infection. The child will have an enlarged spleen, is hypotensive, pale and in pain. The reticulocyte counts are elevated and the Hb decreased.

Aplastic crisis

This may result from a folic acid deficiency, an infection or a toxic event which affects the bone marrow. An aplastic crisis means that the blood cell production cycle is reduced and can result in very low Hb levels.

Infectious crisis

Because of multiple small splenic infarctions resulting in impaired immune response, patients with sickle cell are more at risk of meningitis, pneumonia, osteomyelitis, urinary tract infections and septicaemias.

Nursing care and management

These children and their families need urgent and sympathetic, symptomatic attention when admitted in crisis. They may need a rapid track to a high dependency area for ease of observation and monitoring. This may be reassuring or may result in elevated anxiety depending on the family's previous exposure and experience of the health services. The child needs assessment of cardio-respiratory function to identify the presence of respiratory distress/failure and eliminate the possibility of shock. The management of pain is of primary importance and the child may require morphine. These children respond well to patient controlled analgesic and often have significant insight into their condition and what works best for them. These views ought to be respected.

They need vascular access and are typically dehydrated. They will require a fluid bolus in line with the hospital protocols, an example of which is 20 mL/kg of normal saline and maintenance of 50% in excess of the usual rate. A strict fluid balance chart needs to be maintained and the urinary output measured. They frequently need urgent blood transfusions to decrease the concentration of the sickled red cells and complete exchanges might be required in severe cases.

Hypoxia is frequently a precipitating cause so the administration of supplementary oxygen by whichever means is tolerated best by the child is beneficial. The child's respiratory function and saturations need to be monitored. Respiratory support in the form of CPAP may be required to maintain good oxygenation.

Antibiotics and antimicrobial management are administered intravenously. Initially these are broad spectrum and then may be changed to target the causative organism as identified by blood culture or lumbar puncture.

Splenectomy

The spleen is vital for the removal of non-opsonised material from the circulation. An individual without a functioning spleen is at risk of invasion by encapsulated micro-organisms. Removal is best not done as an emergency but may be required for acute sequestration as this is a life-threatening condition.

Bone marrow transplant

This is the only cure for sickle cell disease, but can only be safely carried out if the child has an human leukocyte antigen (HLA)-identical sibling who can donate bone marrow. The cure rate is about 90%, but there is a small risk of fatal transplant-related complications. Further therapies may emerge with research on the stem cell.

Lifestyle and effective discharge

Once the acute phase is over, there is an opportunity for health promotion and identification of the cause of the trigger of the crisis. A review should be done of vaccination uptake and the child's compliance with medications such as prophylactic antibiotic therapy and hydroxyurea.

Complications

Between 5 and 10% of children will develop cerebral disease stroke, sub-arachnoid haemorrhage and cranial nerve palsies. Priapism is a painful and persistent erection of the penis owing to vaso-occlusion of the corpus cavernosum which needs urgent referral to the urologists to prevent impotence.

Thrombocytopenia

Thrombocytes are essential for the formation of blood clots as part of a body defence mechanism to prevent haemorrhage in response to minor trauma. Thrombocytopenia is a reduction in the number of circulating platelets (normal value 150 000–350 000/mL). There are a variety of causes:

- Congenital as a result of an autoimmune process or an infection before birth
- Inherited as a result of an X-linked recessive disease such as Wiskott–Aldrich syndrome
- Secondary as a result of leukaemia or Fanconi's anaemia
- Acquired as a result of infection (by herpes simplex, cytomegalovirus, mumps, etc.). Or it could be a toxic insult as a result of ingestion of quinine, aspirin, alcohol, some antibiotics and a range of other drugs such as digoxin

Investigation

Thrombocytopenia needs to be investigated as it is difficult to differentiate from the early presentation of haemolytic uraemic syndrome (see Chapter 8) and idiopathic thrombocytopenia.

Signs and symptoms of idiopathic thrombocytopenia

Idiopathic means cause unknown, and because of the role thrombocytes play in blood clotting the signs and symptoms of the disorder include bleeding and purpura (tiny pin-prick haemorrhages just under the skin which resemble a rash).

Treatment

In children, acute idiopathic thrombocytopenia may occur suddenly, require no treatment and spontaneously resolve. In adolescents it may take a more chronic form and require treatment for years. Treatments are supportive and include the use of steroids. These are usually given orally in the form of prednisolone. They are taken over several weeks and need to be withdrawn slowly. Immunoglobulin (IgG) may be given if a sudden increase in platelets is required to see the individual over a crisis point such as pregnancy. The exact mechanism of how this therapy works is unknown, but the IgG may block platelet removal, resulting in an increase. Anti D antibody has also been used to this effect.

Alternative therapies include other immune suppressive drugs such as cyclophosphamide, vincristine and azathioprine. There may need to be lifestyle changes, with contact and high risk sports avoided until the platelet count returns to normal.

In rare cases of chronic idiopathic thrombocytopenia, surgery may be considered and splenectomy performed. This would not usually be considered in children under 5. As one of the functions of the spleen is to remove bacteria from the blood, individuals who have a splenectomy have to take prophylaxis antibiotic all their lives.

Chapter 13

PLAY FOR THE INFANT AND CHILD IN THE HIGH DEPENDENCY UNIT

Tina Clegg

Introduction

This chapter aims to introduce the children's nurse to the complex developmental needs of children in the high dependency unit (HDU). The chapter illustrates the complexities faced by the child and family who experience a short- or long-term stay in an HDU. For some, their admission is as a result of a newly acquired condition; others have a long-term need for high dependency care. The chapter also shows how the environment is potentially damaging and how appropriate stimulation can be built into the child's day. As always the parents and families should be regarded as partners in care. The way a child is accepted and accommodated into the family is crucial to the ongoing development of the individual and the health of the entire family.

Rudlof and Levene (2006) state that the 'The fundamental objective of paediatrics is to guide children safely and happily through childhood so that they will become healthy, well adjusted, normal young adults – to enable them to achieve their maximum potential physically, intellectually, psychologically and socially'.

Children are complex in their needs. Advances in medical and nursing care have resulted in increasing numbers surviving their traumas. They may spend a considerable amount of time in a High Dependency Unit during their formative years of

childhood or adolescence. These experiences are far from the normal that would be enjoyed following the birth of a family member. The stimulation, touch, sounds and smells of a hospital, coupled with medical and nursing interventions and the separation from home, family and school are powerful influences on children and their families.

The developmental and play needs of children are an essential element of hospital care. Sick children will experience many disadvantages in their play and their developmental needs. They do not need to have these disadvantages exaggerated by a lack of or inappropriate stimulation which can lead to further delay in play skills, developmental milestones and social interaction. Play that is assessed, organised and evaluated can be one of the ways in which the developmental care and the active participation of the families can be of benefit to all.

Development

Development can be described as a process of continuous change; sometimes it is fast-paced and obvious and, at other times, it is slow and difficult to see. Developmental change is not haphazard but proceeds in an orderly fashion throughout life. The entire child's knowledge about the world comes through the six senses, sight, hearing, taste, smell and touch. The sixth sense is proprioception that tells the infant about the location of the mobile parts of the body, the legs and hands and their relationship to the rest of the body (Sylva 1990).

Hospital experiences affect subsequent development in profound and long-lasting ways. Developmental care encompasses all care procedures as well as social and physical aspects in the neonatal unit (NNU) or HDU. A child's physiological parameters and behavioural expressions in response to stimuli can be seen as a constant and reliable guide for caregivers (Peters 1999). A plan of play and developmental care can then be formulated and implemented to meet the needs of the individual child. This will enhance each child's opportunities without becoming a source of stress.

For older children the effects also include the loss of independence, communication skills and choice. Children will experience loss, grief and fear. These elements must be included in the care plan. A consistent approach in delivering any care plan is essential to the wellbeing of a child.

In the HDU a child's world is restricted to what is provided by adults. These may be positive and negative experiences as well as the influences that adults have on the environment – temperature, light, noise, smell, taste, handling and positioning. All children are individuals and will present a variety of challenges and opportunities to the healthcare team looking after them.

Play

Play, as a single concept, is exceptionally difficult to define but has come to be recognised as a normal and essential requirement for a child's wellbeing and development. It is the primary medium through which children learn and make sense of their environment (OMEP 1989). The works of Freud, Groos, Piaget and Erikson offer the reader an opportunity to study the philosophies of play in more depth.

Article 31 of the UN Convention on the Rights of the Child states that every child has the right to rest and leisure, and to engage in play and recreational activities appropriate to the age of the child. The Children Act (1989) recognises that children's needs for good quality play opportunities change as they grow up, but they need such opportunities throughout childhood in order to reach and maintain their optimum development and wellbeing.

The National Service Framework for Children and Young People provides a clear statement on the provision of play services throughout the NHS and recognises that a child in hospital should have daily access to a play specialist.

Children need play that provides suitable opportunities to strengthen the body, improve the mind, develop personality and acquire social competence. Play is therefore as necessary for a child as food, warmth and protective care (Sheridan 1997).

Providing play can cause anxiety and confusion in the healthcare team and parents. The interaction between a child and the child's medical, nursing and developmental needs has to be balanced with the child's responses and behavioural changes. These need to be documented by all carers so that a clear picture of toleration and behavioural changes is presented.

Developing play skills and play programmes

Play stimulates a variety of skills – physical, cognitive, social and personal. It is essential that a developmental assessment of the child is undertaken. This will form the basis of any planned play intervention undertaken by the play specialist and care-giving team.

All aspects of a child's development need to be included when planning play sessions – sequences of development, current skills and losses, and the primary need for communication. This information is then linked to the current medical and nursing needs of the child to provide a play plan that will be evaluated and developed as the child's needs or skills change. This plan may reflect the continuing developmental losses or improvements that the child is experiencing.

Such a programme should be based on theory, be dynamic in nature and respect the child's unique behavioural organisation, maternal/child interaction and parenting needs (Wolke 1991).

Play specialists use play programmes that are care plans for play and developmental sequencing. Like nursing care, many different models can be used, but this needs to be based on the nursing notes and be accessible to the healthcare team.

As the parents are partners in care and have access to the care plans, the play programmes will need to be phrased sensitively and diplomatically. They are written after assessing the stage of the child's development. Care must be taken that this is written in a positive format and based on what the child has already achieved developmentally. Regular reviews of the progression made and new developmental targets are essential as progress will take place even if this is slow or at times regressed due to the child's medical condition. Evaluations of each play session need to be made so that a clear picture of the play input and developmental progress can be recorded. Parents should be encouraged to record their input into the evaluation, thereby gaining a sense of pride, and see the importance of their contribution to their child's wellbeing.

The play specialist may introduce a diary in which the child, caregivers and family write the life story of the child. This provides a positive sequenced record of the child and family's hospital journey, the highs and lows of the admission and is important when working post procedurally with the child and siblings.

Therapeutic play

A skilled play specialist will provide developmental based and evaluated therapeutic play sessions with the child and/or family. This will include play preparation, distraction and post-procedural play.

Play preparation uses a variety of tools including books, photographs, dolls and medical equipment and specifically made toys to prepare, explore and inform the child about a nursing or medical procedure or their current medical condition. Through preparation, the child is aware of why, how and what will happen to them. An honest approach is required that builds the child's trust and confidence in the caregivers and the information they are given. The preparation needs to be timely, designed to meet the individual needs of the child and be clear on the information that is to be provided. Several sessions may be required for children who are experiencing complex and long-term hospitalisation.

Distraction play works to the plan made in preparation play to identify and use coping strategies with the child while the procedure is carried out. Strategies to provide an alternative focus from the medical or nursing intervention include the use of books, bubbles and interactive toys that the child has made some choices about using.

Post-procedural play allows children to work through their experiences of hospitalisation and medical and nursing interventions using role play with medical equipment or toys to share their thoughts, ideas and emotions concerning their care, condition and treatment. This is very skilful play and needs to be managed carefully so that the child's misconceptions and fears can be managed in a proactive way.

Children have to have a system in place so that they can effectively communicate their needs, desires and fears. This will need to be individualised to the child and may involve the use of computer systems, pointing pictures, sign language or Makaton. The system chosen must be consistently used by all caregivers and the family.

Working with parents

Hospitalisation can be a stressful and distressing time, not only for the child, but also for parents and families. The parents' feelings of disempowerment, isolation and fear should not be underestimated (Action for Sick Children 1989).

The most common worry that mothers have about the future relates to their child's development (Reid 2000). Parents are very keen to support the developmental progression of their children. One of the primary objectives of play specialists should be to encourage parents to be involved in their child's play and to understand the value and consistency of care that only the parents can give (Reynolds 1993). It is important to involve parents in all aspects of play, right from the early discussion of the need. The parents should be involved with the assessment of play needs, planning and implementing of play activities, evaluating and recording of play as well as monitoring the developmental progression. As partners in care they can have an active part in the delivery of play and help promote a normalising activity.

Play specialists can be involved in introducing siblings to the newly changed child. Using their skills, they can prepare the siblings for the alien and sometimes distressing world of the HDU as well as the events and procedures that the family will share. They can work with the sick child to develop play opportunities that will eventually form part of the child's play experiences. Hospital visits should be a positive experience for siblings.

Siblings can be jealous and resentful of those who they perceive as taking what is rightfully theirs or who have things they themselves want (O'Hagen and Smith 1993). Siblings are in a very vulnerable position when a sick child is cared for on an NNU or HDU. Little time or preparation will have been given to them and their needs. Many may not be able to visit or take an active part with the new family member, but they will be aware of the distress around them.

In the HDU, the physiological stress responses are being relentlessly re-activated due to over-handling, painful procedures and changes in temperature. In most cases, there is little positive input given to counteract the negative stimuli that these sick children receive. All infants need some form of positive touch during their day (Bond 1999).

Bond (1999) cites the Adamson Macede study on positive tactile touch and showed that when compared to a control group, children in this study at the age of 7 years scored higher in all measures of intelligence and achievement. It was felt that touch therapy helped to reduce the stress of the NNU and to promote healthy brain development. This is also important for older children.

The model of 'gentle human touch' with infants and children is the placing of hands to contain the head and lower back and buttocks or abdomen, taking care only to provide support not intermittent stimulation. The results of this study indicated few detrimental effects and suggested that, in the short term, infants had less behavioural distress, more quiet sleep and less motor activity during procedures (Harrison 1996).

Parental involvement in touch programmes can be beneficial. It may help to bring parents and infants closer, improve handling skills, self-esteem and positive thinking. It may also help to allay feelings of guilt and helplessness (Bond 1999). Parents may instinctively want to stroke their infant, but the infant may not be able to tolerate so much stimulation. Holding offers a more appropriate way of touching that is rewarding and enjoyable to both the infant and the parent.

Rest is an important feature of normal growth and development. Ensuring periods of undisturbed time is significant for high-risk children. More than 4 hours without interaction is abnormal and periods of less than 1 hour are insufficient to complete the sleep cycle (Fenwick et al. 1999).

Quiet time

It is important to reduce the environmental disturbances that can affect the child whenever possible. Environmental modifications such as reducing noxious stimulation (light and sound) and the promotion of supported positioning and minimal handling are all key factors in stress reduction (Boxwell 2000). Hospitals are dangerous places to be, especially if you are small and sick! They are brightly lit, noisy, and full of high-tech equipment and dangerous organisms. Steps by the care team to introduce quiet periods and, with infants, not using the incubator surfaces as worktops are beneficial to all in this environment.

Multicultural awareness

An awareness and understanding of cultural factors and backgrounds is important as they may have an influence and impact on parenting styles and attitude to play. Play resources must reflect the cultural diversity of the client group so that parents and siblings can fully participate with enjoyment and confidence in the play sessions.

Transitional care

More and more children are being discharged to the community on home ventilation or with other complex care packages. The play specialist is an essential part of the discharge planning and implementation package.

Children will need to have a play programme that reflects their current developmental, communication and play skills. Referral to community play services is essential if the child is going to be able to fully integrate into community play resources.

On discharge, the parents will be confident about the developmental play required and their abilities to provide this. Parents' knowledge of child development and play will be enhanced along with good play skills.

For the child who has experienced a long stay in hospital, a transitional play programme will be required. Home may not be a concept that the child is familiar with and, in the same way that we prepare children for a hospital admission, we may need to prepare the child for the home environment, routine, bedroom, the caregivers and sharing space and time with other family members.

Hospital play specialists

The Department of Health recommended in 1991 that there should be provision for play in all areas of the hospital where children are found and that a play specialist should be employed. The National Service Framework for Children, Young People and Maternity Services provides clear guidance on the provision of play services throughout the NHS. Hospital play specialists, with their training, are in a unique position to meet the play needs of children and to work towards achieving their full potential in partnership with the healthcare team and family.

It is essential that play specialists work as part of the overall healthcare team and liaise closely with other staff members. There must be consultation on treatment plans, procedures and diagnostic implications so that a play programme can be designed to suit the individual child (Action for Sick Children 1989). Play specialists have the skills to observe a child and monitor development, behavioural organisation and emotional state.

Play safety

The safety of the child is paramount both in medical and play terms. Toys need to be cleaned and inspected on a daily basis in order to meet safety and infection control regulations. This process must be monitored regularly to ensure that the high standards are maintained.

Play space in the incubator, cot, chair or floor needs to be provided so that monitoring equipment is not compromised or a hazard to anyone in the area. Close liaison with medical and nursing staff regarding play activities and times needs to be negotiated.

Chapter 14

TRANSPORTATION OF THE ACUTELY ILL CHILD

Michaela Dixon, Marian Perrott and Gill West

Introduction

This chapter focuses on the practicalities of transport. While there is overlap with many of the previous chapters in this book, this has been written as a stand-alone text. Most nurses do not transport acutely unwell children in their daily practice because, since the reorganisation of children's intensive care services in the late 1990s, transport/retrieval teams have been established to provide a service dedicated to the movement of critically ill infants and children between local hospitals and the tertiary or lead centres for paediatric intensive care units (PICUs) (DH 1997). The majority of critically ill children requiring inter-hospital transfer are now moved under the care of these teams.

There is a small group of critically ill children who require immediate transfer to a specialist centre, e.g. children requiring immediate neurosurgical intervention, who cannot wait for the arrival of a retrieval/transport team due to the time-critical nature of their condition. The responsibility for the transfer of these children will rest with the local team of doctors and nurses. Support and advice in these instances is always available from the specialist centre and the retrieval/transport team within the locality. In addition most retrieval/transport services have websites where guidelines and management strategies can be accessed at any time.

A significant number of less critically ill children are transferred every day between hospitals for ongoing management, and the responsibility for the safe transfer of these children often lies with nursing staff from the child's original hospital. In addition to inter-hospital transfers, acutely unwell children are transported round hospital sites every day between clinical areas and from clinical areas to X-ray departments and theatres. The preparation and practice for transferring these children should not differ greatly from the preparation required to transfer a child from one hospital to another. It is very easy to be comfortable within a familiar environment, but if the transfer involves using a lift or moving from one building to another, e.g. then anticipation of potential problems apart from deterioration in the clinical condition of the child is essential.

There is a large body of literature available relating to the transport/transfer of the critically ill neonate and/or child and the use of specialised teams, but currently there is a lack of literature relating to the transfer of the acutely unwell rather than the critically ill child. While the principles of transport are essentially the same across the whole age spectrum there are some very important considerations which must be applied within each specific age group.

Principles for safe transport

- Children are affected by critical illness differently, both physiologically and psychologically, from adults.

- There needs to be a structured approach to transfer/transport.
- Preparation is the key to a safe transfer/transport.
- Children should receive the same standard of care during transfer/transport as they had in their clinical area.
- Take everything you could need with you (that you can safely use).

Intra-hospital transfer

Transfer of the highly dependent infant/child may be from a PICU to a high dependency unit (HDU) or a ward area or between other clinical areas depending on the medical and nursing needs of the child and the availability of services within each hospital.

The mnemonic 'TRANSFER' (see Table 14.1) can be used in ensuring a structured approach to transfer whether it is from a PICU, HDU or ward area.

Safe transfer/transport begins with full assessment of the child (Table 14.1).

Inter-hospital transfer

As discussed previously there are a small number of children who will require urgent transfer which will need to be undertaken by staff in the referring centre. Key priorities for this process are outlined in Table 14.2 and while there are many similarities between the intra- and inter-hospital transfer process there are a number of additional considerations to be taken into account when leaving the safety of a familiar environment.

Practicalities of transfer/transport

Equipment

While it may seem a very obvious point to make, it is important to ensure that all the equipment used for transfer is kept fully charged and ready for use. There is nothing more frustrating than finding the piece of equipment needed with little or no battery life left. It is also important that practitioners are familiar with the pumps and monitors used within their clinical areas. Most clinical areas now have specific pieces of equipment used for transfer.

Monitoring

A minimum level of monitoring is required for all children. This normally incorporates the same monitoring the child is receiving in the clinical area prior to moving and should include:

- ECG/respirations
- Saturations
- Non-invasive BP

Additional monitoring is determined by the child's clinical condition as well as the nature and duration of the transfer. For the child who is receiving more intensive/invasive interventions the following should be considered:

- Core-peripheral temperature monitoring
- Arterial line (for invasive BP monitoring and blood gas analysis)

If the child is intubated and ventilated, then the use of an $ETCO_2$ monitor is also recommended particularly if the child does not have arterial monitoring.

Calculation of oxygen required

A spontaneously breathing child receiving oxygen therapy via a face mask at 15 L/min will use more oxygen than a child who is intubated and mechanically ventilated.

Two questions need to be answered.

How much will this child require?
It is possible to calculate approximately how much oxygen will be required by using a simple calculation (Table 14.3).

Table 14.1 A structured approach to intra-hospital 'TRANSFER'.

'TRANSFER'	Notes/considerations
Timing	Communication is essential between ward areas, the site co-ordinator (where applicable), members of the multi-disciplinary team (MDT) and the child and family to ensure a co-ordinated approach Arrange as early as possible to facilitate discharge planning. Whenever possible the transfer should occur in day-time hours for minimal disruption to the ward, child and family
Resources	Ensure the availability of staff to facilitate safe transfer The child's allocated nurse should wherever possible accompany the child as this will maintain effective communication Any additional staff required to ensure safe transfer, e.g. porters, should where possible receive prior notice
Assessment: Airway Breathing Circulation Disability Exposure	Full assessment should be undertaken prior to the child being moved. This allows for a structured assessment which includes the method and percentage of oxygen administration, location of feeding lines, chest drains, urinary catheters, intravenous lines and any other devices Ensure that infusions have the appropriate amount in syringe for safe transfer and to continue infusing for a period of time after transfer is complete (normally 2 hours as a minimum) There should always be emergency equipment available (which may be safely used by staff involved in transfer) The minimum monitoring recommended during intra-hospital transfer is a saturation monitor which will normally display heart rate and saturations
Notes	Child should have at least one name band stating name, date of birth and registration number If any known allergies then child should have a red name band on and an allergy alert must be clearly identified on notes All appropriate documentation should be completed and up to date Ensure that child's name, date of birth and registration number are entered on all documentation Documentation should include a transfer sheet and discharge summary. All prescription sheets should be up to date and appropriately completed
Safety	Prior to transfer, staff on the receiving ward may require additional training (e.g. in the case of a child who is receiving ongoing ventilatory support or the child with a tracheostomy) Check amount of air/oxygen in cylinders is adequate to complete the journey Check cot sides are in working order Ensure drains and intravenous lines are securely fixed to prevent disconnection
Family	The child's parents/primary care givers should be informed and continually kept updated on transfer The family should be given full contact details of the new ward
Equipment	Ensure equipment for transfer is in working order There should be enough battery life on equipment to reach destination
Report	Handover is recommended from nurse to nurse prior to transfer to facilitate preparation of bedspace prior to child's arrival Discus fluid balance and status and examination of line sites Ensure timing and details of transfer are entered into ward record book or computer system to complete the record trail

How much oxygen is available

Oxygen cylinders are available in a number of sizes which are referred to according to their allocated letter. The most commonly encountered cylinders for transfer are CD and E size cylinders. F size cylinders are the large cylinders normally found on the bottom of trolleys in theatre recovery, in emergency departments and are those carried by paramedic ambulances (Table 14.4).

Table 14.2 Assessment and preparation for transport.

Assessment	Notes/consideration
Airway Does the child need his/her airway protected before leaving? If intubated: • Correct size/length of endotracheal tube (ETT) • Chest X-ray for confirmation of placement • ETT securely strapped • Suction catheters available (correct size) • Humidity available (HME)	If the child is at risk of not maintaining a patent airway, intubation may be required, e.g. • Significant airway obstruction • Progressive respiratory failure • Comatose child/child with altering level of consciousness
Breathing Full assessment of respiratory status Spontaneously breathing child: • Oxygen supplies (see below) • Emergency equipment available Ventilated child: • Type of ventilator to be used (available within the locality) • Use of sedation (and muscle relaxants if required) • Blood gas sampling – capillary or arterial blood gas dependent upon arterial access	Ensure that child's respiratory status is stable prior to transfer or that appropriate levels of support have been instituted before leaving clinical area Ensure that child is receiving adequate levels of analgesia and sedation before considering the use of muscle relaxants
Circulation Assessment of haemodynamic status Ensure working IV access – minimum of two peripheral IVs or central venous access Baseline biochemistry and haematology results available for transfer to another hospital	If child is haemodynamically unstable there may be a need for inotropic support which should be started before leaving where possible A second (working) IV cannula is important to ensure that child continues to receive any IV infusions without having to interrupt the transfer process to site a new cannula
Disability Baseline neurological observations using age-appropriate assessment tools Child secured to avoid movement during transfer	If child has suspected or known raised intracranial pressure ensure that mannitol is available as it may be required should child deteriorate neurologically during transfer For inter-hospital transfers, CT scan prior to leaving base site where possible
Exposure Transport incubator Bubble wrap/gamgee Warming mattress/space blanket Keep ambulance warm while waiting, especially in winter – keep back doors closed Clothing – using the child's own hat, gloves, socks, blankets and babygro/pyjamas	Infants and small children who are acutely unwell have difficulty in maintaining their body temperature. The effects of cold stress on the neonate are well documented and will adversely affect clinical stability of the child (see section on 'Thermoregulation') Heat may be lost in a number of different ways such as conduction, evaporation, radiation and convection Using the child's own clothing and blankets can provide a degree of reassurance for parents
Glucose Monitor blood glucose prior to leaving and in transit if journey time is greater than 2 hours (1 hour if child has had previous blood glucose instability)	The acutely ill child will have increased metabolic demands and will utilise glycogen stores rapidly to meet these needs

Table 14.3 Calculations for oxygen requirements for transfer.

Respiratory requirements	Method for calculating oxygen
Self-ventilating child	Number of litres per minute × duration of journey
Ventilated child	Tidal volume in millilitres × number of breaths per minute × duration of journey
Estimate tidal volume at 10 mL/kg	Example: 10 kg child receiving 20 breaths per minute and a 1-hour journey: 10 mL × 10 kg = 100 × 20 breaths = 2000 mL 2000 mL = 2 L/minute × 60 minute = 120 L

Table 14.4 Oxygen cylinder capacities.

Cylinder type (letter)	Number of litres of oxygen
CD	460
E	680
F	1360
G	3400

BOC Medical (2007) at www.vitalair.co.uk.

Documentation

Clear and informative documentation is important particularly when transferring a child between hospitals but also for transfer within the same hospital site. Poor communication and a lack of preparation have been proven to increase the risk of adverse events occurring when moving acutely unwell children (Moss *et al.* 2005). An integrated comprehensive document such as the one designed by the South West Regional High Dependency Group in 2006 (Appendix 3) provides all the essential information required and has the added benefit of familiarity as all the hospitals in the region were involved in its development. This collaborative approach, working across Trusts, can only serve to improve communication between centres and therefore the service provided for children and their families.

Family

Parents are very important in a child's life, just as children are very precious to parents. There is considerable discussion and divided opinion about parents travelling in the ambulance with their child and ultimately it is likely to be the decision of the accompanying medical staff or the ambulance service (for insurance and vehicle capacity reasons). There are some circumstances where a parent must accompany the child, e.g. when a child may not survive the journey but for whom transfer is unavoidable or in the case of a child who is likely to be aware of and distressed by the absence of a parent in the ambulance.

Top tip

Do not allow parents to leave the hospital until the child is also ready to leave as this may lead to heightened anxieties for parents if for some reason the child's departure is delayed after they have left.

If parents are not accompanying the child in the ambulance it is important that they are fully informed regarding the child's progress and the plans for the child on arrival at the receiving centre. The parents should also have contact details for the child's destination as well as directions and a map if possible.

Additionally ensure that the parents know not to attempt to travel at speed behind the transferring ambulance as this can be very dangerous not only for them but also for the child and personnel travelling in the ambulance.

If preparation is the key to a safe transfer/transport then the final stage in this process is a final check before leaving the clinical area. This can be used for either internal or external transfers (see the next section).

Quick checklist for departure

- Is the airway protected?
- Is breathing satisfactory?
- Is circulation satisfactory?
- Is everything secure, including the child?
- Is emergency equipment available?

Top tip

Before leaving, think Warm, Pink, Sweet and all will be neat.

Adverse events

The potential problems or complications associated with a transport or transfer may be categorised as follows:

Personnel
Equipment
Child
Other

Neonatal transport – specific considerations

The safest way to transfer an infant is *in utero*, as there is a better outcome for this group of infants compared to those transferred *ex utero* (Fowlie *et al.* 2004). There will, however, be times when this is not possible. This includes advanced preterm labour or maternal ill health precluding safe transfer of the mother, or the necessity of having to transfer the baby to a specialist centre for ongoing care, e.g. a cardiac or surgical centre. There are a number of areas that require additional consideration specific to the neonate, along with all the other considerations discussed with regard to paediatric transportation. 'The ethos of neonatal transport care is to keep the infant stable and preferably, improve the clinical status of the infant' (Fowlie *et al.* 2004).

Practicalities of transferring a newborn infant

Thermoregulation

The need to keep infants warm has its base in historical practice; however, during the nineteenth century the level of mortality associated with hypothermia in the newborn became apparent (Woods *et al.* 2006). The regulation of temperature in newborns is greatly affected by gestational age and their size relative to surface area. This requires careful consideration when transporting neonates. Within the neonatal unit environment, incubators have double walls to minimise heat loss by radiation and are capable of providing high humidity to reduce heat loss by evaporation.

Although transport incubators are also double walled, thermoregulation still poses a challenge when transporting the newborn. Figure 14.1 outlines the effect of cold stress on the body, and how it may contribute to the deterioration of an infant during transportation by increasing ventilatory and glucose requirements (Wright 2000). To reduce the possibility of cold stress being a factor during neonatal transport, it is vital that a normal body temperature is achieved before transferring the infant into the transport incubator. Normal temperature for the newborn is 36.5–37.5°C (WHO 1997).

The transport incubator should be preheated to reduce heat loss by conduction and the time that the incubator is opened should be kept to the minimum possible. This can be achieved by transferring all of the monitoring onto the transport monitor and the infusions onto the transport infusion devices before the child is lifted into the transport incubator. If the door has to be open for any length of time while the baby is secured and settled, cover the infant with a warm blanket to reduce heat loss by convection. The use of rolls around infants will not only secure them but also reduce the heat loss by radiation. Any transparent covering over the baby should allow clear visibility of the intravenous and intra-arterial lines, the baby's colour and chest wall

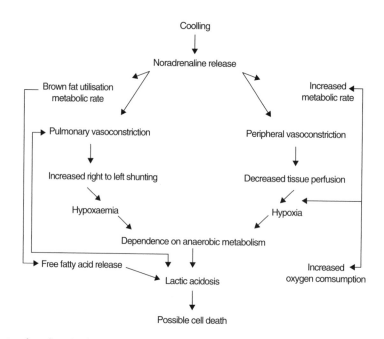

Figure 14.1 Effects of cooling in the neonate. Adapted from Lynam (1992).

movement, and should not cover the head unless the baby is ventilated.

Heated gel mattresses are also a useful tool for keeping smaller infants warm, and also provide some protection from vibration during transportation (Braithwaite 2000; Buckland *et al.* 2003; Fowlie *et al.* 2004). With bigger and more mature infants, the transport incubator may cause them to overheat, so care should be taken with them, and even if they are well babies returning to their original hospital, their temperature should be monitored and the incubator temperature adjusted accordingly.

Medical history

As well as the usual patient history that is taken and documented prior to transfer, there are some other pieces of information that are important for the team to know and be able to convey to the receiving unit. This includes a full antenatal history from early pregnancy through to any problems during delivery. The mother's previous obstetric history should also be obtained. Factors such as scan results, especially if there are discrepancies between the calculated gestational age from last menstrual period (LMP) and scan dates, placental doppler studies and the condition of the placenta after delivery may affect the ongoing treatment of the child. Mode of delivery and any CTG abnormalities, length of time the membranes were ruptured, and the administration of maternal antibiotics, and any history of maternal infection or group B *Streptococcus* carrier status (if known) are also important to know, and this information should be documented in the baby's notes and referral letters.

Communication

This is a vital part of transferring any patient; however, with neonatal transportation there are additional areas that need to be considered. The neonatal team needs to consider the health and location of the parents, especially the mother, who may be undergoing medical treatment within the maternity unit herself (Willman 1997). There are implications for bonding as there will be times when the mother has not yet seen her infant. If this is the case then this needs to be rectified before the infant is moved to another hospital. If the mother is not able to visit the unit before the infant is moved, then the transport team should try to take the infant to visit her on route to the ambulance.

Whenever possible time should be allowed for the mother to see and touch her infant. Before transfer the team should ensure that photographs are taken and personal details such as the infant's birth weight recorded. It is also important to ensure that both parents understand why transfer is necessary and are given explanations of treatment so far, and the likely management on arrival at the receiving hospital and, most importantly, are given the opportunity to ask questions (Leslie and Middleton 1995). They will also need to be given the contact details for the receiving hospital including phone numbers, as well as directions of how to get there. Hopefully, the father will be able to go to the receiving hospital and will see the infant on arrival. It is unusual to allow parents to travel in the ambulance with the team due to limited space.

The midwifery staff should be informed that the infant is being transferred so they can provide additional support for the parents. They also need to know where the infant is being transferred to so that they can make the arrangements for the ongoing care of the mother. The primary aim is to transfer the mother to the maternity services of the receiving hospital once well enough to travel. If there is going to be a delay in transferring the mother, the midwifery staff need to ascertain her

Table 14.5 Departure checklist for neonatal transport.

Check	Notes/considerations
Airway	ETT secure and not kinked Good air entry
Breathing	Check SpO_2 and respiratory rate Synchrony with the ventilator
Circulation	Arterial line transduced and BP satisfactory Baby well perfused
Vascular access	All lines visible and sites satisfactory Check perfusion distal to arterial line site
Documentation	Referral letter, copies of X-rays and scans with baby Parents' contact numbers Date of neonatal screening/ Guthrie test
Identification	Two name bands *in situ* on infant Cot card from incubator
Maternal blood sample	Required for cross matching
Breast milk	Keep frozen in a cool bag
Toys/belongings for baby	
Clinical trial information	If infant has been entered into a clinical trial, relevant information/ trial details need to accompany the infant

wishes regarding breast feeding and get her lactation established by the use of a breast pump or by manual expression. The milk needs to be stored in the deep freeze until it can be taken to the receiving hospital.

Another area of communication with the maternity staff is the necessity of obtaining a sample of blood from the mother for cross matching. This goes with the transport team and is sent to the blood bank at the receiving hospital for cross matching blood for the baby should a transfusion be required. Ensure that it is correctly labelled before leaving the hospital, or the receiving hospital blood bank will not accept it for processing.

Consent

As with all areas of treatment, there will be times when consent needs to be obtained for procedures to be performed or to permit the inclusion of the infant into clinical trials. Within neonatal care, there are some legalities as to who may give consent. There was a section added to the Children Act (1989) which related to unmarried fathers which was enacted in 2003. The Adoption and Children Act 2002, Statutory Instrument No. 3079 (C. 117) meant that unmarried fathers automatically acquired parental responsibilities if both parents jointly registered the birth of the child and the father's name appeared on the birth certificate. However, a newborn infant will not yet be registered and the sole responsibility for consent lies with the mother. This has implications if the mother and infant are in separate hospitals.

When dealing with mothers less than 16 years of age, Gillick competency needs to be taken into consideration. Although the involvement of the biological father and the grandparents may be appropriate, social services support may need to be sought (Leigh and Rennie 2005). Additionally where the parents, married or not, have learning difficulties which result in concern that they lack the capacity to make decisions on behalf of their infant, the Mental Capacity Act (2005) allows for full recourse to the courts to act on their behalf and in their best interests.

Neonatal transfer checklist

Before leaving the safety of the neonatal unit and beginning the transportation, a last-minute check of everything is vital. A summary of the checks is shown in Table 14.5.

Table 14.6 gives the outlying treatment for some specific conditions that require infants to be transferred during the neonatal period. It is worth noting that with congenital abnormalities, there may be more than one condition present so it is important to evaluate each of these during stabilisation.

Table 14.6 Summary of clinical conditions in neonates requiring specific considerations.

Abnormality/condition	Problem	Action	Rationale
Upper GI tract anomalies including oesophageal atresia and tracheoesophageal fistula	Excessive secretions unable to enter the stomach, increasing risk of aspiration	Insertion of large-bore nasogastric tube (NGT) (8 Fg) or Repogle tube into pouch Irrigate with 0.9%NaCl Aspirate NGT or Repogle tube regularly and suction oropharynx as required	Allows for drainage of thick secretions Loosens secretions Reduces risk of aspiration Nurse prone to allowing increased drainage
	Increased amount of air entering stomach, causing increased pressure on the diaphragm and increased respiratory problems	Avoid positive pressure ventilation if possible Keep baby settled	Air takes the line of least resistance and so will enter stomach through fistula. Positive pressure ventilation increases air flow in the trachea
	Unable to maintain hydration and blood glucose by enteral feeding	Commence intravenous infusion (IVI) 10% dextrose, monitoring blood glucose and hydration	Allows for adequate hydration and glucose for metabolism
Abdominal obstruction including duodenal, jejunal and ileal atresia, Hirschprung's disease, imperforate anus, malrotation, strangulated hernia and distended abdomen	Non-patent gastro-intestinal tract	Insertion, on free drainage of large-bore NGT (8 Fg). Aspirate regularly	Allows for decompression of the bowel
	Unable to maintain hydration and blood glucose by enteral feeding	IVI 10% dextrose, monitoring blood glucose and hydration	Allows for adequate hydration and glucose for metabolism

(Continued)

Table 14.6 Continued.

Abnormality/condition	Problem	Action	Rationale
Abdominal wall defects including gastroschisis, omphalocele and cloacal exstrophy	Exposed viscera, increasing risk of infection	Cover exposed viscera with food-grade 'cling film'	Allows for visualisation of exposed viscera without handling Reduces risk of contamination Reduces fluid loss and heat loss from evaporation
	Risk of compromise to blood supply	Ensure that viscera is supported and not twisted, observing colour and perfusion	If bowel is unsupported, the blood supply may become compromised as the mesenteric artery could become occluded
	Increased loss of fluid from exposed tissue	Commence IVI 10% dextrose, monitoring output. Measure blood pressure regularly, replacing with colloid if losses excessive	Allows for adequate hydration and glucose for metabolism Hypotension could be secondary to fluid loss, and should be replaced with colloid for volume
	Increased loss of temperature from evaporation	Nurse in thermal neutral environment and monitor temperature continuously	Minimise energy expenditure through temperature regulation Continuous monitoring allows for adjustment to incubator temperature
Diaphragmatic hernia	Poor respiratory function secondary to underdeveloped lungs from herniation of abdominal contents into chest cavity	Intubation without using bag-valve-mask	Minimises amount of air entering stomach, causing abdominal distension and further compromising oxygenation
		Use analgesia and paralysis	Allows for easier intubation and maximises control over ventilation
		Insert large-bore NGT (8 Fg), on free drainage and regularly aspirated	Allows for stomach decompression

Condition	Problem	Action	Rationale
Necrotising entercolitis (NEC)	Abdominal distension	Insert large-bore NGT (6 or 8 Fg) on free drainage and regularly aspirated	Allows for decompression of the stomach. May not get 8 Fg inserted in preterm babies
	Pain	Nurse supine and administer analgesia	Allows for observation of abdomen and is less uncomfortable for baby
	Inadequate ventilatory effort	May need ventilatory support	Due to systemic effects of sepsis, respiratory depressive effects of strong analgesics and diaphragmatic embarrassment from distended abdomen
Respiratory conditions including surfactant deficiency or insufficiency, meconium aspiration syndrome and pneumonia	Respiratory compromise due to pathology	Intubate and ventilate	Allows for mechanical ventilation and administration of exogenous surfactant
		Monitor all physiological parameters	Monitors effectiveness of ventilation and systemic effects of disease process, allowing for treatment
	Discomfort from intubation and handling	Administer analgesia/sedation, monitoring effectiveness, consider paralysis if baby very unsettled	Minimises discomfort from procedures and handling. Stops baby from 'fighting' the ventilator, reducing the risks of mechanical ventilation, allowing for greater control of ventilation
Upper airway anomalies including cleft lip and palate, micrognathia, Pierre–Robin syndrome, choanal atresia	Infant unable to maintain airway	Use Guedel airway for choanal atresia and nasopharyngeal prong for cleft palate and micrognathia	Allows air to pass through nasopharyngeal passages without need to intubate
		Monitor respiratory effectiveness	Ensures that adequate ventilation is achieved
		Nurse prone (cleft palate and micrognathia)	Allows tongue to fall forward out of pharynx

(Continued)

Table 14.6 Continued.

Abnormality/condition	Problem	Action	Rationale
Air leak syndromes, e.g. pneumothorax, pneumopericardium	Sudden deterioration of general condition from air accumulation	Insertion of chest drain, checking for lung re-expansion by chest X-ray prior to moving baby	Optimise condition of baby prior to moving
	Moving baby with chest drain *in situ*	Ensure that drain is securely fixed	Minimises risk of drain slipping
		Have a bladder syringe readily available or three-way stop-cock in chest drain tubing	Allows for drainage of re-accumulation of air in transit if baby suddenly deteriorates
		Administer analgesia, consider paralysis in agitated, ventilated babies	Reduces pain and discomfort. Paralysis reduces risk of asynchrony with ventilator
		Use a Heimlich (flutter) valve rather than underwater seal drain	No risk of water entering chest cavity and reduces risk of drain being caught and becoming dislodged
Congenital heart defects	Compromised circulation	May need to accept lower SpO_2 reading than normal	Administration of O_2 either has no effect on oxygenation or promotes closure of ductus arteriosus which may be enabling mixing of blood at cardiac level in certain heart anomalies
		May need ventilatory support	
	Administration of prostaglandins in duct-dependent circulation	Ensure that baby is monitored carefully during transfer	A side effect of prostin, especially in higher doses, is apnoea (see Chapter 4)
			Other side effects of prostin include hypotension, hyperthermia and bleeding abnormalities

Condition	Consideration	Action	Rationale
Neurological conditions including hypoxic ischaemic encephalopathy (HIE) and neonatal seizures	Systemic effects of acute or chronic hypoxia	Ventilate as necessary, considering use of sedation and muscle relaxants	Maintains airway, especially during seizures. Sedation and muscle relaxants will help reduce the complications of intubation in a large or mature baby
	Use of anti-convulsants	Large doses of anti-convulsants may cause respiratory depression	Ventilate if respiratory depression noted
	Use of inotropes to support systemic blood pressure	Ensure that you have satisfactory blood pressure monitoring, preferably by invasive methods	Use of cuff blood pressure monitoring may be inaccurate due to interference from movement during transfer. Monitoring allows for dose adjustment as necessary
		Preferably administer via central access	Peripheral administration of inotropes via peripheral veins causes localised vaso-constriction and reduces circulation to the limb
	Increased seizure activity by overstimulation during transfer	Insulate incubator as much as possible from noise and light, though still allowing for continuous observation of infant. Consider carefully the use of lights and sirens during transfer	Minimises sensory stimulation which can induce seizure activity
Neural tube defects, including meningocoele and meningomyelocoele	Protruding meninges and/or spinal cord through spinal lesion which may or may not be covered with a sac	Cover with food-grade cling film	Reduces risk of infection by reducing exposure to contaminants while allowing for observation for irritation or CSF leakage
		Nurse baby prone with head raised	Reduces pressure on the sac, minimising risk of rupture and, encourages urine and faeces to drain away from lesion

Adapted from: Braithwaite (2000), Wright (2000), Bates and Balistreri (2002), Fanaroff and Martin (2002), Buckland et al. (2003), Weir (2003), Bissaker et al. (2004), Berseth and Poenaru (2005), Stringer et al. (2005), Knight and Washington (2006), Paige and Moe (2006), Roaten et al. (2006)

Chapter 15

ONGOING CARE AND MANAGEMENT

Janet Murphy, Doreen Crawford and Michaela Dixon

Introduction

The aim of this chapter is to consider some of the management challenges that the care of a highly dependent child and his or her family can bring to the health care team. The areas that will be reviewed are discharge planning for the child with complex care needs into the community, safeguarding the child, spirituality and bereavement.

Any one of these topics would justify a whole chapter or indeed a whole book being written about them. This chapter provides an overview, it is not intended to be prescriptive and many of the points considered will not apply to all children as there will be individual needs and variation.

Discharge planning for children with complex care needs

Discharge planning for the highly dependent child is an essential element of the child's care and should be considered and planned for almost at the point of admission in order that discharge is achieved in a planned, timely and safe manner.

It is currently estimated that there are approximately 6000 technology-dependent children in the UK (DH 2007), although there is no reliable mechanism of national data collection to ascertain exact figures of the number of children

with high dependency needs who are receiving or need to receive complex care in the community. It is anticipated that with continued advances in neonatal and paediatric intensive care therapies more children will survive critical illness, congenital abnormalities and trauma. The demand for high dependency care in the community will increase.

The term 'technological need' is usually applied to children who require long-term oxygen therapy, parenteral nutrition and/or management of tracheostomies. However, there is a growing population of children who require long-term ventilator support. This means any child who is medically stable but continues to need support for breathing following at least 3 months of attempted weaning (Jardine and Wallis 1998). This growing number of children who require complex care raises a number of issues for the children and families involved and for those engaged in service provision.

Environment

Many medically stable children who require complex care needs and, in particular, long-term ventilation are being cared for in an acute hospital setting while waiting for discharge packages to be established. Many of these children are nursed in paediatric intensive care units (PICU) or on high dependency units (HDU) whilst others are cared for in isolation in cubicle areas on wards. It is estimated that approximately 12% of total beds available for PICU admissions are occupied by this group of children (Fraser *et al.* 1997). There is evidence that demonstrates positive improvements in children's physical, emotional, psychological and social dimensions when their health care is managed at home (Bradley *et al.* 1995; McKenzie 2000).

Resources

Many children with high dependency/complex care needs are nursed in PICU while waiting for their community care packages to be established. This has financial and resource implications. It is estimated that the cost of nursing a patient in a PICU is at least £1700 per day. Costs of community packages vary considerably depending on the individual child's needs but are not as costly as inappropriate stay on a PICU. From a service point of view, where paediatric intensive care beds are at a premium, this can result in cancelled operations, refused admissions and often necessitates families travelling many miles to the nearest available unit. More importantly, however, is the impact that being cared for in inappropriate areas has on the child and family. Research studies have shown that the emotional, social and psychological needs of these children are not being met (Gemke *et al.* 1995; Noyes 2000; Margolan *et al.* 2004). Intensive care units are known to have a higher mortality rate than any other hospital environment by the very nature of their admissions. Nursing of 'medically fit' children in these environments is inappropriate to their global development and wellbeing.

Policy directives

There have been many governmental directives and policies over the last seven decades which clearly state that the best place for children to be cared for is in their own homes (Platt Report 1959; Children Act 1989; NSF 2004). The NSF Foreword written by the then Secretary of State for Health, John Reid, stated that the NSF advocated a shift with services being designed and delivered around the needs of the child.

The core standards of the NSF can be applied to any child and young person who requires complex care in the community, but Standard 8 is particularly specific to this group of children and their families. This referred to children and adolescents who were disabled or who had complex health needs for co-ordinated, high quality child and family-centred services which were to be based on assessed needs. The ethos is to promote social inclusion and where possible enable them and their families to live ordinary lives.

Overview of discharge planning

Discharge planning for this group of children is complex, challenging, time consuming and often requires the establishment of complex multi-agency care packages between health, education, local authorities and social care.

There are no national (and, in many areas, local) guidelines or policies regarding inter-agency responsibilities. This often results in confusion, with no clear lines of responsibility. Funding for care packages can vary according to where the child resides and this can result in an inequitable level of service being provided to the children and their families.

Although there are some good examples of cross-disciplinary working and communication between various agencies with the use of excellent assessment tools and nursing dependency scores, there are many regions that have no agreed method or tool to assess the level of care input required. One of the benefits of using these tools appears to be improved multi-agency communication and planning leading to improved discharge planning. Lewis and Noyes (2007) suggest key areas for planning to facilitate and improve discharge planning (Table 15.1).

Table 15.1 Key goals for discharge planning.

Components	Actions
Funding	Funding decisions need to be agreed as early as possible across all agencies so that discharge plans and discharge are not delayed. Some regions now have inter-agency funding
Training	Parents will need to be trained and taught the necessary skills for caring for their children at home. This should include equipment use and resuscitation. If possible at least two family members should be trained. A care team will need to be established and trained appropriate to the care needs of the individual child. The use of competency documents will aid assessment and training
Communication	Early liaison is essential across all agencies involved in order to meet the needs of the child and family. The child, parents and appropriate family members should, wherever possible, be involved, valued and consulted in discharge planning
Lead professional for discharge planning	Discharge planning will be more successful if the organisation has a key professional whose responsibility is to take the lead role, or whose role it is to advise and share expertise with others. This person needs to be involved, experienced and proactive in discharge meetings to help ensure that the meetings are focused and well managed
Documentation	Explicit and accurate documentation of all stages of discharge planning is essential in ensuring every aspect is covered. A number of discharge checklists have been developed that can be adapted and used for individual cases
Resources	An awareness of the services and facilities available in the community that the child will be discharged to is important in order to have a realistic expectation of the services across health, education, housing and social care that are available
Equipment	The decision as to what equipment will be needed in the home environment will need to be made by the clinician. This has the potential to delay discharge as new equipment may need to be trialled. Once decided there may be further delays in agreeing funding streams, procurement and training of staff. Consideration will need to be given over duplication of essential equipment in case of equipment failure

Adapted from Lewis and Noyes (2007).

Stop and think

Most equipment will require electricity and batteries. Installation of an uninterruptible power supply (UPS) should be considered to cater for failure of the mains electrical supply.

Parents

It is essential that parents and family are included from the very beginning in the discharge process. The role of the parents and family in helping to care for their child at home is generally assumed (Lewis and Noyes 2007).

Parents will differ in what care they are able or willing to undertake and what level of support they will need to achieve and maintain this.

Consideration needs to be given regarding the emotional, physical and psychological ability of parents to be able to take a proactive part in their child's home care and it should not be assumed that all parents will be able to do so. Negotiation between all the agencies involved and the parents is essential to reach a realistic and agreed discharge care package which should be confirmed both verbally and by written communication, a copy of which should be given to the parents. The use of assessment tools for all children with complex care needs should help ensure equity, to be able to offer as much as possible to one child and family without disadvantaging another. Parents will often feel very anxious about caring for their child at home. A strategy should always be agreed as to the action that parents should take, together with relevant contact numbers if they should need any advice or support. Children being discharged home requiring ongoing ventilation will normally have open access arrangements in place, where they can be re-admitted directly to the HDU/PICU from home at any time of the day or night.

Carers

The recruitment and training of staff to care for children with complex care needs in the community should commence as soon as funding streams have been established. There appear to be regional differences in how this is undertaken. Some regions have a centralised team which looks after the child whilst in hospital and then through to discharge while local community teams are being set up. These teams may also be instrumental in the training of the carers. Other practices are to train carers for individual children. They are trained either by hospital staff or by continuing care teams. Variation also exists in the number of children that community carers are expected and able to care for, with some care teams caring for one child whilst others may care for two or three children on a rotational basis. Families are heavily reliant on carers to keep their children safely at home. Unfortunately some children will need to be re-admitted to hospital, not because of a medical need but because their care package has broken down due to carer illness or the non retention of carers.

Respite care for family members

Consideration and agreement needs to be given during discharge planning for the provision of respite care for the families of these children. Although there are some centres and hospices that will admit the child with complex care needs for respite, it is usually with the understanding that the trained carers come and look after the child. If respite is to occur in the family home it is usually dependent upon another family member being able and willing to come and stay at home with the child while the carers continue to

perform the care. Sadly, sometimes the only way a family can get any respite is for the child to be re-admitted into a hospital environment with their carers carrying out the care.

Resources

Department of Health, National Service Framework for Children: www.dh.gov.uk/en/policyandguidance/index.htm

Long-term ventilation working party: www.longtermventilation.co.uk

Successful discharge

Discharging children with complex care needs into the community requires organised and systematic multi-agency planning. Discharge planning appears to take varying lengths of time, from months to years in some children's cases, depending on the nature of the care package required and the facilities available within their area. Examples of good practice need to be adapted and used nationally to ensure that these children and their families receive appropriately timed and planned discharge so they can be cared for in their home environment, which, for the majority of children, is where they should be.

Holistic care

Children with complex needs are not seen as extensions of their technology; they are, first and foremost, children with individual likes and preferences. Frequently these needs are physical and are obviously met, but other needs are for comfort, play and development and this adds pleasure to parenting and gives job satisfaction to the art of caring. Other needs such as those of a spiritual dimension can be more challenging to meet and can be less easy to address. However, these needs must also be considered if the claim of holistic care is made.

Spiritual care

Like high dependency care, spiritual care is hard to define but equally essential. Defining what is meant by spirituality is problematic; it seems to mean many things to many people. Some of the difficulties in definition could be attributed to Western mainstream cultural perspectives (Thompson 2002). This is where 'spiritual' was regarded as synonymous with an organised religion or a belief system. Because spirituality was linked so closely with religion, many professionals in the past found it difficult to separate the ritual and trappings of Judo–Christian religion from the concept of spirituality. This is a very narrow focus and unless religion is separated from spirituality it could be difficult to ensure that agnostics and atheists from any culture also receive a spiritual consideration in their care.

There is a tendency to tick a box assigning the child to a particular religion and this may mean that, as far as this child is concerned, he/she is pigeonholed and labelled. This might be convenient, but it might not address individual's needs. This is especially true of children where the assumption is that they will share the same beliefs of their parents or that their parents will provide for their spiritual needs. Arguably by merging spirituality and religion and by making these assumptions there is a risk of not performing our duty of care. As a result, this core aspect of care is passed on to overstretched and pressured pastoral services, or thrust upon relatives, friends and family who might be under stress.

The literature regarding spirituality is largely philosophical in nature and interpretation and application is not straightforward, but the theme running through it is that 'it is a settled state, an emotional contentment, a peace, harmony and balance'. This can be achieved through religion but not exclusively so and the way one child finds comfort and answer to spiritual distress might not work for another. In the absence of consensus it could be stated that spirituality is many things to many people, but importantly spirituality is so individual that what one person understands it to be might not make sense to another.

Assessment of spiritual need

McSherry and Ross (2002) considered some of the dilemmas concerning the assessment, timing and comprehensiveness of the assessment process. For nurses there is the added dimension of developmental awareness and the family's needs to take into account. McSherry and Ross (2002) briefly considered the dangers of utilising a tool to assess spiritual needs, recognising the difficulties in practice. No tool is perfect and a tool is only as good as its users. Nurses are familiar with tools. Scores are used for 'measuring' pain and tissue risk; if the appropriate tool is not developed which nurses understand (and feel empathy and ownership towards), such a practice will be given lip service and the tool will occupy a folder at the foot of the cot or reside in the office. Another facet of the assessment process is who is ideally equipped to undertake it. Given the workload of the average nurse the question could be asked as to the scope and willingness to take this on. It is the essence of holistic nursing, but the cynic might reflect on how would it be costed and commissioned?

Assessment of a child's spiritual needs related to developmental awareness

There are several developmental theories that could be used to assess a child's developmental awareness. One of the more familiar is that of Piaget who considered that there were stages in development, and for convenience these are replicated below:

- Sensory-motor
- Pre-operational
- Concrete operational
- Formal operational
- Abstract

There are many criticisms of Piaget and a full critique will not be considered here. Piaget considered there to be ages related to stages; however, when children are highly dependent, chronically or terminally ill, they may have lacked the opportunity to develop normally. Additionally in some areas of development, because of different life experiences, they may seem more mature than their peers. Nurses also have to care for children with learning disabilities and those with extraordinary needs. Given this, a rigid age-related delineation is less helpful; however, as a framework to aid the understanding of cognition this work remains valuable.

Sensory motor. An infant, in the early sensory-motor stage, could only react to perceived visceral and imposed environmental stimulus. In the absence of cognitive capacity, there is no concept of the spiritual and any spiritual work done would be performed to meet the needs of the family. The soothing and comfort of the infant is of paramount importance. Tactile comfort, control of symptoms and controlled distraction can be utilised to bring about a calm, peaceful state of being.

A later sensory motor stage could mean that the nurse is working with an individual who is egocentric but has no concept of time or finality. This child is vocal but unable to verbalise feelings. Anything useful is seen as working and alive. Some of the care situations and requirements may come to be disliked, such as the re-passing of a nasogastric tube (NGT) and could be seen by the child as punishment. Developing cognition may result in a child who will accept assurances at face value and will accept fantasy and story-type explanations. The child's apparent irrational fears may indicate the iceberg of the developing subconscious and to achieve success nurses will need to work closely with the parents.

The concrete stage. During the concrete stage a child may have decentralised but is still driven by self-interest. These children are aware of the past and can worry about the future. They might challenge story and fantasy explanations and although able to articulate their feelings might not have the vocabulary to best explain what is felt. They are also developing some consideration for others and may not ask for fear of trespassing on what is obviously painful to their parents. Equally so, they may use words to hurt and punish others as they perceive that they themselves are being punished. This stage is characterised by feelings of good and bad, black and white, punishment and guilt. The tactile is still very important and artwork is valuable for working through difficult emotions. The parents are still major forces of power in these children's lives, but there can be flash points and frictions where the child feels differently compared to the parents.

Formal operations. During the formal operations stage there are developed problem-solving skills and children are certainly interested in the spiritual. They may dwell on hypothetical concepts and may try to bargain and negotiate away the feared experience. Although their comprehension and vocabulary are near that of the adult, their life experiences are not and they may struggle with spiritual work. Although seemingly mature they may regress to a point where they felt secure and the nurse may need to stay alert to the behavioural cues which might give this away. Acceptance and life review are possible and for many children it is not the death event but the process of life-threatening illness that is so frightening. These children have struggled for independence and control and spiritual work should try to offer elements of choice to reflect this.

Meeting spiritual needs in the mature child, young person and family

When planning spiritual care, with the aim of achieving spiritual balance, a range of resources and techniques can be employed. Govier (2000) suggested assessment on the basis of reason, reflection, religion, relationships and restoration.

These have to be tailored to the individual and are unlikely to fit the belief system of the carers. Those who provide such care must exert caution not to impose elements of what they think and feel on the patient. Sometimes this can be achieved through a recognised religion or a process of mediation. Other times, spiritual balance can be following a supported life review with a trusted friend or counsellor where the individual accepts what he/she has achieved and been responsible for. Some patients may need expert help to perform guided image work to uncover what their fears are and provide them with the tools to address them.

In many cases all that is required is the allocation of time on the part of the carers. Nurses need to have the time and the willingness to sit and share with the patient either in quiet companionship or to reminisce and discuss points that are important to the child. By investing time and portraying unconditional positive regard the carers are making a statement that the patient is seen as worthy and what he or she says has value and meaning. This boost to self-esteem and the comfort of being cared for is as important as the physical care.

Evaluating spiritual care

When evaluating the success of nursing care sometimes a needs cycle can be identified, with the patients needs in one area being met then resulting in other areas of need being identified. This is also true of spiritual care. When working with individuals our actions can help them to accept adversity and cope with change. Spirituality fosters a positive, calm, peaceful, harmonious state of mind and this can be evaluated. When working with a family in distress it may be harder for them to simultaneously reach coping strategies and positive states together. This might have implications for when the family leaves the direct care of the nurse and disengages from the hospital or hospice setting. McSherry and Ross (2002) identify the need for discharge to be a seamless

service and they clearly feel that continuity of care is important.

The risks of delivering spiritual care

Dealing with patients in spiritual distress can be emotionally draining for the staff involved and we have to acknowledge our own needs. Wright (2001) felt that the very ordinary experiences in life could deepen personal awareness, facilitate learning and expand the consciousness. Perhaps so, but letting off steam, recreational diversion, co-counselling and time out can also be of immense value. Many large institutions have staff counselling services built in to occupational health. Managers and senior clinicians need to foster a good team spirit and a caring staff environment where the staff can feel valued and secure in expressing how they feel. Managers need to be alert to any sick patterns that may be developing, as well as stress and burn-out in staff. For smaller teams, perhaps on agency contracts or individually appointed, these facilities and support networks may not be available and the onus is on individuals to be aware of their own mental health needs and to monitor changes in their behaviour patterns which may indicate stress.

The dying child and his or her family

For most children in HD areas the outcome will be positive. However, a few children, for a variety of reasons, will die. Some of these children will not respond to treatment, others will exhaust treatment options; in some cases the emphasis on treatment may change from aggressive or sustaining to palliative. For some the burden of life and survival will become so great that decisions are made to withdraw aggressive means of support, affording the child a dignified and peaceful death. These are circumstances where the death can be anticipated and although there are many legal and ethical implications to be considered, they are not considered here.

The context of death in childhood has changed remarkably in the past few decades with advances in healthcare technology and the change to the family structure, meaning that it has become a rarer (but not a rare) event which most commonly occurs in a hospital setting rather than in the home. This reflects what has become the societal norm, but if children and their families were given choices they may well choose different options such as home or hospice.

The death of a child is one of the most devastating experiences a parent can have (RCPCH 2004), and the loss of a child impacts not only on the individual parents but also on the family, local community and wider society (Riches and Dawson 2000; Fletcher 2002). This text provides an overview of some of the important considerations for staff involved in the death of a child in the acute hospital setting. It provides a reference tool of the practicalities involved while acknowledging that local and national policies and guidance have been developed with great care and attention to detail. This text is not intended to replace any established guidance available to practitioners.

Parents and the family

Parental grief is complex, non-linear and ongoing (Arnold *et al.* 2005). Compared to other family deaths, the grief felt by parents is severe and long lasting due in part to the nature of the parent–child relationship and the societal context and expectations of death. There are many theories around grief and bereavement which may be applied to parental grieving and these are constantly being reviewed to develop understanding amongst healthcare providers, allowing for better support and help. What is becoming apparent through research being undertaken is that the traditional stages or models of grief through which it was expected an individual would transition, arriving finally at a resolution, are too simplistic in their approach to fully explain the parental grief experience, and as noted previously grief is a complex and highly individual process (Kavanaugh and Moro 2006).

Factors that can influence grieving

There are many factors that can influence grief behaviour (Laakso and Paunonen-Ilmonen 2001; Dent and Stewart 2004; Kavanaugh and Moro 2006). These include:

- Age
- Personality
- Life experiences
- Previous experience
- Family and cultural background
- Strength of religious faith
- Availability of support
- Circumstances in which the death takes place
- Level of preparation
- Gender

Maternal grief has been extensively researched and the intensity of the grief experience is documented in many studies; however, discussion continues as to whether it is the intensity or the level of demonstration of maternal grief that may explain the perceived differences between a mother's and father's grief. The grief of fathers may well be complicated by societal expectations of their role as provider and protector of the family unit (Riches and Dawson 2000). Often staff and other family members can inadvertently reinforce these restrictions on fathers through their actions, e.g. by discussing details of the practicalities of registering a child's death with the father alone rather than with both parents.

Grandparents are in the unique and unenviable position of experiencing the death of a grandchild and watching their own child suffer at the same time. They may be overwhelmed by feelings of helplessness and seek advice about ways in which they may support their child (Dent and Stewart 2004). Individual family dynamics and other factors such as the health of the individuals determines the degree to which grandparents may be actively involved in supporting their child through their bereavement, but consideration should be given to the needs of grandparents particularly when they are present around the time of the child's death.

Siblings

The effects of the death of a child on their surviving siblings is an area where there is growing awareness and research; however, the evidence base is still limited in comparison to that of the effects of child's death on parents (Riches and Dawes 2000; Dent and Stewart 2004). Bereaved children not only lose their sibling and the sense of normality that they have known up to that point in their lives but also may suffer from the reaction of their parents (Giovanola 2005). Parents may become so immersed in their grief that the siblings are temporarily overlooked. Some of the issues practitioners should consider when talking with and caring for siblings are as follows:

- Children's perception of death, like their ability to comprehend the spiritual, depends on their age and stage of cognitive development.
- The language used to tell children about death can influence the way in which children manage death; it is important that terms such as 'gone to sleep' or 'lost' are not used due to their ambiguity and potential for misinterpretation.
- Parents are given the most support; children may be forgotten, or asked to support parents.
- Parents may wish to protect their surviving children from experiencing the death of their sibling but by doing so can make them feel excluded.
- The death of a sibling makes a child aware of his or her own mortality depending on age and cognitive development.
- Sometimes a younger child on reaching the age at which an older sibling died can become very apprehensive or fearful, particularly if he/she

was excluded rather than included at the time of the sibling's death.
- Surviving children can express their grief in many ways, including behavioural disturbances.
- Parents can compare aspects of their surviving child unfavourably with that of the dead child.
- For many children, measuring up to a dead sibling may seem an impossible task; surviving children may demonstrate low self-esteem and this may persist for years after the death.
- The surviving sibling's nursery/school should be made aware of the bereavement suffered.

The impact of death on staff

Caring for parents and families at the time of and after a child's death is a complex and challenging aspect for the team and one that is a vital part of the process of bereavement. Yoder (1994) noted that nurses have a critical role in supporting the bereaved family through their abilities to assess and respond to parents' needs regardless of the circumstances of the child's death and this view is reinforced throughout the literature. Care at the time of a child's death lays the foundations for the family over the following months and years (Davies 2004; Dent and Stewart 2004; RCPCH 2004; Schott et al. 2007). It is acknowledged that providing the level of support required by bereaved parents is very stressful for the staff involved (Papadatou 2001; Baren and Mahon 2003; Moules and Ramsay 2008).

Skills for working with bereaved families are as follows:

- Listening is one of the greatest skills and forms the foundation that supports the care that can be offered to the child's parents, siblings and other family members.
- The ability to keep an open mind and never make assumptions about the experience of the bereaved family members.
- The ability to accept grief reactions – there are no rights or wrongs for parents who have just

seen their child die; grief will manifest itself in a myriad of diverse and complex ways.

- An awareness of their own understanding and experiences of grief and bereavement and an acknowledgement that this has the potential to influence their responses to dealing with the death of a child.
- The ability to avoid imposing their own beliefs or ideas on parents through their actions or reactions.
- The ability to accept and seek support and guidance from more senior staff – ideally there should be two members of nursing staff involved in managing a child's death, one of whom should be experienced.
- The ability to reflect on the situation at the end of a shift where there has been the death of a child. It is good to take a few moments with other staff involved to review the events.

It is also important that staff have the opportunity for a more formal debriefing at a date that is suitable to those involved. The benefits of staff support following the death of a child should not be underestimated.

Care of the child after death

It is important that as much respect and care is shown for the child after death as before. Caring for the child after death involves preparing the child's body or helping and supporting the child's parents in completing some of the rituals surrounding death. Part of the ritual process of washing and dressing the child in their own clothes may in a small way contribute to a re-establishing of the parenting role, which for many parents will have been fractured by the illness and hospitalisation of their child.

Key considerations include:

- Whenever possible, removing all invasive lines, catheters, drains and tubes. (On very rare occasions it may not be possible to remove all invasive lines – in these instances there should be scope for minimising their presence)
- Applying clean dressings to any wounds
- Washing and dressing the child or assisting the child's parents to undertake this
- With parental permission, taking hand- and/or footprints along with photographs and a lock of hair. If parents do not wish to take these tokens of remembrance with them at this time, they should be stored in the child's medical notes
- Providing a private, peaceful environment where the parents and family members can spend time with the child; this may be a cubicle within the clinical area or a specific room dedicated for this purpose. It is important that parents and family members are able to spend time with the child without the presence of the healthcare team but that they know the nurse is readily accessible at all times

Ritual and custom

After a child has died there may be particular rituals or customs that need to be observed according to the child's and/or parents' faith or beliefs. Even though a child and family may be part of a particular faith, it does not necessarily mean that they practise or follow all tenets of the faith. Establishing good communication and being honest with parents if there is uncertainty about how to care for the child after death should prevent mistakes being made which may serve to heighten parental distress. A summary of some of the key factors for consideration is shown in Table 15.2; however, this list is not exhaustive and covers only some of the many faiths and belief systems practised in today's society.

Post-mortem examination (PM)

There may be instances where a PM examination may be of benefit to the parents in determining a cause of death or identifying/confirming an underlying diagnosis which may have implications for

Table 15.2 Specific considerations according to various faiths.

Faith	Considerations
Buddhism	No specific practices to be undertaken after death other than those requested by parents No religious objections to post mortem (PM) or organ donation Child will usually be cremated (cremation form will need completing)
Christianity	No specific practices to be undertaken after death other than those requested by parents No religious objections to PM or organ donation Child may be either buried or cremated according to parental wishes (cremation form will need completing if necessary)
Christian Scientist	If child is a girl it is preferred that female staff are involved in handling the child No other specific practices unless requested by parents Organ donation usually not acceptable (parents should, however, be given the option in a sensitive manner that recognises their beliefs) Cremation is usually preferred but it is individual family choice (cremation form will need completing)
Hinduism	Rituals/ practices around the time of death: • A priest tying a thread around the child's wrist or neck and the sprinkling of water from the Ganges over the child's body After death: • The child's body must not be touched by non-Hindus without the specific permission of the parents • If a non-Hindu is required to touch the child's body then gloves must be worn at all times • The child's eyes must be closed and any religious objects such as the threads applied at the time of death and/or jewellery must not be removed • The child's body should be wrapped in a plain sheet • There are no religious objections to organ donation • PM is usually refused unless required for legal reasons • If PM is carried out after death, rituals will be carried out after the procedure has been completed • Funerals usually occur within 24 hours of death; infants and young children may be buried but older children are normally cremated (cremation form will need completing)
Islam (Muslim faith)	Rituals/practices around the time of death: • A dying child should be able to lie with their face towards Mecca, which often necessitates moving the child's bed (many hospitals now have markers indicating the direction) After death: • The child's body must not be touched by non-Muslims unless it is absolutely necessary, in which case gloves must be worn • The child's head should be turned towards his or her right shoulder • A sheet should be used which covers the whole child • The child's hair must not be cut and nor should the child be washed by members of staff • The child's eyes should be closed and if necessary the lower jaw bandaged to ensure the child's mouth remains closed • Organ donation is according to the individual family's wishes • PM is discouraged unless legally required; it may be a source of distress to families • Funerals usually occur within 24 hours of death and will involve burial, as cremation is not acceptable within the faith • Parents may wish to return the child's body to the family's original home country for burial

(Continued)

Table 15.2 Continued.

Faith	Considerations
Jehovah's Witnesses	No specific practices to be undertaken after death other than those requested by parents No religious objections to PM or organ donation Child may be either buried or cremated according to parental wishes (cremation form will need completing if necessary)
Judaism	No specific practices around the time of death After death: • Within the Orthodox faith a feather is placed over the child's mouth and nose and left in place for about 8 min to confirm the absence of breath and therefore death • Wherever possible a rabbi's presence is important to the family • The child's eyes and mouth should be closed and the arms moved to lie beside the body • The child should be wrapped in a sheet and not touched until a Jewish undertaker arrives • A family member (not necessarily the parents) normally stays with the child after death until the body is taken to the undertakers • PM is not allowed unless it is for legal reasons within the orthodox faith • Organ donation is not permitted on religious ground within the orthodox faith, but less orthodox Jews and those within the Reformist movement and other tenets may consider the possibility • Funerals usually occur as soon as possible after death and if possible within 24 hours with the exception of during the Sabbath • Orthodox Jews will always have a burial for the child but other Jews may wish for cremation
Sikhism	No specific practices around the time of death After death: • There are no objections to the child being touched by non-Sikhs • The child's eyes and mouth should be closed • The family normally prepares the child's body after death • If the family is not able to prepare the child's body then staff of the same gender should wash the child's body • The symbols associated with the five K's should not be disturbed nor should any jewellery be removed • The child's body but not the face should be covered with a plain sheet • No religious objections to PM or organ donation • Funerals usually occur within 24 hours of death were possible and will involve burial for neonates and cremation for all other children

surviving children or if the parents were to have another child in the future. Seeking consent for PM is a process that should be unhurried, honest and geared towards helping parents to reach the decision that is right for them (Schott *et al.* 2007). This should be done by a member of the medical team responsible for the child's care and it is appropriate that a member of the nursing team should also be present for these discussions. Once parents have reached their decision, whatever it is, then that decision must be respected. If parents decide that a PM would be right for them, full informed consent must be obtained.

Reporting of deaths to the coroner

There are a number of cases in which the death of a child must be referred to the coroner who will then decide whether the child should undergo PM. If the coroner decides that PM is warranted then parental permission is not required and nor can the parents refuse to allow the PM to take place. The responsibility of reporting or referring a case to the coroner normally lies with the medical staff, although in some instances senior nursing staff may undertake this role (this is normally only in emergency departments).

Instances in which a death should be reported to the coroner include where:

- There is an element of suspicion surrounding the circumstances of the death or a history of violence
- The death may be linked to an accident, no matter when it occurred
- The death may be related to a medical procedure or treatment
- The death occurred during an operation before recovery from anaesthesia or may be related to anaesthesia
- Death occurred within 3 months of an invasive operation

Written information for parents

Booklets that provide parents with written information about the practicalities of managing their child's death can be invaluable. They act to reinforce verbal information given to parents at the time but which may very easily be forgotten or in some cases misheard. These booklets can also act as a guide for staff who do not have much experience in managing a child's death, by reminding them of the information parents need to be given. Many centres now have such booklets available; however, advice and support can always be sought from either local acute hospital children's services, tertiary centres or external agencies such as the Child Bereavement Trust. The availability of the booklet in appropriate languages should also be a consideration. Advice can always be gained from the leaders or representatives of a child's faith or community where appropriate, which may overcome translation difficulties.

Checklists and documentation

A comprehensive checklist which identifies the child's details, family structure, parental contact details, all the personnel involved at the time of death along with the important tasks that need

to be done after the death of a child is essential to ensure that nothing is missed that may cause further distress to the child's parents and family (PICS 2002). There is no set format for the checklist; however, there should be a place for a signature of the person responsible for carrying out each of the tasks and where staff are unable to complete all the checks, e.g. at night and weekends, there should be space for the name of the person the remaining tasks are allocated to. The checklists can be divided into medical and nursing responsibilities; however, the approach to the care of bereaved parents and the family must be one of a cohesive team.

Key medical responsibilities include:

- Ensuring the child's medical records are up to date and completed (with cause of death where possible)
- Where necessary referring to the coroner
- If not for coroner's referral or PM and where appropriate, discussion regarding hospital PM and outcome should be documented in medical records
- Obtaining consent for hospital PM (use of correct consent form)
- Where appropriate, discussion regarding organ donation for transplant purposes – outcome should be documented in medical records
- If parents wish to go ahead with organ donation, contacting the transplant co-ordinator
- Contacting the child's GP and referring consultant

Key nursing responsibilities include:

- At parent's request only, informing other family members
- After discussion with parents, informing the child's nursery or school, making a note of the name of the person contacted
- Contacting referring ward/hospital if the child was transferred in
- Contacting the child's health visitor (and where necessary liaison health visitor) and any

community nursing teams who may have been involved in the child's care

- Where appropriate, informing the chaplain and/or other support workers who may have been involved with the child and family
- Explaining the booklet of information and helping the parents identify the formalities that need to be completed, such as registering the child's death (and sometimes in the case of newborn infants, the child's birth), finding a funeral director (staff should not recommend individual funeral directors but should guide parents as to where they may find a funeral director)
- Ensuring any hospital appointments pending for the child are cancelled to avoid parents receiving reminder letters

Organ donation

As indicated in other chapters in this book there is a shortage of suitable size organs and more children on the waiting list die than receive transplants. The subject of organ donation for transplant is a sensitive issue that should be raised by the medical staff involved in the care of the child with the support of nursing staff. Experienced senior nurses may also be responsible for initiating discussions with parents. While it is a difficult topic to broach when parents are facing the death or imminent death of their own child it is noted in literature that parents are appreciative of having the opportunity to consider donation even if they decide against it as an option (PICS 2002; Dent and Stewart 2004).

Taking a child home after death

Unless a child's death is to be investigated by the coroner or the child has died from an infectious disease (advice should be sought from local infection control teams if there is any uncertainty) parents are entitled to take their child home directly from the hospital after death should they wish to do so. This does not happen very often;

however, staff have a responsibility to make parents aware that it is possible. It is important that parents do not feel rushed into making a decision or that they are being asked to leave. Before the parents leave the hospital with their child the following steps need to have been completed:

- All invasive lines must have been removed and waterproof dressing applied to wound sites.
- The death certificate should be completed and handed to the parents.
- Parents need to be made aware that they have to register the child's death within 5 days.
- Advice should be given about the practicalities of keeping the child in a cool environment once he/she is at home and the need to make contact and arrangements with a funeral director as soon as possible.

Useful resources

Child Death Helpline – www.childdeathhelpline.org.uk

Child Bereavement Charity (Trust) – www.child-bereavement.org.uk

Child Bereavement Network – www.childhood-bereavementnetwork.org.uk

Stillbirth and Neonatal Death Charity – www.uk-sands.org

Winston's Wish – www.winstonswish.org.uk

The Compassionate Friends – www.tcf.org.uk

CRUSE – www.crusebereavementcare.org.uk

These websites are provided as potential resources only – it is the responsibility of the practitioner to visit the sites and assess their suitability before providing them to parents and children.

Safeguarding children

The term 'safeguarding children' means protecting children from maltreatment, preventing impairment of children's health or development, and ensuring that children are growing up in circumstances consistent with the provision of safe and effective care (Working Together to Safeguard Children, HM Government 2006). In a modern and developed country, it would be reasonable to believe that a child's safety and development would be paramount. Unfortunately this is not so, and some children in the UK remain at risk (Healthcare Commission 2007). This remains the case despite a number of high profile and distressing enquiries into services which for one reason or another failed to safeguard children (Laming 2000; Kennedy 2001).

The HD child at risk

Children remain at risk whether in the hospital or the community. Arguably HD infants and children are at increased risk owing to their unique and special circumstances and the potentially complex nature of their relationships with family, carers, close friends and acquaintances. They are more at risk owing to the number of interventions they require and there are also special circumstances that may apply to some members of this group of children more than any other, in that they may be more at risk through unlicenced medications, emerging supportive technology and clinical trials.

The Health Care Commission Report (2007)

Although there are existing national and local guidelines for the protection and safety of children, the Health Care Commission (2007) identified areas of improvement, with respect to developing networks for planned surgical intervention, for example, and the management of pain. The commission reiterated the hospital standard to be achieved for the maintenance of life support in serious emergencies.

This hospital standard states that every acute hospital providing emergency care, inpatient care or surgery must secure and maintain a rota for the resuscitation of very sick children. Staff should be trained and experienced in advanced

Table 15.3 Assessment framework for safeguarding children.

Domain	Areas for consideration
Child's developmental needs	Health, education, emotional and behavioural development, identity, family and social relationships, social presentation, self-care skills
Family and environmental factors	Family history and functioning, wider family, housing, employment, income, family's social integration, community resources
Parenting capacity	Basic care, ensuring safety, emotional warmth, stimulation, guidance and boundaries, stability

Adapted from Working Together to Safeguard Children, HM Government (2006).

paediatric life support (APLS) or its equivalent. Moreover these staff should be able to recognise the symptoms of life-threatening illnesses, such as meningitis, and start emergency treatment to resuscitate and stabilise the child, including managing the airway.

The staff should have back-up and support from a consultant who can attend within a short time.

Specific strategies to keep children safe

The common assessment framework
In addition, a common assessment framework was developed as a guide for inter-agency working to safeguard children and promote the welfare of children (see Table 15.3). This created a clear pathway to be followed in the event of any concern and pulled together strands from the Children Act (2004) and the National Service Framework for Children (2004).

The ethos behind these legislative frameworks is encapsulated in the NSF (2004) which states that all children should have the best opportunity

Table 15.4 Staff training for safeguarding children.

Level of training	Target audience	Content
Level 1	All staff on induction	Recognise and respond to concern for a child in need. Appreciate own role and that of others. Communicate and act appropriately within national and local guidelines to safeguard children. Be familiar with available services.
Level 2	Compulsory for all staff working directly with children	Revisits level 1 + increased knowledge around process. Increased awareness of national and local policies. Awareness of local safeguarding children board (LSCB). Knowledge of forms/process
Level 3	Senior practitioners	Level 1&2 + Some elements of level 2 but to a higher level. Specifically focus on issues within the child protection field
Level 4	Senior practitioners (nurses and doctors) in child protection area	Risk management. Managing conflict. Update of relevant practice/research within safeguarding arena
Level 5	Lead professionals in child protection. Named doctors/ nurses	Level 4 + political awareness. Strategic developments in protection and safeguarding children

to achieve their full potential and to be healthy, stay safe, to enjoy and achieve, to make a positive contribution and to achieve economic wellbeing. The principal point here is all children, and this applies to HD children wherever they are cared for as much as well children cared for by family at home.

Ensuring staff are suitable to work with vulnerable children

Nurses have a statutory duty to remain clinically updated and they must adhere to NMC regulations in order to remain on the professional register. Healthcare assistants, teacher support workers, volunteers and nursery nurses have as yet no statutory obligation.

However, organisations providing services for children have a statutory responsibility in ensuring personnel are safe to work with children and their families and in training staff at an appropriate level. All healthcare professionals who have contact with children require an enhanced police check which is performed by the criminal records bureau. In addition all employees should have relevant training on safeguarding children. The level of training is usually decided locally. An example of training given by a Children's Foundation Trust is illustrated in Table 15.4.

Reviewing strategies for safeguarding children

When reviewing strategies for safeguarding children it is tempting to focus on the macro-strategies – the major legislative frameworks. However, if safeguarding children is everybody's business it is important to not lose sight of the smaller activities that nurses caring for HD children can do. Thus close adherence to infection control policy, keeping up to date with the latest NICE guidelines, keeping an eye on the National Patient Safety Agency (NPSA) guidelines, maintaining a child-friendly perspective, remaining vigilant and following one's common sense (if something sounds unsafe, looks unsafe, feels unsafe – it probably is!) are all important strategies.

APPENDIX 1

Daily check list for equipment in high dependency areas.

	M	T	W	T	F	S	S
Dry white board and markers APLS/good practice algorithms Organised emergency trolley Printed drug doses/tape Clock							
Monitoring equipment ECG monitor/defibrillator with paediatric paddles 0–400 J and hardcopy capabilities Pulse oximeter (adult/paediatric probes) Blood pressure cuffs (infant, child, adult, thigh) A method of measuring core temperature, covering both hypo- and hyperthermia (e.g. rectal, tympanic membrane, naso-pharyngial thermometer) Otoscope, ophthalmoscope, stethoscope Cardiopulmonary monitor with capability to monitor invasive arterial and central venous pressure Non-invasive blood pressure monitoring (infant, child, adult cuffs) Portable capnograph Arterial/capillary blood glucose monitor (desirable) Access to blood gas machine Access to 12 lead ECG							
Airway control/ventilation equipment Bag-valve-mask device: paediatric (500 mL) and adult (1000/2000 mL) with oxygen reservoir Infant, child and adult masks Oxygen delivery device with flow meter Clear oxygen masks, standard and non-rebreathing (neonatal, infant, child, adult) Nasal cannula (infant, child, adult) Oral airways (sizes 0–5) Suction devices – catheters (6–14 Fg yankauer tip) Nasal airways (infant, child, adult)							

	M	T	W	T	F	S	S
Nasogastric tubes (sizes 6–16 Fg)							
Laryngoscope handle and blades: curved 2,3; straight or Miller 0,1,2,3							
Endotracheal tubes: uncuffed (2.5–5.5), cuffed (6.0–9.0)							
Stylets for endotracheal tubes (paediatric, adult)							
Lubricant, water soluble							
Magill forceps (various sizes)							
Laryngeal masks (size 0–3) (desirable)							
Tracheal guide (desirable)							
Tracheostomy tubes (shiley sizes 0–6) (desirable)							
Oxygen blender							
Paediatric ventilators (desirable)							
Chest drain set							
Cricoidotomy set (desirable)							
Vascular access							
Butterflies (19–25 gauge)							
Needles (18–27 gauge)							
Intraosseous needles							
Catheters for intravenous lines (16–24 gauge)							
IV administration sets and extension tubing with calibrated chambers							
Paediatric infusion pumps							
Syringe drivers							
IV fluids							
Lumbar puncture set							
Urinary catheters (Foley 6–14 Fg)							
Fracture immobilisation (desirable)							
Cervical collar – hard and soft (desirable)							
Spinal board (child/adult)							
Femur splint (desirable)							
Extremity splints							
Miscellaneous							
Weighing scale							
Heating source (for infant warming)							

Devised from NHS (2004) Appendix 5; available from http://www.perinatal.nhs.uk/manners/Standards.pdf.

APPENDIX 2

Normal values

	Pre-term	Neonatal
Neonatal electrolyte and urea ranges		
Sodium (Na) mmol/L	130–140	130–145
Potassium (K) mmol/L	4.5–7.0	4.0–6.0
Chloride (Cl) mmol/L	90–115	92–110
Calcium (Ca) mmol/L	1.9–2.8	2.0–2.9
Phosphate (PO_4) mmol/L	1.1–2.6	1.8–3.0
Magnesium (Mg) mmol/L	0.62–1.27	0.7–1.15
Glucose mmol/L	2.0–5.5	2.5–5.5
Creatinine μmol/L	50–120	55–150
Urea mmol/L	1.5–6.7	2.0–5.2

Blood gas values	
pH	7.3–7.4
$PaCO_2$	4.6–6.0 kPa (35–45 mmHg)
PaO_2	7.3–12 kPa (55–90 mmHg)
Bicarbonate	18–25 μmol/L
Base excess	−2 to +2

APPENDIX 3

TRANSFER DOCUMENT

| PLEASE AFFIX |
| PATIENT'S ADDRESSOGRAPH |

Patient's weight ....

Date: ....   Time: ....

   1. Discussion with receiving unit / Name of staff member ....

   2. Handover provided ....

   3. Departure time ....

Mode of transport:

Ambulance	☐	Hospital transport	☐
Para-medic ambulance	☐	Own transport	☐
Other			☐

Destination: ....

Receiving doctor: ....   Tel. no: ....

Receiving nurse: ....   Tel. no: ....

Accompanying staff / Family:

Dr: ....

Nurse: ....

Parent / Carer / Other: ....

Contact details of parent / carer / other: ....

Current care issues: 1. ....

                            2. ....

                            3. ....

Principle reason for transfer:

SWPHDG 2006

SOUTH WEST REGIONAL PAEDIATRIC HIGH DEPENDENCY GROUP

OBSERVATIONS

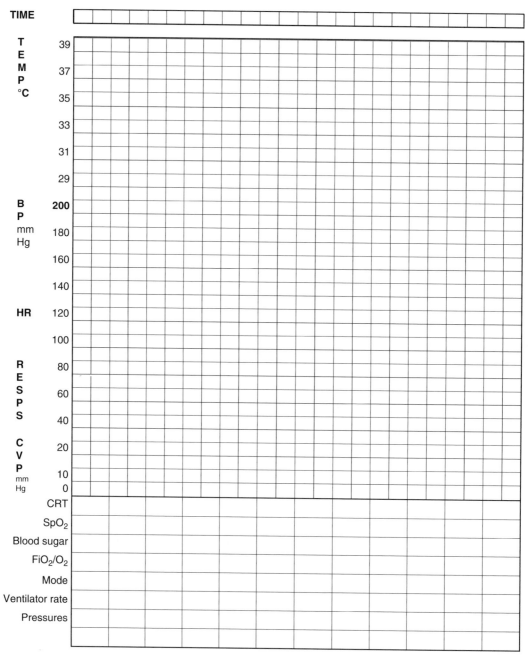

SWPHDG 2006

SOUTH WEST REGIONAL PAEDIATRIC HIGH DEPENDENCY GROUP

NEURO OBS:		Glasgow Coma Scale (4–15 yrs)								Children's Coma Scale (<4 yrs)								TIME
C O M A S C A L E	Eyes Open	Spontaneously	4							Spontaneously	4							Eyes closed by swelling = C
		To speech	3							To speech	3							
		To pain	2							To pain	2							
		No response	1							No response	1							
	Best Motor Response	Obeys verbal commands	6							Obeys verbal commands	6							Usually the best arm response
		Localises pain	5							Localises pain	5							
		Flexion to pain	4							Withdraws in response	4							
		Abnormal flexion	3							Abnormal flexion	3							
		Extension to pain	2							Abnormal extension	2							
		No response	1							No response	1							
	Best Verbal Response	Orientated & converses	5							Smiles, orientated to sounds, follows objects, interacts	5							Endotracheal tube or tracheostomy =T
		Disorientated & converses	4							Crying / Interacts Consolable Inappropriate	4							
		Inappropriate words	3							Inconsistently Moaning Consolable	3							
		Incomprehensible sounds	2							Inconsolable Irritable	2							
		No response	1							No response No response	1							
PUPILS	Right	Size								Size								+ reacts - no reaction c eyes closed
		Reaction								Reaction								
	Left	Size								Size								
		Reaction								Reaction								

FLUIDS

	TIME										
IN T A K E											
	TOTAL										
O U T P U T	Urine										
	TOTAL										
	BALANCE										

TRANSFER EVALUATION FORM

Airway / C-Spine   **E**nvironment

Breathing   **F**amily

Circulation   **G**lucose

Disability

Other Comments ....

....

Signed: ....   Date: ....

SWPHDG 2006

SOUTH WEST REGIONAL PAEDIATRIC HIGH DEPENDENCY GROUP

TRANSFER CHECK LIST

SELF-INFLATING AMBU BAG - INF / PAED / ADULT ☐

OXYGEN / AIR CYLINDERS
× 2 / × 3 E SIZE (× 1 WITH VENT VALVE)
PORTABLE CYLINDER FROM BEDSPACE ☐

PORTABLE SUCTION
APPROPRIATE SUCTION CATHETERS ☐

ECG MONITOR
POWER PACK AND LEAD
ETCO2 MONITOR APPROPRIATE CABLES ☐☐

THERMOMETER ☐

FACE MASKS
NEO / INFANT / CHILD / SML & LGE ADULT ☐

GREEN TUBING ☐

NEBULISER SET + TUBING ☐

STETHOSCOPE ☐

YANKEUR × 2 ☐

GUEDEL AIRWAYS SIZES (×1 of each):
4 / 3 / 2 / 1 / 0 / 00 / 000 ☐

**ELASTOPLAST / ASSORTED TAPE /
PLASTERS** ☐

SYRINGE PUMPS ☐

VOLUMETRIC PUMP ☐

DRUG BAG
INOTROPES / RESUS DRUGS
SEDATION
MISCELLANEOUS ☐☐☐

INTRA-OSSEOUS NEEDLE ☐

IV CANNULAS (e.g. Neoflon, Medicut, etc.) ☐

ASSORTED IV BUNGS / STERETS ☐

FOR INTUBATED CHILDREN

VENTILATOR ☐

ETT 2.5–8.5 UNCUFFED / CUFFED ☐

STYLET SIZES
12 × 2
2.2 × 1 ☐☐

ENDOTRACHEAL TAPE ☐

LARYNGOSCOPE BULBS × 2 SPARE ☐

AQUAGEL × 2 ☐

MAGILLS:
1 SMALL
1 LARGE ☐☐

SYRINGES
50ML
10ML / 5ML LEURLOCK ☐

NORMAL SYRINGES
10ML / 5ML / 2ML / 1ML ☐

INSULIN SYRINGES ☐

GLUCOSE MONITOR ☐

IV EXTENSION LINES ☐

3 WAY TAPS / T-PIECE ☐

SPACE BLANKET ☐

DRUG LABELS ☐

SCISSORS / FORCEPS ☐

NG TUBE & LITMUS PAPER ☐

GLOVES 6.0–8.5 ☐

GAUZE × 2 ☐

**SURGISILK 3/0 / SURGICAL BLADES /
SUTURE CUTTER** ☐

GAMGEE / BUBBLE WRAP ☐

BATTERIES (Appropriate for equipment) ☐

FAMILY - INFORMED / CONSENT / DIRECTIONS ☐

COPIES OF NOTES / X-RAYS / REF. LETTER ☐

RESTRAINT IN TRANSPORT ☐

ACCEPTING HOSPITAL AWARE OF DEPART. ☐

STAFF - FOOD & DRINK / MONEY / PHONE ☐

ARRANGEMENT FOR RETURNING STAFF ☐

LARYNGOSCOPE HANDLES × 2 ☐

FLEXIBLE CATHETER MOUNT ☐

ANGLE PIECE ☐

LARYNGOSCOPE BLADES:
1 × SHORT STRAIGHT
1 × LONG STRAIGHT
1 × SHORT CURVED
1 × LONG CURVED ☐☐☐☐

OTHER: .... ☐

OTHER: .... ☐

SWPHDG 2006

SOUTH WEST REGIONAL PAEDIATRIC HIGH DEPENDENCY GROUP

NURSING REFERRAL FORM - TRANSFER OF PATIENTS

Home
 	
From   Ward
 	
       Ward tel. no.
 	
       Hospital
	To:
	
	Hosp. no:

Surname: Forenames:	Age: Religion: D.O.B.
Home address: Tel. no:	Discharge address:
Consultant: Social worker: General practitioner: Address: Health visitor (HV): HV informed of transfer: Yes / No Other:	Next of kin: Address: Relationship: Tel. no:
Date of admission: Date of transfer:	Relatives notified of transfer: Yes / No

SWPHDG 2006

SOUTH WEST REGIONAL PAEDIATRIC HIGH DEPENDENCY GROUP

Diagnosis and Brief Summary of Patient's condition
Other comments *(e.g. allergies, special disabilities, pre-existent conditions, etc.)*

Nursing requirements *(Including special diets, feeding and dressings)*

Drugs and medicines

Family information

Follow-up treatments and appointments

Date   1. ....   Time ....   Place ....

Date   2. ....   Time ....   Place ....

What arrangements have been made for transport? ....

Please photocopy and keep
1 copy in notes

Signature ....

Designation ....

Date ....

REFERENCES, FURTHER READING AND RESOURCES

Aaronson, P.I., Ward, J.P.T. and Wiener, C.M. (2003) *The Cardiovascular System at a Glance*, 2nd edn. Oxford, UK: Blackwell Publishing.

Abdulla, R., Blew, G. and Holterman, M.J. (2004) Cardiovascular embryology. *Pediatric Embryology* **25** (3), 191–200.

Action for Sick Children (1989) *A Collection of Essays on Children's Healthcare London*. London: HMSO, pp. 10–20.

Adomat, R. and Hicks, C. (2003) Measuring nursing workload in intensive care: an observational study using closed circuit video cameras. *Journal of Advanced Nursing* **42** (4), 402–412.

Advanced Life Support Group (2005a) *Advanced Paediatric Life Support: The Practical Approach*, 4th edn. London/Oxford, UK: BMJ Books/Blackwell Publishing.

Advanced Paediatric Life Support Group (APLS) (2005b) *Advanced Paediatric Life Support: The Practical Approach*, 4th edn. London: BMJ Publishing Group.

Alexander, J.W. (1999) Is early enteral feeding of benefit? *Intensive Care Medicine* **25** (2), 129–130.

Alexander, S. (1996) Peritoneal dialysis. In: *Replacement of Renal Function by Dialysis*, 4th edn. Boston: Kluwer Academic Publishers.

Altman, A.J. and Fu, C. (2006) Chronic leukaemia's of childhood. In Pizzo, P.A. and Poplack, D.G. (editors) *Principles and Practice of Paediatric Oncology*, 5th edn. Philadelphia, USA: Lippincott Williams & Wilkins, pp. 645–673.

Anand, K. and Hall, R. (2006) Pharmacological therapy for analgesia and sedation in the newborn. *Archives of Disease in Childhood* **91** (6), 448–453.

Anter, A.M. and Bondok, R.S. (2004) Peripheral venous pressure is an alternative to central venous pressure in paediatric surgery patients. *Acta Anaesthesiologica Scandinavica* **48** (9), 1399–6576.

Antonarakis, E.S. and Hain, R.D.W. (2004) Nausea and vomiting associated with cancer chemotherapy: drug management in theory and practice. *Archives of Disease in Childhood* **89** (9), 877–880.

Arafat, M. and Mattoo, T.K. (1999) Measurement of blood pressure in children: recommendations and perceptions on Cuff Selection. *Pediatrics* **104** (3), 30. Available at http://pediatrics.aappublications. org/cgi/content/full/104/3/e30#Discussion. Accessed 5/10/06.

Arnold, J., Bushman, G.P. and Cushman, L.F. (2005) Exploring parental grief: combining quantitative and qualitative measures. *Archives of Psychiatric Nursing* **19** (6), 245–255.

Arrowsmith, J. and Campbell, C. (2000) A comparison of local anaesthetics for venepuncture. *Archives of Disease in Childhood* **82** (4), 309–310.

Audit Commission (1999) *Critical to Success: the Place of Efficient and Effective Critical Care Services within the Acute Hospital*. London: Audit Commission.

Australia and New Zealand Burn Association (2006). Emergency management of severe burns. *UK Course Manual*, 10th edn. ANZBA.

Aziz, H.F., Martin, J.B. and Moore, J.J. (1999) The pediatric disposable end tidal carbon dioxide role in endotracheal intubation in newborns. *Journal of Perinatology* **19** (2), 110–113.

Babl, F., Munro, J., Kainey, G. *et al.* (2006) Scope for improvement hospital wide sedation practice at a children's hospital. *Archives of Disease in Childhood* **91** (8), 716–717.

Baggaley, A. (2001) *Human Body*. London: Dorling Kindersley.

Baker, C. (2004) Preventing ICU syndrome in Children. *Paediatric Nurse* **16** (10), 32–35.

Ball, C., Walker, G., Harper, P., Sanders, D. and McElligott, M. (2004) Moving on from "patient dependency" and "nursing workload" to managing risk in critical care. *Intensive and Critical Care Nursing* **20** (5), 62–68.

Ball, J. and Bindley, R. (2006) *Clinical Handbook for Pediatric Nursing*. New Jersey, USA: Pearson Prentice Hall.

Baren, J.M. and Mahon, M. (2003) End-of-life issues in the Pediatric Emergency Department. *Clinical Pediatric Emergency Medicine* **4** (4), 265–272.

Barker, R.A., Barasi, S. and Neal, M.J. (2003) *Neuroscience at a Glance*, 2nd edn. Oxford, UK: Blackwell Publishing.

Barrow, R. and Herndon, D. (2007) History of treatment of burns. In Herndon, D. (editor) *Total Burn Care*, 3rd edn. Philadelphia, USA: Elsevier Saunders.

Bartlett, E.M. (2000) Temperature measurement: why and how in intensive care. *Nursing Standard* 14 (44), 39–43.

Barua, P. and Bhowmick, B. (2005) Hypodermoclysis; a victim of historical prejudice. *Age and Aging* 34 (3), 215–217.

Bates, M.D. and Balistreri, W.F. (2002) The neonatal gastrointestinal tract. In Fanaroff, A.A. and Martin, R.J. (editors) *Neonatal and Perinatal Medicine*, 7th edn. London: Mosby.

Baur, P. (2001) High dependency care – an ill-defined concept? *Nursing in Critical Care* 6 (1), 40–47.

Beath, S.V. (2003) Hepatic function and physiology in the newborn. *Seminars in Neonatology* 8 (2), 337–346.

Bechard, L.J., Adiv, O.E., Jaksic, T. and Duggan, C. (2006) Nutritional supportive care. In Pizzo, P.A. and Poplack, D.G. (editors) *Principles and Practice of Pediatric Oncology*, 5th edn. Philadelphia, USA: Lippincott Williams & Wilkins, pp. 1330–1347.

Beeson, M. (2007) Superior vena cava syndrome. www.emedicine.com/emerg/topic651 (Last accessed October, 2007).

Beiri, D., Reeve, R., Champion, G. et al. (1990) The faces pain scale for the self assessment of the severity of pain experienced by children; development, initial validation and preliminary investigation for ratio scale properties. *Pain* 41 (2), 139–150.

Bell, F. (2002) Assessment and management of the child with nephrotic syndrome. *Paediatric Nursing* 14 (1), 37–42.

Belliene, C., Cordelli, D., Raffaelli, M. et al. (2006) Analgesic effect of watching TV during venepuncture. *Archives of Disease in Childhood* 91 (12), 1015–1017.

Bennett, L. (2005) Understanding sickle cell disorders. *Nursing Standard* 19 (32), 52–61.

Bennett, M. (2003a) Guidelines for sedation of the critically ill child. *Paediatric Nurse* 15 (9), 14–18.

Bennett, M. (2003b) Sleep and rest in PICU. *Paediatric Nurse* 15 (1), 3–6.

Bennett-Rees, N. and Soanes, L. (1999) Complications of bone marrow transplant. In Gibson and Evans, M. (editors) *Paediatric Oncology* London: Whurr Publishers, pp. 225–241.

Berde, C.B., Billett, A.L. and Collins, J. (2006) Symptom management in supportive care. In Pizzo, P.A. and Poplack, D.G. (editors) *Principles and Practice of Pediatric Oncology*, 5th edn. Philadelphia, USA: Lippincott Williams & Wilkins, pp. 1348–1379.

Berger, M.M., Spertini, F., Shenkin, A. et al. (1998) Trace element supplementation modulates pulmonary infection rates after major burns: a double-blind, placebo-controlled trial. *American Journal of Clinical Nutrition* 68 (2), 365–371.

Berseth, C.L. and Poenaru, D. (2005) Necrotizing enterocolitis and short bowel syndrome. In Taeusch, H.W., Ballard, R.A. and Gleason, C.A. (editors) *Avery's Diseases of the Newborn*, 8th edn. Philadelphia, USA: Elsevier Saunders.

Beyer, J. and Wells, N. (1989) The assessment of pain in children. *Pediatric Clinics of North America* 36 (4), 837–854.

Birmingham Children's Hospital Paediatric Laboratory Medicine Handbook (2001) August. Birmingham Children's Hospital NHS Trust.

Bissaker, S., Hindley, C., Gaillard, E. and Shaw, N.J. (2004) Respiratory status of infants being transported with respiratory distress syndrome: the effect of pretransfer advice, stabilisation and the transport itself. *Journal of Neonatal Nursing* 10 (3), 96–98.

Blows, W.T. (2004) *The Biological Basis of Nursing: Clinical Observations*. London: Routledge.

BNF (2007) *BNF for Children*. London: BMJ Publishing Group.

Bond, C. (1999) Positive touch and massage for the neonate needing; a means of reducing stress. *Journal of Neonatal Nursing* 5 (5), 16–20.

Bonica, J. (1990) Evolution and the current status of pain programs. *Journal of Pain and Symptom Management* 5 (6), 368–374.

Boxwell, G. (editor) (2000) Neonatal intensive care nursing. *Developmentally Focused Nursing Care*. UK: Routledge.

Bradford Community Children's Team (2002) *Continuing Care Needs Assessment Tool*, 1st edn. Bradford City: NHS Primary Care Trust.

Bradley, R.H., Parette, H.P. and Bierliet, A. (1995) Families of young technology dependent children and the social worker. *Social Work in Pediatrics* 21 (1), 23–27.

Braithwaite, I. (2000) Issues in neonatal transport: improving safety for patients and staff. *Journal of Neonatal Nursing* 6 (2), 65–69.

Brant, J.M. (2002) Rasburicase: an innovative new treatment for hyperuricemia associated with tumor lysis syndrome. *Clinical Journal of Oncology Nursing* 6 (1), 12–16.

Breitfield, P.P. and Meyer, W.H. (2005) Rhabdomyosarcoma: new windows of opportunity. *Oncologist* 10 (7), 518–527.

British Committee for Standards in Haematology (2003) Guidelines for the use of platelet transfusion. *British Journal of Haematology* 122 (1), 10–23.

British National Formulary for Children (BNFC) (2006) London: BMJ Books.

British National Formulary for Children (BNFC) (2007) London: BMJ Publishing Group. Available from www.bnfc.org/bnfc/

British Society For Paediatric Endocrinology and Diabetes (BSPED) (2004) *Recommended DKA Guidelines.* Available online at www.bsped.org.uk.

Brown, C.G. and Wingard, J. (2004) Clinical consequences of oral mucositis. *Seminars in Oncology Nursing* 20 (10), 16–21.

Brown, P. (1999) Nutrition and cancer. *Medsurg Nursing* 8 (6), 333–348.

Broyer, M., Selwood, N. and Brunner, F. (1998) Minimal changes and focal segmental glomerular sclerosis. In Davidson, A.M., Cameron, J.S., Grunfeld, J.P. *et al.* (editors) *Oxford Textbook of Clinical Nephrology,* 2nd edn., Vol. 1. Oxford: Oxford University Press.

Bruce, E. and Franck, L. (2000) Self administered nitrous oxide (Entonox) for the management of procedural pain. *Paediatric Nursing* 12 (7), 15–19.

Buckland, L., Austin, N., Jackson, A. and Inder, T. (2003) Excessive exposure of sick neonates to sound during transport. *Archives of Disease in Childhood Fetal and Neonatal* 88 (6), F513–F518.

Butcher, D. (2004) Pharmacological techniques for managing acute pain in emergency departments. *Emergency Nurse* 12 (1), 26–35.

Cairo, M.S. and Bishop, M. (2004) Tumour lysis syndrome; new therapeutic strategies and classification. *British Journal of Haematology* 127 (1), 3–11.

Campbell, D. (2003) How acute renal failure puts the brakes on kidney function. *Nursing* 33 (1), 59–63.

Campbell, S. (2007) The need for a global response to antimicrobial resistance. *Nursing Standard* 21 (44), 35–40.

Campbell, T. (2000) Central venous catheter management in patients with cancer. *International Journal of Palliative Nursing* 6 (7), 331–337.

Cancer Research UK (2007) Learn about cancer. Radiotherapy. http://info.cancerresearchuk.org/cancerandresearch/learnaboutcancer/treatment/radiotherapy/ (Last accessed 29/10/07).

Carbajal, R., Soocramanien, V., Couderc, S. *et al.* (2003) Analgesic effect of breast feeding in term neonates. *British Medical Journal* 236 (1136), 13.

Carli, M., Cecchetto, G., Sotti, G., Alaggio, R. and Stevens, M.G.S. (2004) Soft tissue sarcomas. In Pinkerton, R., Plowman, P.N. and Pieters, R. (editors) *Paediatric Oncology,* 3rd edn., Chapter 17. London: Arnold, pp. 339–371.

Carney, N.A., Chesnut, R. and Kochanek, P.M. (2003) Guidelines for the acute medical management of severe traumatic brain injury in infants, children and adolescents. *Pediatric Critical Care Medicine* 4 (Suppl 3), S1.

Chamley, C.A., Carson, P., Randall, D. *et al.* (2005) *Developmental Anatomy and Physiology of Children – A Practical Approach.* Edinburgh: Elsevier Churchill Livingstone.

Chandler, T. (2000) Oxygen saturation monitoring. *Paediatric Nursing* 12 (8) 37–42.

Children's Act England (1989) London: HMSO.

Children's Cancer and Leukemia Group (CCLG) (2007) *Children's Cancer and Leukaemia Group.* www.cclg.org.uk (Last accessed November, 2007).

Colby-Graham, M. and Chordas, C. (2003) The childhood leukaemia's. *Journal of Pediatric Nursing* 18 (2), 87–95.

Cole, E. (2007) Measuring central venous pressure. *Nursing Standard* 22 (7), 40–42.

Coles, L., Glasper, A., Fitzgerald, C. *et al.* (2007) Measuring compliance to the NSF for children and young people in one English Strategic Health Authority. *Journal of Children's and Young People's Nursing* 1 (1), 7–15.

Collins, M., Phillips, S., Dougherty, L. *et al.* (2006) A structured learning programme for venepuncture and cannulation. *Nursing Standard* 20 (26), 34–39.

Constanzo, L.S. (2006) *Physiology,* 3rd edn. Philadelphia, USA: Elsevier Mosby.

Cook, P. (1999) Supporting the staff. In *Supporting Sick Children and their Families.* London: Ballière-Tindall.

Crawford, D. (1994) Expert care in anxious times: nursing care of neonates with jaundice. *Child Health* 1 (6), 225–231.

Creedon, A. (2005) Healthcare workers hand decontamination practices – compliance with recommended guidelines. *Journal of Advanced Nursing* **51** (3), 208–216.

Cronin, K., Butler, P., McHugh, M. and Edwards G. (1996) A 1 year prospective study of burns in an Irish paediatric burns unit. *Burns* **22** (3), 221–224.

Cropper, J. (2003) Post operative urine retention in children. *Paediatric Nurse* **15** (7), 15–18.

Cunningham, R.S. and Bell, R. (2000) Nutrition in cancer: an overview. *Seminars in Oncology Nursing* **16** (2), 90–98.

Curley, M.A.Q. and Moloney-Harmon, P.A. (2001) *Critical Care Nursing of Infants and Children*, 2nd edn. Philadelphia, USA: WB Saunders Company.

Currie, J. (2006) Management of chronic pain in children. *Archives of Disease in Childhood* **91** (4), 111–114.

Davies, J. and Hassell, L. (2007) *Children in Intensive Care: A Survival Guide*, 2nd edn. London: Churchill Livingstone.

Davies, R. (2004) New understandings of parental grief: literature review. *Journal of Advanced Nursing* **46** (5), 506–513.

Davis, J. and Hassell, L. (2001) Children in intensive care. *A Nurse's Survival Guide*. Edinburgh: Churchill Livingstone.

Davis, M.A., Gruskin, K.D., Chiang, V.W. and Manzi, S. (2005) *Signs and Symptoms in Pediatrics: Urgent and Emergent Care*. Philadelphia, USA: Elsevier Mosby.

Day, H. (2005) Classifying High Dependency Care. Available online http://www.picupt.nhs.uk/_Rainbow/Documents/f27ae6b2-c6e1–4062–80b0–ba5206ea8969.doc (Last accessed 7/11/07).

Day, H., Allen, Z. and Llewellyn, L. (2005) High dependency care: a model for development. *Paediatric Nursing* **17** (3), 24–28.

de Lima, J., Lloyd-Thomas, A., Howard, R. *et al.* (1996) Infant and neonatal pain, anaesthetists perceptions and prescribing patterns. *British Medical Journal* **313** (7060), 787–788.

Debeukelaer, M. Batisky, D.L. and Melber, S.L. (1999) Acute dialysis in children. In Henrich, W. (editor) *Principles and Practice of Dialysis*, 2nd edn. Maryland: Williams & Wilkins.

Den Broeder, E., Lippins, R.J., van't Hof, M., Tolboom, J.J., Sengers, R.C. and Staveren, W.A. (2000) Association between the change in nutritional status in response to tube feeding and the occurrence of infections in children with solid tumour. *Pediatric Hematology* **17** (7), 567–575.

Den Broeder, E., Lippens, R.J., van't Hof, M.A. *et al.* (2000) Nasogastric tube feeding in children with cancer: the effect of two different formulas on weight, body composition and serum protein concentrations. *Journal of Parenteral and Enteral Nutrition* **24** (6), 351–359.

Dent, A. and Stewart, A. (2004) *Sudden Death in Childhood – Support for the Bereaved Family*. Edinburgh, UK: Butterworth Heinemann.

Department for Education and Skills/Department of Health (DH) (2004) National service framework for children, young people and maternity services. *Disabled Children and Young People and those with Complex Care Needs*. London: DH.

Department of Health (DH) (1989) *The Children's Act*. London: HMSO.

Department of Health (DH) (1996) *Guidelines on Admission to and Discharge from Intensive Care and High Dependency have been Utilized Care Units*. London: NHS Executive.

Department of Health (DH) (1997a) *Paediatric Intensive Care: "A Framework for the Future"*. London: DH.

Department of Health (DH) (1997b) *A Bridge to the Future: Nursing Standards, Education and Workforce Planning in Paediatric Intensive Care*. London: DH.

Department of Health (DH) (2000) *Comprehensive Critical Care: A Review of Adult Critical Care Services*. London: DH.

Department of Health (DH) (2001) *High Dependency Care for Children – Report of an Expert Advisory Group for Department of Health*. London: DH.

Department of Health (DH) (2003) Getting the right start: the national service framework for children, young people and maternity services. *Hospital Standards*. London: HMSO.

Department of Health (DH) (2005) *Saving Lives: The Delivery Programme to Reduce Healthcare Associated Infections (HCAI) Including MRSA*. London: The Stationary Office.

Department of Health (DH) (2006a) *The Acutely or Critically Sick or Injured Child in the District General Hospital: a Team Response*. London: DH.

Department of Health (DH) (2006b) *The Health Act – Code of Practice for the Prevention and Control of Healthcare Associated Infections*. London: The Stationary Office.

Department of Health (DH) (2007a) *A Simple Guide to Clostridium Difficile*. London: The Stationary Office.

Department of Health (DH) (2007b) *Making Every Young Person with Diabetes Matter: Report of the Children and Young People with Diabetes Working Group*. Available online at www.dh.gov.uk/publications/

Department of Health (DH) (2007c) *Making it Better for Children and Young People. Clinical Case for Change*. Report by Shelia Shribman, National Clinical Director for children, young people and maternity services. London: DH Publications.

Department of Health (DH) (2007d) *Uniforms and Workwear: An Evidence Base for Developing Local Policy*. www.dh.gov.uk/en/Publicationsandstatistics/Publications/PublicationsPolicyAndGuidance/DH_078433/

Department of Health (DH) and Modernization Agency (2003) *The National Outreach Report*. London: DH.

Department of Health (DH) and Department for Education and Skills (2004) *National Service Framework for Children, Young People and Maternity Services*. Available online at www.dh.gov.uk/en/Policyandguidance/

Department of Health Critical Care Outreach (2003) *Progress in Developing Services*. London: NHS Modernisation Agency.

Dibble, S.L., Luce, J., Cooper, B.A. *et al*. (2007) Acupressure for chemotherapy-induced nausea and vomiting: a randomized clinical trial. *Oncology Nursing Forum* 34 (4), 813–820.

Doman, M. and Browning, R. (2001) Gap? What gap? Celebrating collaboration between education and practice. *Paediatric Nursing* 13 (9), 34–37.

Doman, M., Prowse, M. and Webb, C. (2004) Exploring nurses' experiences of providing high dependency care in children's wards. *Journal of Child Health Care* 8 (3), 180–197.

Douglas, G., Nicol, F. and Robertson, C. (2005) *McLeod's Clinical Examination*. London: Churchill Livingston.

Dowling, M. (2004) Pain assessment in children with neurological impairment. *Paediatric Nurse* 16 (3), 37–40.

Duerden, B.I. (2007) Confronting infection in the English National Health Service. *Journal of Hospital Infection* 65 (S2), 23–26.

Duncan, H. (2007) Typical values of blood substances. Unpublished materials in use at BCH.

Edwards, E., O'Toole, M. and Wallis, C. (2004) Sending children home on tracheostomy dependent ventilation: pitfalls and outcomes. *Archives of Disease in Childhood* 89 (3), 251–255.

Eilers, J., Berger, A.M. and Petersen, M.C. (1988) Development, testing, and application of the oral assessment guide. *Oncology Nursing Forum* 15 (3), 325–330.

Engleberg, N.C., DiRita, V. and Dermody, T. (2007) *Schaechters Mechanisms of Microbial Disease*. Philadelphia, USA: Lippincott, Williams & Wilkins.

Farrington, M. (2007) Infection control education: how to make an impact – tools for the job. *Journal of Hospital Infection* 65 (S2), 128–132.

Fearon, D.M. and Steele, D.W. (2002) End-tidal carbon dioxide predicts the presences and severity of acidosis in children with diabetes. *Academic Emergency Medicine* 9 (12), 1373–1408.

Fenwick, J., Barclay, L. and Schmied, V. (1999) Activities and interactions in Level II nurseries. A report of an ethnographic study. *The Journal of Perinatal and Neonatal Nursing* 3 (1), 53–65.

Feusner, J. and Hastings, C. (2002) Recombinant human erythropoietin in pediatric oncology: a review. *Medical Pediatric Oncology* 39 (4), 463–468.

Finlay, B. and McFadden, G. (2006) Anti-immunology: evasion of the host immune system by bacterial and viral pathogens. *Cell* 124 (4), 767–782.

Fitzgerald, M. (1995) *Foetal Pain an Update of Current Scientific Knowledge*. London: DH.

Flamant, F., Rodary, C., Rey, A. *et al*. (1998) Treatment of non-metastatic rhabdomyosarcomas in childhood and adolescence. Results of the second study of the International Society of Paediatric Oncology: MMT84. *European Journal of Cancer* 34 (7), 1050–1062.

Flemming, K. and Randle, J. (2006) Toys a friend or foe? A study of infection risk in a paediatric intensive care unit. *Paediatric Nursing* 18 (4), 14–18.

Fletcher, P.N. (2002) Experiences in family bereavement. *Family and Community Health* 25 (1), 57–70.

Flombaum, C.D. (2000) Metabolic emergencies in the cancer patient. *Seminars in Oncology* 27 (3), 332–334.

Flounders, J.A. and Ott, B.B. (2003) Oncology emergency modules: spinal cord compression. *Oncology Nursing Forum* 30 (1). File://C:DOCUME~1/PKarmaz\LOCALS~1\Temp\K1DGK7R3.htm (Last accessed 14/02/06).

Fowlie, P.W., Booth, P. and Skeoch, C.H. (2004) The ABC of preterm birth: moving the preterm infant. *British Medical Journal* 329 (7471), 904–906.

Fraise, A.P. (2007) Decontamination of the environment. *Journal of Hospital Infection* 65 (S2), 58–59.

Franklin, C. and Mathew, J. (1994) Developing strategies to prevent in hospital cardiac arrest: analysing responses of physicians and nurses in the hours before the event. *Critical Care Medicine* 22 (4), 244–247.

Fraser, J. Mok, Q. and Tasker, R. (1997) Survey of occupancy of paediatric intensive care units by children who are dependent on ventilators. *British Medical Journal* 315 (7104), 347–348.

Garfield, M., Jeffrey, R. and Ridley, S. (2000) An assessment of the staffing level required for a high dependency unit. *Anaesthesia* 55 (9), 137–143.

Garland, L. and Kenny, G. (2006) Family nursing and the management of pain in children. *Paediatric Nursing* 18 (6), 18–20.

Garretson, S. (2005) Haemodynamic monitoring; arterial catheters. *Nursing Standard* 19 (31), 55–64.

Gausche-Hill, M., Fuchs, S. and Yamamoto, L. (2006) APLS The Pediatric Emergency Medicine Resource. *Medical Emergencies*, Chapter 13. Boston: Jones and Bartlett.

Gemke, R., Van Bonsel, G. and Vaught, J. (1995) Long term survival and state of health after paediatric intensive care. *Archives of Disease in Childhood* 73 (2), 196–201.

Gibney, J., Marinos, E., Ljungquist, O. and Dowsett, J. (editors) (2005) Pediatric nutrition. *Clinical Nutrition*, Chapter 22. Williams, A. Oxford: Blackwell Publishing.

Gibson, F. and Nelson, W. (2000). Mouth care for children with cancer. *Paediatric Nursing* 12 (1), 18–22.

Gibson, J. (1997) Focus of nursing in critical and acute care settings: prevention or cure? *Intensive and Critical Care Nursing* 13 (5), 163–166.

Gill, D. and O'Brien, N. (2005) *Paediatric Clinical Examination Made Easy*. Edinburgh: Churchill Livingstone.

Gillman, M.W. and Cook, N.R. (1995) Blood pressure measurement in childhood epidemiological studies. *Circulation* 92, 1049–1057.

Giovanola, J. (2005) Sibling involvement at the end of life. *Journal of Pediatric Oncology Nursing* 22 (4), 222–226.

Giuliano, K.K. and Higgins, T.L. (2005) New generation pulse oximetry in the care of critically ill patients. *American Journal of Critical Care* 14 (1), 26–37.

Glasper, A. and Richardson, J. (editors) (2006) *A Textbook of Children's and Young Peoples Nursing*. Edinburgh: Elsevier, Churchill Livingstone.

Glasper, E.A., Mc Ewing, G. and Richardson, J. (2007) *Oxford Handbook of Children's and Young People's Nursing*. Oxford: Oxford University Press.

Glendinning, C. and Kirk, S. (2000) High-tech care: high-skilled parents. *Paediatric Nursing* 12 (6), 25–27.

Glenny, A. (2006) Mouth care for children and young people with cancer: evidence-based guidelines. *UKCCSG-PONF Mouth Care Group*.

Glover, V. and Fisk, N. (1996) Do foetuses feel pain. *British Medical Journal* 313 (7060), 796.

Goldhill, D.R., White, S.A. and Sumner, A. (1999a) Physiological values and procedures in the 24 h before ICU admission from the ward. *Anaesthesia* 54 (5), 529–534.

Goldhill, D.R., Worthington, L., Mulcahy, A., Tarling, M. and Sumner, A. (1999b) The patient at risk team: identifying and managing seriously ill ward patients. *Anaesthesia* 54 (6), 853–860.

Gollop, R. (2002) Burns aftercare and scar management. In Bosworth, B.C. (editor) *Burn Trauma, Management and Nursing Care*, 2nd edn. London, UK: Whurr Publishers.

Gomez. L., Martino, R. and Rolston, K.V. (1998) Neutropenic enterocolitis: spectrum of the disease and comparison of definite and possible causes. *Clinical Infection and Disease* 27 (2), 695–699.

Gosling, P., Rothe, H., Sheehan, T. and Hubbard, L.D. (1995) Serum copper and zinc concentrations in patients with burns in relation to burn surface area. *Journal of Burn Care and Rehabilitation* 16, 481–486.

Gould, D.J., Chudleigh, J., Drey, N.S. and Morajelo, D. (2007) Measuring handwashing performance in health service audits and research studies. *Journal of Hospital Infection* 66, 109–115.

Gray, J. (2002) Conscious sedation of children in A&E. *Emergency Nurse* 9 (8), 26–31.

Gray, L., Watt, L. and Blass, E.M. (2000) Skin to skin contact is analgesics in healthy newborns. *Pediatrics* 105 (1), 110–111.

Great Ormond Street Hospital (2005a) Paediatric dependency and acuity scoring tool. Available online http://www.picupt.nhs.uk/_Rainbow/Documents/Dependency%20acuity%20category%20guidance%20revised_1.pdf (Last accessed 7/11/07).

Great Ormond Street Hospital (2005b) Children's services patient acuity and dependency levels. Available online http://www.picupt.nhs.uk/_Rainbow/Documents/Childrens%20Services%20patient%20acuity%20and%20dependency%20levels.pdf (Last accessed 7/11/07).

Great Ormond Street Hospital NHS Trust (2005) Clinical procedure guidelines – arterial line management. Available online http://www.gosh.nhs.uk/clinical_information/clinical_guidelines/downloads/Arterial_Lines_Management.pdf (Last accessed 5/6/07).

Great Ormond Street Hospital NHS Trust (2006) Clinical Procedure Guidelines – Blood sampling; Neonatal Capillary. Available online http://www.ich.ucl.ac.uk/clinical_information/clinical_guidelines/downloads/Blood%20Sampling%20Neonatal%20Capillary%202006.pdf (Last accessed 5/6/07).

Gregory, M., Bunchman, T.E. and Brophy, P.D. (2004) Continuous renal replacement therapies for children with acute renal failure and metabolic disorders. In Warady, B.A., Schaefer, F.S., Fine, R.N. and Alexander, S.R. (editors) *Paediatric Dialysis*, Chapter 34. Netherlands: Kluwer Academic Publishers, pp. 567–585.

Griffiths, H. and Gallimore, D. (2005) Positioning critically ill patients in hospital. *Nursing Standard* 19 (42), 56–64.

Haas, F. (2003) Management of malignant spinal cord compression. *Nursing Times* 99 (15), 32–34.

Haines, C. (2005) Acutely ill children within ward areas – care provision and possible development strategies. *Nursing in Critical Care* 10 (2), 98–104.

Haines, C. and Pedley, S. (2007) Cardiac surgical nursing. In Chambers, M.A. and Jones, S. (editors) *Surgical Nursing of Children*. Edinburgh: Butterworth Heinemann.

Haines, C., Perrott, M. and Weir, P. (2006) Promoting care for acutely ill children – development and evaluation of a paediatric early warning tool. *Intensive and Critical Care Nursing* 22 (4), 73–81.

Hall, J. (2002) Paediatric pain assessment. *Emergency Nurse* 10 (6), 31–33.

Hall, J. and Horsley, M. (2007) Diagnosis and management of patients with *Clostridium difficile*-associated diarrhoea. *Nursing Standard* 21 (46), 49–56.

Hallett, A. (2004) Narratives of therapeutic touch. *Nursing Standard* 15 (19), 33–37.

Hamilton, H. (2006a) Complications associated with venous access devices, part 1. *Nursing Standard* 20 (26), 43–49.

Hamilton, H. (2006b) Complications associated with venous access devices, part 2. *Nursing Standard* 20 (27), 59–65.

Hankins, C.L. Tang, X.Q. and Phillips, A. (2006) Hot beverage burns: an 11 year experience of the Yorkshire Regional Burns Centre. *Burns* 32 (1), 87–91.

Hanumadass, M. and Ramakrishnan, M. (2005) *The Art and Science of Burn Wound Management*. Tunbridge Wells, UK: Anshan.

Haouari, N., Wood, C. and Griffiths, G. (1995) The analgesic effect of sucrose in full term infants. *British Medical Journal* 310 (6993), 1498–1500.

Haque, K.N. (2007) Defining common infections in children and neonates. *Journal of Hospital Infection* 65 (S2), 110–114.

Hargrave, D.R., Messahel, B. and Plowman, P.N. (2004) Tumours of the central nervous system. In Pinkerton, R., Plowman, P.N. and Pieters, R. (editors) *Paediatric Oncology*, 3rd edn. London: Arnold, pp. 287– 322.

Harrison, M. (1996) Foetal surgery. *American Journal of Obstetrics and Gynaecology* 174 (4), 1225–1264.

Hart, C.A. and Thompson, A.P.J. (2006) Meningococcal disease and its management in children. *British Medical Journal* 333 (7570), 685–690.

Hart, S. (2007) Using an aseptic technique to reduce the risk of infection. *Nursing Standard* 21 (47), 43–48.

Hastings, C.A., Lubin, B.H. and Feusner, J. (2006) Hematologic supportive care for children with cancer. In Pizzo, P.A. and Poplack, D.G. (editors) *Principles and Practice of Pediatric Oncology*, 5th edn. Philadelphia, USA: Lippincott Williams & Wilkins, pp. 1231–1268.

Haut, C. (2005) Oncological emergencies in the PICU. *AACN Clinical Issues* 16 (2), 232–245.

Hazinski, M. (1992) *Nursing Care of the Critically Ill Child*, 2nd edn. London: Mosby.

Healthcare Commission (2007a) *The Healthcare Commission Annual Report*. London: Commission for Healthcare Audit and Inspection.

Healthcare Commission (2007b) *Commission for Healthcare Audit and Inspection; Improving Services for Children in Hospital*. London: Health Care Commission.

Herban, H.N. and Sullivan, L.M. (2004) *Management Guidelines for Nurse Practitioners working with Children and Adolescents*, 2nd edn. Philadelphia, USA: F.A. Davis Company.

Hestor, N., Foster, R. and Kirsstenson, R. (1990) Measurement of pain in children generalizability and validity of the pain ladder and the poker chip tool. In Tyler, D. and Krane, E. (editors) *Paediatric Pain – Advances of Pain Research and Therapy*. USA: Raven Press.

Hettiaratachy, S. and Dziewulski, P. (2004) ABC of burns: pathophysiology and types of burns. *British Medical Journal* **328**, 1427–1429.

Hettiaratachy, S., Papini, R. and Dziewulski, P. (2005) *ABC of Burns*. London, UK: *British Medical Journal* and Blackwell Publishers.

Hettiaratchy, S. and Papini, R. (2004) ABC of burns: initial management of a major burn; II – assessment and resuscitation. *British Medical Journal* **329** (7457), 101–103.

Heyderman, R.S., Ben-Shlomo, Y., Brennan, C.A. and Somerset, M. (2004) The incidence and mortality for meningococcal disease associated with area deprivation: an ecological study of hospital episode statistics. *Archives of Disease in Childhood* **89** (2), 1064–1068.

Hicks, C., Von Baeyer, C., Spafford, P. *et al.* (2001) The faces pain scale revised, towards a common metric in paediatric pain measurement. *Pain* **93** (2), 173–183.

Higdon, M.L. (2006) Treatment of oncologic emergencies. *American Family Physician* **74** (11), 1873–1880.

Higgins, C. (2000) *Understanding Laboratory Investigations – a Text for Nurses and Healthcare Professionals*. Abingdon: Blackwell Science.

Hockenberry, M.J. and Wong, D. (2003a) Health promotion of the infant and family. In Wong, D.L., Hockenberry, M.J., Wilson, D., Winkelstein, M.L. and Kline, N.E. (editors) *Wong's Nursing Care of Infants and Children*, Chapter 12. St Louis: Mosby.

Hockenberry, M.J. and Wong, D. (2003b) The child with hematologic or immunologic dysfunction. In Wong, D.L., Hockenberry, M.J., Wilson, D., Winkelstein, M.L. and Kline, N.E. (editors) *Wong's Nursing Care of Infants and Children*, Chapter 35. St Louis: Mosby.

Hockenberry, M.J., Wilson, D., Winklestein, M. and Kline, N. (2003) *Wong's Nursing Care of Infants and Children*, 7th edn. St Louis: Mosby.

Hoffbrand, A. and Pettir, J. (1997) *Essential Haematology*, 3rd edn. London: Blackwell Science.

Hogan, C.M. (1998) The nurse's role in diarrhoea management. *Oncology Nurses Forum* **25** (5), 879–886.

Hon, K.E., Leung, A., Chik, W., Chu, C.C., Cheung, K. and Fok, T. (2005) Critical airway obstruction, superior vena cava syndrome, and spontaneous cardiac arrest in a child with acute leukaemia. *Pediatric Emergency Care* **21** (12), 844–846.

Hopkins, M. (1999a) The nature of radiotherapy. In Gibson, F. and Evans, M. (editors) *Paediatric Oncology. Acute Nursing Care*, Chapter 20. London: Whurr Publishers, pp. 395–404.

Hopkins, M. (1999b) Administration of radiotherapy. In Gibson, F. and Evans, M. (editors) *Paediatric Oncology. Acute Nursing Care*, Chapter 21. London: Whurr Publishers, pp. 405–432.

Hopkins, S.J. (1999) *Drugs and Pharmacology for Nurses*, 13th edn. Edinburgh: Churchill Livingstone.

Horne, C. and Derrico, D. (1999) Mastering ABG's. *American Journal of Nursing* **99** (8), 26–33.

Horrox, F. (2002) *Manual of Neonatal and Paediatric Congenital Heart Disease*. London, UK: Whurr Publishing.

Imperial-Perez, F. and McRae, M. (2002) Arterial pressure monitoring. *Critical Care Nurse* **19** (2), 105–107.

Investigation of Neonatal Conjugated Hyperbilirubinaemia. Accessed from http://bspghan.org.uk. Posted on website July 2007.

International Guidelines for Neonatal Resuscitation (2000) An excerpt from the Guidelines 2000 for CPR and ECC. International Consensus in Science. Circulation. **102** (Suppl), 343–357.

Jackson, D. (1953) The diagnosis of the depth of burning. In Herndon, D. (editor) *Total Burn Care*, 3rd edn. *British Journal of Surgery* **40**, 588–596. China: Elsevier Saunders.

Jain, Y., Laxman, S.A. and Kataria, R. (2000) Neutropenic enterocolitis in children with acute lymphoblastic leukaemia. *Pediatric Haematology and Oncology* **17**, 99–103.

James, D. (1998) Foetal medicine. *British Medical Journal* **316** (7144), 1580–1583.

Janzekovic, Z. (1977) The treatment of burns. *Burns* **4**, 61–66.

Jardine, E. and Wallis, C. (1998) Core guidelines for the discharge home of the child on long term assisted ventilation in the United Kingdom. *Thorax* **53** (9), 762–767.

Jeha, S. (2001) Tumor lysis syndrome. *Seminars in Hematology* **38** (4, Suppl 10), 4–8.

Jenkins, G. Kemnitz, C. and Tortora, G. (2006) *Anatomy and Physiology from Science to Life*, 1st edn. USA: Wiley.

Jenkins, M.E., Gottschlich, M.M. and Warden, G.D. (1994) Enteral feeding during operative procedures. *Journal of Burn Care and Rehabilitation* 15 (2), 199–205.

Jennet, B. (1990) Is intensive care worthwhile? *Care of the Critically Ill* 6 (2), 85–88.

Jevon, P. (2004) *Paediatric Advanced Life Support – a Practical Guide*. Edinburgh: Butterworth Heinemann.

Jevon, P. and Ewens, B. (2005) *Monitoring the Critically Ill Patient*. Oxford: Blackwell Science.

Johnston, C. and Stevens, B. (1996) *Experience in a Neonatal Intensive Care Unit Affects Pain Response* 98 (5), 925–930.

Joint planning and commissioning framework for children, young people and maternity services: http://icn.csip.org.uk/_library/Resources/ICN/Joint_Planning_and_Commissioning_Framework.pdf/

Jones, D.P., Mahmoud, H. and Chesney, R.W. (1995) Tumor lysis syndrome: pathogenesis and management. *Pediatric Nephrology* 127 (1), 206–212.

Joseph, M. and Tayar, R. (2005) Spinal cord compression requires early detection. *European Journal of Palliative Care* 12 (4), 141–143.

Kallab, A.M. (2005) Superior vena cava syndrome. *Emedicine*. http://www.emedicine.com/me/topic2208.htm (Last accessed 29/06/07).

Kavanaugh, K. and Moro, T. (2006) Supporting parents after stillbirth or newborn death. *American Journal of Nursing* 106 (9), 74–79.

Kelly, D.A. (2002) Managing liver failure. *Postgraduate Medical Journal* 78 (925), 660–667.

Kelly, D.A. (2004) *Useful Investigations in the Assessment of Liver Disease: Diseases of the Liver and Biliary System in Children*, 2nd edn. Oxford: Blackwell Publishing.

Kelnar, C.J. (1995) *The Sick Newborn Baby*, 3rd edn. London: Balliere Tindall.

Kemper, K. (2001) Complementary and alternative therapies for children: does it work? *Archives of Disease in Childhood* 84 (1), 6–9.

Kemper, K. and Sarah, R. (2000) On pins and needles pediatric pain patients experience with acupuncture. *Pediatrics* 105 (4), 941–947.

Kennebeck, S.S. (2005) Tumors of the mediastinum. *Clinical Pediatric Emergency Medicine* 6, 156–164.

Kennedy, I. (2001) Learning from Bristol. The Bristol Royal Infirmary Inquiry. http://www.bristol-inquiry.org.uk/final_report/report/

Kenner, C. and Lott, J.W. (2003) *Comprehensive Neonatal Nursing – a Physiological Perspective*, 3rd edn. Philadelphia, USA: Elsevier Saunders.

Khan, M. and Younger, G. (2007) Promoting safe administration of subcutaneous infusions. *Nursing Standard* 21 (31), 50–56.

King, N. (2002) Nursing care if the child with neutropenic enterocolitis. *Journal of Pediatric Oncology Nursing* 19 (6), 198–204.

Knight, S.E. and Washington, R.L. (2006) Cardiovascular diseases and surgical interventions. In Merenstein, G.B. and Gardner, S.L. (editors) *Handbook of Neonatal Intensive Care*, 6th edn. Philadelphia, USA: Mosby Elsevier.

Kobler, K., Limbo, R. and Kavanaugh, K. (2007) *Meaningful Moments: the Use of Ritual in Perinatal and Pediatric Death Maternal and Child Nursing* 32 (5), 288–295.

Kodali, B.S. (2001) *Capnography – A Comprehensive Educational Website*. Updated March 2007. www.capnography.com/ (Last accessed 3/5/07).

Kopotic, R.J. and Linder, W. (2002) Assessing high risk infants in the delivery room with pulse oximetry. *Anaesthesia and Analgesia* 94 (Suppl), 31–36.

Kornblau, S.M., Mitchell, E., Rubin, J., Trotta, P. and Vakes, E. (1998) Recommended guidelines for the treatment of chemotherapy-induced diarrhea. *Journal of Clinical Oncology* 16 (9), 3169–3178.

Kushner, B.H. and Cheung, N.V. (2005) Neuroblastoma – from genetic profiles to clinical challenge. *New England Journal of Medicine* 353 (21), 2215–2217.

Kwok, Y., Tibbs, P.A. and Patchell, R.A. (2006) Clinical approach to metastasis epidural spinal cord compression. *Hematology/Oncology Clinics of North America* 20 (6), 1297–1305.

Kydd, A. (2007) The NHS may get the best deal on its housekeeping but at what cost to care? *Nursing Times* 103 (34), 12.

Laakso, H. and Paunonne-Ilmonen, M. (2001) Mother's grief following the death of a child. *Journal of Advanced Nursing* 36 (1), 69–77.

Laight, S., Currie, M. and Davis, N. (2005) Cardiac care. In Sheppard, M. and Wright, M. (editors) *Principles and Practice of High Dependency Nursing*, 2nd edn. Edinburgh: Bailliere Tindall/Elsevier.

Lawrence, J. (1991) Bacterial infection of wounds. *Wound Management* 1, 13–15.

Lee, A., Highfield, E., Berde, C.B. and Kemper, K.J. (1999) Survey of acupuncturists practice characteristics and paediatric care. *Western Journal of Medicine* 171 (3), 153–157.

Lee, A., Bishop, B., Hillman, K.M. and Daffurn, K. (1995) The medical emergency team. *Anaesthesia and Intensive Care* 23 (5), 183–186.

Lee, S., Ralston, H., Drey, E. *et al.* (2005) Foetal pain a systemic and multidisciplinary review of the evidence. *Journal of the American Medical Association* **294** (8), 947–954.

LeGrand, T.S. and Peters, J.I. (1999) Pulse oximetry; advantages and pitfalls. *The Journal of Respiratory Disease* **20** (3), 195–206.

Lehmann, S. (1993) Nutrition support in the hypermetabolic patient. *Critical Care Nursing Clinics of North America* **5** (1), 7–103.

Lehrnbecher, T. and Welte, K. (2002) Haematopoietic growth factors in children with neutropenia. *British Journal of Hematology* **116** (3), 28–56.

Leigh, M.A.M.S. and Rennie, J.M. (2005) The law. In Rennie, J. (editor) *Roberton's Textbook of Neonatology*, 4th edn. China: Elsevier Churchill Livingstone.

Leon, P., Jimenez, M., Barona, P. and Sierrasestimaga, L. (1998) Recombinant human erythropoietin for the treatment of anemia in children with solid malignant tumors. *Medical and Pediatric Oncology* **30** (2), 110–116.

Leslie, A. and Middleton, D. (1995) Give and take in neonatal transport: communication hazards in handover. *Journal of Neonatal Nursing* **1** (5), 27–31.

Levy, M.N., Koeppen, B.M. and Stanton, B.A. (2006) *Berne and Levy Principles of Physiology*, 4th edn. Philadelphia, USA: Elsevier Mosby.

Lewis, M. and Noyes, J. (2007) Discharge management for children with complex needs. *Paediatric Nursing* **19** (4), 26–30.

Lim, E., Bennett, P. and Beilby, J. (2003) Sample preparation in patients receiving uric acid oxidase (rasburicase) therapy. *Clinical Chemistry* **49** (8), 1417.

Linton, M. (2000) Endotracheal tube suctioning. In Sinha, S.K. and Donn, S.M. (editors) *Manual of Neonatal Respiratory Care*. New York: Futura.

Lissauer, T. and Clayden, G. (2005) *Illustrated Textbook of Paediatrics*. London: Mosby.

Lissauer, T. and Clayden, G. (editors) (2007) Haematological disorders. In *Illustrated Textbook of Paediatrics*, 3rd edn, Chapter 22. Edinburgh, UK: Mosby Elsevier.

Llewellyn, N. and Moriarty, A. (2007) The national paediatric epidural audit. *Paediatric Anaesthesia* **17** (6), 520–533.

London, M.L., Ladewig, P.W., Ball, J.W. and Bindler, R.C. (2006) *Maternal and Child Nursing Care*, 2nd edn. New Jersey, USA: Pearson and Prentice Hall.

Lote, C.J. (2000) *Principles of Renal Physiology*, 4th edn. Netherlands: Kluwer Academic Publishers.

Lowis, S.P., Goulder, N. and Oakhill, A. (2004) Caring for the child with cancer. In Pinkerton, R., Plowman, P.N. and Pieters, R. (editors) *Paediatric Oncology*, 3rd edn., Chapter 34, pp. 623–649.

Lymphoma Information Network (2007) http://www.lymphomainfo.net/childhood/hodgkins.html/ (Last accessed November 2007).

Lynam, L.E. (1992) It isn't just the lungs: a case presentation. *Neonatal Network* **11** (3), 65–68.

MacGregor, J. (2000) *Introduction to the Anatomy and Physiology of Children*. London: Routledge.

MacGregor, J. (2003) *Introduction to the Anatomy and Physiology of Children*. London: Routledge.

MacGregor, R., Evans, D., Sugdem, D. *et al.* (1998) Outcome at 5–6 years of prematurely born children who received morphine as neonates. *Archives of Disease in Children, Foetal and Neonatal Edition* **79** (1), 40–43.

Mackechnie, C. and Simpson, R. (2006) Traceable calibration for blood pressure and temperature monitoring. *Nursing Standard* **21** (11), 42–47.

Mackintosh, M. (2006) Transporting critically ill patients: new opportunities for nurses. *Nursing Standard* **20** (36), 46–48.

Mader, S. (2007) *Human Biology*, 10th edn. New York: McGraw Hill Higher Education.

Mantle, F. (2001) Hypnosis in the management of eczema in children. *Nursing Standard* **5** (15), 41–44.

Mareib, E.N. (2004) *Human Anatomy and Physiology*, 6th edn. San Francisco: Pearson/Benjamin-Cummings.

Margolan, H., Fraser, J. and Lenton, S. (2004) Parental experience of services when their child requires long-term ventilation. Implications for commissioning and providing services. *Child: Care, Health and Development* **30** (3) 257–264.

Marshall, W. (2002) *Clinical Chemistry*, 4th edn. London: Mosby.

Martin, S.A. (1992) The ABC of pediatric LFTs. *Pediatric Nursing* **18** (5), 445–449.

Mathews, J., McGrath, P. and Pigeon, H. (1993) Assessment and measurement of pain in children. In Schechter, N.L., Berde, C.B. and Yaster, M. (editors) *Pain in Infants, Children and Adolescents*, Chapter 8. USA: Williams & Wilkins.

Mc Conkey, R., Barr, O. and Baxter, R. (2007) Complex needs the nursing response to children and YP with complex physical health care needs. Department of Health Social Services and Public Safety, Institute of Nurse Research, University of Ulster.

McArdle, J. (1999) Understanding oesophageal varices. *Nursing Standard* **14** (9), 46–54.

McArthur, C.D. (2003) AARC Clinical Practice Guideline capnography/capnometry during mechanical ventilation – revision and update. *Respiratory Care* **48** (5), 534–539.

McCaffery, M. (1980) Understanding your patients pain. *Nursing* **10** (9), 26–31.

McCance, K. and Huether, S. (2002) *Pathophysiology: the Biologic Basis for Disease in Adults and Children*, 4th edn. Missouri: Mosby.

McCance, K. and Huether, S. (2006) *Pathophysiology the Biologic Basis for Disease in Adults and Children*, 5th edn., Chapter 15. St Louis, USA: Elsevier Mosby.

McCann, L. and Newell, S. (2006) Survey of paediatric complementary and alternative medicine use in health and chronic illness. *Archives of Disease in Childhood* **91** (2), 173–174.

McCloskey, D.J. (2002) Catheter-related thrombosis in pediatrics. *Pediatric Nursing* **28** (2), 97–106.

McConnell, E.A. (2002) Prevent the spread of *Clostridium difficile. Nursing* **32** (8), 24–26.

McCullough, K.D. and McDonald, G.B. (2003) Neutropenic enterocolitis. *Current Treatment Options in Infectious Diseases* **5**, 367–375.

McDonald, J. (1999) SPQ Elective Report. *Specialist Practitioner Qualification in Critical Care Nursing.* Edinburgh: The Lothian University Hospitals NHS Trust.

McDowell, H.P., Messahel, B. and Oberlin, O. (2004) Hodgkin's disease. In Pinkerton, R., Ploughman, P.N. and Pieters, R. (editors) *Paediatric Oncology*, 3rd edn. London: Arnold, pp. 267–282.

McGhee, B.H. and Bridges, E.J. (2002) Monitoring arterial blood pressure – what you may not know. *Critical Care Nurse* **22** (2), 60–79.

McKenzie, M. (2000) Chemotherapy standards for hospital in the home: how useful? *Australian Journal of Advanced Nursing* **17**, 8–13.

McKiernan, P.J. (2004) The acutely ill child. In Kelly, D.A. (editor) *Diseases of the Liver and Biliary System in Children*, 2nd edn. Massachusetts: Blackwell Publishing.

McMahon, K., Decker, G. and Ottery, F.D. *et al.* (1998) Integrating proactive nutritional assessment in clinical practices to prevent complications and cost. *Seminars in Oncology* **25** (2, Suppl 6), 20–27.

McQuilan, P., Pilkington, S., Allan, A. *et al.* (1998) Confidential inquiry into quality of care before admission to intensive care. *British Medical Journal* **316** (7148), 1853–1858.

McSherry, W. and Ross, L. (2002) Dilemmas of spiritual assessment. Considerations for nursing practice. *Journal of Advanced Nursing* **38** (5), 479–488.

Meadow, R. and Newell, S. (2002) *Lecture Notes on Paediatrics*, 7th edn. Oxford, UK: Blackwell Publishing.

Medical and Health Products Regulatory Agency (2001a) DA 2001(04) – The Use of Central Intravenous Access in Neonatal Parenteral Feeding. Available onlinehttp://www.mhra.gov.uk/home/idcplg?IdcService=SS_GET_PAGE&useSecondary=true&ssDocName=CON008910&ssTargetNodeId=573/ (Last accessed 5/6/07).

Medical and Health Products Regulatory Agency (2001b) Safety Notice 08 – Tissue Necrosis Caused by Pulse Oximeter Probes. Available onlinehttp://www.mhra.gov.uk/home/idcplg?IdcService=SS_GET_PAGE&useSecondary=true&ssDocName=CON008841&ssTargetNodeId=420/ (Last accessed 30/4/07).

Medical and Healthcare Products Regulatory Agency (2005a) *MHRA 04144 Thermometer Review UK Market Survey.* London: DH.

Medical and Healthcare Products Regulatory Agency (2005b) *Report of the Independent Advisory Group on Blood Pressure Monitoring in Clinical Practice.* London: DH.

Medical Devices Alert (2006) Risk assessment safer practice recommendation. *National Patient Safety Agency NHS.* London

Melamud, M., Palekar, R. and Singh, A. (2006) Retinoblastoma. *American Family Physician* **73** (6), 1039–1044.

Melhuish, S. and Payne, H. (2006) Nurses attitude to pain management during routine venepuncture in young children. *Paediatric Nursing* **18** (2), 20–23.

Melzack, R. and Wall, P.D. (1965) Pain mechanisms a new theory. *Science* **150** (699), 971–978.

Mendham, J. (2004) Gabapentin for treating itching produced by burns and wound healing in children: a pilot study. *Burns* **30** (8), 851–853.

Mental Capacity Act (2005) (*c.9*). London: HMSO. Available online http://www.opsi.gov.uk/acts/en2005/2005en09.htm/

Mercier, C. and Blond, M. (1996) Epidemiological survey of childhood burn injuries in France. *Burns* **22** (1), 29–34.

Merestein, G. and Gardner, S.L. (2002) *Handbook of Neonatal Intensive Care*, 5th edn. St Louis: Mosby.

Merkel, S., Voepel-Lewis, T. and Shayevitz, S. (1997) The FLACC a behavioural scale for scoring post operative pain in young children. *Pediatric Nursing* **23** (3), 293–297.

Mermel, L.A. (2007) Prevention of central venous catheter-related infections: what works other than impregnated or coated catheters? *Journal of Hospital Infection* **65** (S2), 30–33.

Metheny, N. (2000) *Fluid and Electrolyte Balance, Nursing Considerations*, 4th edn. New York, NY: Lippincott.

Metzger, M.L. and Dome, J.S. (2005) Current therapy for Wilm's tumor. *Oncologist* **10** (10), 815–826.

Meyer, W., Patterson, D. and Jaco, M. (2007) Management of pain and other discomforts in burned patients. In Herndon, D. (editor) *Total Burn Care*, 3rd edn. Philadelphia, USA: Saunders Elsevier.

Molley, E.J. and Deakins, K. (2006) Are carbon dioxide detectors useful in neonates? *Archives of Disease in Childhood Fetal & Neonatal Edition* **91** (4), F295–F298.

Monaghan, A. (2005) Detecting and managing deterioration in children. *Paediatric Nursing* **17** (1), 32–35.

Montgomery, S., Ehlin, A. and Sacker, A. (2006) Breast feeding and resilience against psychosocial stress. *Archives of Disease in Childhood* **91** (12), 990–994.

Moore, K.L. and Persaud, T.V.N. (2003) *Before We Are Born – Essentials of Embryology and Birth Defects*. China: Elsevier Saunders.

Moore, T. and Woodrow, P. (2004) *High Dependency Nursing Care: Observation, Intervention and Support*. London: Routledge.

Morgan, G. (2003) Chemotherapy and the cell cycle. *Cancer Nursing Practice* **15** (21), 27–30.

Morgan, P. (2000) Cellular effects of cancer chemotherapy administration. *Journal of Intravenous Nursing* **23** (1), 44–51.

Moss, S.J., Embleton, N.D. and Fenton, A.C. (2005) Towards safer neonatal transport: the importance of critical incident review. *Archives of Diseases in Childhood* **90** (7), 729–732.

Moules, T. and Ramsey, J. (1998) *Textbook of Children's Nursing*. London: Stanly Thornes.

Moules, T. and Ramsay, J. (2008) *The Textbook of Children's and Young People's Nursing*, 2nd edn. Oxford, UK: Blackwell Publishing.

Mower, W.R., Sachs, C., Nicklin, E.L. and Baraff, L.J. (1997) Pulse oximetry as the fifth paediatric vital sign. *Pediatrics* **99** (5), 678–681.

Moyles, J. (1999) Pulse oximetry. *Journal of Neonatal Nursing* **5**, 2.

Muehlbauer, P.M. and Schwartzentruber, D.J. (2003) Cancer vaccines. *Seminars in Oncology Nursing* **19** (3), 206–216.

Muller, N. and Bryan, A. (1979) Chest wall mechanics and respiratory muscles in infants. *Pediatric Clinics of North America* **26** (3), 503–516.

Nagler, J., Wright, R.O. and Krauss, B. (2006) End tidal carbon dioxide as a measure of acidosis among children with gastroenteritis. *Pediatrics* **118** (1), 260–267.

Naikoba, S. and Hayward, A. (2001) The effectiveness of interventions aimed at increasing handwashing in healthcare-associated infections in healthcare workers – a systematic review. *Journal of Hospital Infection* **47** (3), 173–180.

National Burn Care Review Committee (2001) *Standards and Strategy for Burn Care; a Review of Burn Care in the British Isles*. Available online www.bapras.org.uk/UploadFiles/National%20 Burn%20Care%20Review.pdf/

National Cancer Institute (2007) Available online http://www.cancer.gov/cancertopics/types/ childhoodcancers

National Health Service (2004) West Midlands Strategic Commissioning Group – Standards for the care of critically ill & critically injured children in the West Midlands; West Midlands Specialised Service Agency. Available online http://www.perinatal.nhs. uk/manners/Standards.pdf/ (Last accessed 4/5/07).

National Heath Service (2006) Antenatal and newborn screening programmes. *Sickle Cell Disease in Childhood Standards and Guidelines for Clinical Care*. Available online www.screening.nhs.uk/ sickleandthal/

National Institute for Clinical Excellence (NICE) (2001) *Standard Principles for Prevention of Hospital Acquired Infection*. London: NICE.

National Institute for Clinical Excellence (NICE) (2003) *Infection Control: Preventing Healthcare-Associated Infection in Primary and Community Care*. London: NICE.

National Institute for Health and Clinical Excellence (NICE) (2004) *Clinical Guidelines CG15: Diagnosis and Management of Type 1 Diabetes in Children, Young People and Adults.* Available online www.nice.org.uk/guidance/CG15/

National Institute for Clinical Excellence (NICE) (2006) *Health Technology Appraisal: Entecavir for the Treatment of Chronic Hepatitis B* (Draft Scope-Pre-Referral). London: NICE.

National Institute for Health and Clinical Excellence (NICE) (2007a) *Head Injury: Triage, Assessment, Investigation and Early Management of Head Injury in Infants, Children and Adults* (NICE clinical guideline 56). Available online www.nice.org.uk/CG56/

National Institute for Health and Clinical Excellence (NICE) (2007b) *Feverish Illness in Children – Assessment and Initial Management in Children Younger than 5 Years* (NICE clinical guideline 47). Available online www.nice.org.uk/CG047/

National Service Frameworks (2003/4) National Service Framework for children and young people. *Standards for Children in Hospital.* London: DH.

National Service Frameworks (NSF) (2004) DH policy and guidance.

Neill, S. and Knowles, H. (2004) The biology of child health. *A Reader in Development and Assessment.* Hampshire: Palgrave MacMillian.

NHS Media Release (2006) Antenatal and Newborn Screening Programmes Sickle Cell and Thalassaemia. Embargoed till 20/10/06 skanal@mediastrategy.co.uk

NHS National Needs Assessment (2004) Used for Children who Require Assessment for Long Term Ventilation Requirements in the Community Care. Available online www.longtermventilation.nhs.uk/_Rainbow/Documents/National%20Needs%

NHS Sickle Cell and Thalassaemia Screening Programme. *National Screening Committee Laboratory Newsletter* No. 3 April 2005.

Nichols, J. (2003) Transfusion-transmitted cytomegalovirus infection after receipt of leukoreduced blood products. *Blood* **101**, 4195–4200.

Ninis, N., Phillips, C., Bailey, L. *et al.* (2005) The role of healthcare delivery in the outcome of meningococcal disease in children: case–control study of fatal and non fatal cases. *British Medical Journal* **330** (7505), 1475–1481.

NMC code of conduct now 2008

Norman, L., Anderton, D. and Hubbard, S. (2002) Nutritional care for an individual following burn trauma. In Bosworth B.C. (editor) *Burn Trauma. Management and Nursing Care.* London, UK: Whurr Publishers.

Noyes, J. and Lewis, M. (2005) Care Pathway for the Discharge of Children Requiring Long Term Ventilation in the Community. DH Policy and Guidance.

Noyes, J. (2000) Ventilator-dependent children who spend prolonged periods of time in intensive care units when they no longer have a medical need or want to be there. *Journal of Clinical Nursing* **9**, 774–783.

Noyes, J. and Lewis, M. (2005) *From Hospital to Home: Guidance on Discharge Management and Community Support for Children Using Long-Term Ventilation.* London: Barnardo's. Available online www.barnardos.org.uk/

Nursing and Midwifery Council (2008) *The NMC Code of Conduct; Standards for Performance and Ethics.* London: NMC.

Nursing and Midwifery Council (2007) *Standards for Medicines Management.* London: NMC. Available online www.nmc-uk.org/

Nursing and Midwifery Council (March 2006) *Infection Control A–Z Advice Sheet.*

O'Hagen, M. and Smith M. (1993) *Special Issues in Childcare.* London: Bailliere Tindall.

Organisation Mondiale Pour L'Education Préscolaire (OMEP) (1989) World Organisation for Early Childhood Education. In *Hospital. A Deprived Environment for Children?* The case for hospital play. Play in Hospital.

Osowski, M. (2002) Spinal cord compression: an obstructive oncological emergency. *Topics in Advanced Practice Nursing eJournal* **2** (4), 1–8. Available online http://www.medscape.com/viewarticle/442735/ (Last accessed 19/08/05).

Otaibi, A.A., Barker, C., Anderson, R. and Sigalet, D.L. (2002). Neutropenic entercolitis (typhlitis) after paediatric bone marrow transplant. *Journal of Pediatric Surgery* **37** (5), 770–772.

Paediatric Intensive Care Society (2002) Standards for Bereavement Care. Available from *Paediatric Intensive Care Society* details online at www.ukpics.org/

Paige, P.L. and Moe, P.C. (2006) Neurologic disorders. In Merenstein, G.B. and Gardner, S.L. (editors) *Handbook of Neonatal Intensive Care,* 6th edn. Philadelphia, USA: Mosby Elsevier.

Papadatou, D. (2001) The grieving healthcare provider – variables affecting the professional response to a child's death. *Bereavement Care* **20** (2), 26–29.

Papini, R. (2004) ABC of burns: management of burn injuries of various departments. *British Medical Journal* **329** (7458), 158–160.

Parker, L. (1999) IV devices and related infections: causes and complications. *British Journal of Nursing* 8 (22), 1491–1498.

Patte, C. (2004) Non-Hodgkin's lymphoma. In Pinkerton, R., Ploughman, P.N. and Pieters, R. (editors) *Paediatric Oncology*, 3rd edn. London: Arnold, pp. 254–266.

Payne, R. (2000) *Relaxation Techniques: A Practical Handbook for the Health Professional*. Edinburgh: Churchill Livingstone.

Pearson, G. (2002) *Handbook of Paediatric Intensive Care*. London: W.B. Saunders.

Pellowe, C.M. (2007) Implementing EPIC2 infection control guidelines. *Nursing Times* 103 (33), 30–31.

Perez, A. (2004) Cardiac monitoring mastering the essentials RN 59. In Jevon, P. (editor) *Paediatric Advanced Life Support – A Practical Guide*. Edinburgh: Butterworth Heinemann, pp. 32–39.

Perlstein, P.H., Kotagal U.R., Bolling, C., Steele, R. and Schoettker, P.J. (1999) Evaluation of an evidenced based guideline for bronchiolitis. *Pediatrics* 104 (66), 1334–1341.

Peters, K.L. (1999) Infant handling in NICU does developmental care make a difference. *Journal of Perinatal and Neonatal Nursing* 13 (3), 83–109.

Pizzo, P. (1999) Fever in immunocompromised patients. *The New England Journal of Medicine* 341 (12), 893–900.

Pizzo, P.A. and Poplack, D.G. (1997) *Principles and Practice of Pediatric Oncology*, 3rd edn. USA: Lippincott – Raven Publishers.

Platt Report (1959) Ministry of Health. *Report on the Welfare of Children in Hospital*. London: HMSO.

Plon, S.E. and Peterson, L.E. (1997) Childhood cancer, heredity, and the environment. In Pizzo, P.A. and Poplack, D.G. (editors) *Principles and Practice of Pediatric Oncology*, 3rd edn., Chapter 2. USA: Lippincott – Raven Publishers, pp. 11–36.

Pocock, G. and Richards, C.D. (2006) *Human Physiology – The Basis of Medicine*, 2nd edn. Oxford: Oxford University Press.

Porter, J.C., Leahey, A., Polise, K., Bunin, G. and Manno, C. (1996) Recombinant human erythropoietin reduces the need for erythrocyte and platelet transfusion in pediatric patients with sarcoma: a randomized, double-blind, placebo-controlled trial. *The Journal of Pediatrics* 129 (5), 656–660.

Porth, C. (2004) Disorders of fluid and electrolyte balance. In Matfin, G. and Porth, C. (editors) *Pathophysiology: Concepts of Altered Health States*, 7th edn., Chapter 33. New York: Lippincott Williams & Wilkins.

Proudfoot, C. and Gamble, C. (2006) Site specific skin reactions to amethocaine. *Paediatric Nurse* 19 (5), 26–28.

Pryor, J. and Prasad, S. (2002) *Physiotherapy for Respiratory and Cardiac Problems – Adults and Paediatrics*. Edinburgh: Churchill Livingstone.

Quinn, J. and DeAngelis, L. (2000) Neurological emergencies in the cancer patient. *Seminars in Oncology* 27, 311–321.

RCN guidelines. Available online www.rcn.org.uk/publications/pdf/guidelines/cpg_pain_assessment/ (Last accessed October, 2007).

Rees, L., Webb, A.J.N and Brogan, A.P. (2007) *Paediatric Nephrology*. Oxford: Oxford University Press.

Reid, T. (2000) Maternal identity in preterm birth. *Journal of Child Health Care* 4 (1), 23–29.

Reigle, B.S. and Dienger, M.J. (2003) Sepsis and treatment – induced immunosuppression in the patient with cancer. *Critical Care Nursing Clinical of North America* 15, 109–118.

Reynolds, K. (1993) Let's play, no. 1 baby in hospital. *National Association of Hospital Play Staff*. London: NAHPS.

Rheingold, S.R. and Lange, B.L. (2006) *Pediatric Oncology*, 5th edn. Philadelphia, USA: Lippincott Williams & Wilkins, pp. 1202–1230.

Rich, K. (1999) In hospital cardiac arrest: pre-event variables and nursing response. *Clinical Nurse Specialist* 13 (6), 147–153.

Richardson, A., Douglas, M., Shuttler, R. and Hagland, M.R. (2003) Critical care staff rotation: outcomes of a survey and pilot study. *Nursing in Critical Care* 8 (2), 84–89.

Riches, G. and Dawson, P. (2000) *An Intimate Loneliness – Supporting Bereaved Parents and Siblings*. Buckingham, UK: Open University Press.

Riegel, W. (2003) Continuous replacement therapy in acute renal failure. *Kidney and Blood Pressure Research* 26 (2), 123–127.

Rieger, P.T. (2001) The role of oncology nurses in gene therapy. *Lancet Oncology* 2 (4), 233–238.

Roaten, J.B., Bensard, D.D. and Price, F.N. (2006) Neonatal surgery. In Merenstein, G.B. and Gardner, S.L. (editors) *Handbook of Neonatal Intensive Care*, 6th edn. Philadelphia, USA: Mosby Elsevier.

Robertson, P. and Fritz, J.B. (1996) Gene targeting approaches to the autonomic nervous system. *Journal of Autonomic Nervous System* 61 (1), 1–5.

Royal College of Anaesthetists (2004) Good practice in the management of continuous epidural analgesia in the hospital setting. Available online www.britishpainsociety.org/

Royal College of Anaesthetists and Royal College of Surgeons (1996) *Report of the Joint WorkingpParty on Graduated Patient Care*. London: RCA/RCS.

Royal College of Nursing (RCN) (2003) *Defining Staffing Levels for Children's and Young People's Services*. London: Royal College of Nursing.

Royal College of Nursing (RCN) (2005) *Methicillin-Resistant Staphylococcus aureus: Guidance for Nursing Staff*. London: RCN.

Royal College of Nursing (RCN) (2007) Better at home the need for HDC in the community. Congress paper – Jan Murphy/PNIC. This was overwhelmingly supported by the RCN delegates. Harrogate.

Royal College of Paediatrics and Child Health (2004) *Withholding or Withdrawing Life Sustaining Treatment in Children: A Framework for Practice*, 2nd edn. London, UK: Royal College of Paediatrics and Child Health.

Ruddle, T. (2003) Sedation an overview. *Paediatric Nursing* 15 (1), 38–41.

Rudolph, M. and Levene, M. (1999) Paediatrics and child health. *Health Promotion and Child Health Surveillance*. Oxford: Blackwell Science.

Rushforth, K. (2006) A study of paediatric high dependency care in West, North and East Yorkshire. *A Report of Staffing and Patient Activity*. Jan–Dec 2005. University of Leeds, ISBN 0 85316 171 0.

Rutter, N. (2000) The dermis. *Seminars in Neonatology* 5, 297–302.

Salyer, J.W. (2003) Neonatal and paediatric pulse oximetry. *Respiratory Care* 48 (4), 386–396.

Sander, W., Eshelman, D., Steele, J. *et al.* (2002) Effects of distraction using virtual reality glasses during a lumber puncture in adolescents with cancer. *Oncology Nursing Forum* 29 (1), 8–15.

Sargent, S. (2006) Management of patients with advanced liver cirrhosis. *Nursing Standard* 21 (11), 48–56.

Saria, M.G. and Gosselin-Acom, T.K. (2007) Hematopoietic stem cell transplantation: implications for critical care nurses. *Clinical Journal of Oncology Nursing* 11 (1), 53–63.

Savins, C. (2002) Therapeutic work with children in pain. *Paediatric Nursing* 14 (5), 14–16.

Schierhout, G. and Roberts, I. (1998) Fluid resuscitation with colloid or crystalloid solutions in critically ill patients: a systematic review of randomised trials. *British Medical Journal* 316 (7136), 961–964.

Schott, J., Henley, A. and Kohner, N. (2007) *Pregnancy Loss and the Death of a Baby: Guidelines for Professionals*, 3rd edn. London, UK: Bosun Press (on behalf of Stillbirth & neonatal death charity).

Scrace, J. (2003) Complementary therapies in palliative care of children with cancer: a literature review. *Paediatric Nurse* 15 (3), 36–39.

Secola, R. (2006) Tumor lysis syndrome: nursing management and new therapeutic options. *Advanced Studies in Nursing* 4 (3), 41–48.

Selwood, K. Gibson, F. and Evans, M. (1999) Side effects of chemotherapy. In Gibson, F. and Evans, M. (editors) *Paediatric Oncology. Acute Nursing Care*, Chapter 3. London: Whurr Publishers, pp. 59–128.

Settle, J. (1996) *Principles and Practice of Burns Management*. London, UK: Churchill Livingstone.

Shafford, E.A. and Pritchard, J. (2004) Liver tumours. In Pinkerton, R., Plowman, P.N. and Pieters, R. (editors) *Paediatric Oncology*, 3rd edn. London: Arnold, pp. 448–468.

Shaw, S. (2006) Nursing and supporting patients with chronic pain. *Nursing Standard* 20 (19), 60–65.

Sheppard, M. and Wright, M. (2000) *Principles and Practice of High Dependency Nursing*. Edinburgh: Bailliere Tindall.

Sheppard, M. and Wright, M. (2003) *Principles and Practice of High Dependency Nursing*. Edinburgh: Bailliere Tindall.

Sheridan, M. (1997) *Spontaneous Play in Early Childhood from Birth to Six Years*. London: Routledge.

Siegler, R., Oakes, R. *et al.* (2005) Hemolytic uremic syndrome: pathogenesis, treatment and outcome. *Current Opinion in Pediatrics* 17 (2), 200–204.

Singh, N.C. (1997) *Manual of Pediatric Critical Care*. Philadelphia, USA: WB Saunders and Company.

Singri, N., Ahya, S.N., Levin, M.L. *et al.* (2003) Acute renal failure. *Journal of the American Medical Association* 289 (6), 747–751.

Skills for Health (2007) Awards and Qualifications. Available online www.skillsforhealth.org.uk/page/awards-and-qualifications/

Slater, R. Cantarella, A. Gallella, S. *et al.* (2006) Cortical pain responses in human and infants. *The Journal of Neuroscience* 26 (14), 3662–3666.

Slocombe, A. and Boynes, S. (2005) Malignant spinal cord compression. *Radiology* 11, 293–298.

Smith, O.P. and Hann, I. (2004) Pathology of leukaemia. In Pinkerton, R., Ploughman, P.N. and Pieters, R. (editors) *Paediatric Oncology*, 3rd edn. London: Arnold.

Smith, S.F., Duell, D.J. and Martin, B.C. (2004) *Clinical Nursing Skills, Basic to Advanced*, 6th edn. New Jersey, NJ: Pearson Prentice Hall.

Smith, S. (2001) Evidence based management of constipation in the oncology patient. *European Journal of Oncology Nursing* 5 (1), 18–25.

Society for Cardiological Science and Technology (2005) Clinical Guidelines by Consensus. Number 1 Recording the 12 lead electrocardiogram. Available online http://scst.org.uk/docs/Consensus%20guidelines%20for%20recording%20a%2012%20lead%20ECG.pdf#search=%22performing%2012%20lead%20ECG%22/ (Last accessed 26/09/06).

Starr, S. and Hand, H. (2002) Nursing care of chronic and acute liver failure. *Nursing Standard* 16 (40), 47–55.

Steggal, M. (2007) Acute urinary retention: causes clinical features and patient care. *Nursing Standard* 21 (29), 42–46.

Stevens, B., Yamada, J. and Ohlsson, A. (2003) Sucrose for analgesia in newborn infants undergoing painful procedures. *Cochrane Database Systematic Review* 1, CD001069. www.cochrane.org/reviews.

Streeton, C. and Nolan, T. (1997) Reduction in paediatric burn admissions over 25 years, 1970–1994. *Injury Prevention* 3, 104–109.

Summers, K. (2007) Evidenced based practice; non-invasive blood pressure measurement in children. *Journal of Children's and Young Peoples Nursing* 1 (2), 59–63.

Sung, L., Nathan, P.C., Lange, B., Beyene, J. and Buchanan, R. (2002) Prophylactic granulocyte colony-stimulating factor and granulocyte–macrophage colony stimulating factor decreases febrile neutropenia after chemotherapy in children with cancer: a meta-analysis of randomized controlled trials. *Journal of Clinical Oncology* 22 (16), 3350–3356.

Susseman, N.B. (1996) Fulminant hepatic failure. In Zakim, D. and Boyer, T.D. (editors) *Hepatology: A Text Book of Liver Disease*. St. Louis: Saunders WB, pp. 618–630.

Sylva, K. and Lunt, I. (1990) *Child Development a First Course*. Oxford: Blackwell.

Symonds, R. (2001) Recent advances in radiotherapy. *British Medical Journal* 323 (7321), 1107–1110.

Available online http://www.bmj.com/cgi/content/full/323/7321/1107. (Last accessed 14/10/07).

Taddio, A. and Katz, J. (2005) The effects of early pain experience in neonates on pain responses in infancy and children. *Paediatric Drugs* 7 (4), 245–257.

Taylor, C.M., Chua, C., Howie, A.J. *et al.* (2004) Clinico-pathological findings in diarrhea-negative haemolytic uraemic syndrome. *Paediatric Nephrology* 19, 419–425.

Thalange, N., Holmes, P., Beach, R. and Kinnaird, T. (2006) *Pocket Essentials of Paediatrics*. Edinburgh, UK: Elsevier Saunders.

Thompson, I. (2002) Mental health and spiritual care. *Nursing Standard* 17 (9), 33–38.

Thompson, I. (2004) The management of nausea and vomiting in palliative care. *Nursing Standard* 3 (19), 46–53.

Thorne, L. and Hackwood, H. (2002) Developing critical care skills for nurses in the ward environment: a work based learning approach. *Nursing in Critical Care* 7 (3), 121–125.

Thurgate, C. and Heppell, S. (2005) Needle phobia – changing venepuncture practice in ambulatory care. *Paediatric Nursing* 17 (9), 15–18.

Tobias, J.D. and Johnson, J.O. (2003) Measurement of central venous pressure from a peripheral vein in infants and children. *Pediatric Emergency Care* 19 (6), 428–430.

Tortora, G. and Derrickson, B. (2005) *Principles of Anatomy and Physiology*, 11th edn. London: Wiley.

Trey, C. and Davidson, C.S. (1970) The management of fulminant hepatic failure. *Progress in Liver Disease* 2, 282–298.

Truman, P. (2006) Jaundice in the preterm infant. *Paediatric Nursing* 18 (5), 20–22.

Tume, L. and Bullock, I. (2004) Early warning tools to identify children at risk of deterioration; a discussion. *Paediatric Nursing* 16 (8), 20–23.

Twycross, A. (1997) Nurses perception of pain in children. *Paediatric Nursing* 9 (1), 17–19.

Twycross, A. and Smith, J. (2006) The management of acute pain in children. In Glasper, A. and Richardson, J. (editors) *A Textbook of Children's and Young Peoples Nursing*. UK: Churchill Livingstone Elsevier.

U.S. Food and Drug Administration, National Institute for Occupational Safety and Health, Centers for Disease Control, and the Occupational Safety and Health Administration (1999–2/22/99) Glass

Capillary Tubes; Joint Safety Advisory about potential risks. Available from http://www.cdc.gov/niosh/ Accessed 01.05.07.

Unicef (1995) *The Convention on the Rights of the Child*. London: HMSO.

Vere-Jones, E. (2007) Will the new inspection scheme really help to cut infection rates? *Nursing Times* **103** (24), 9.

Veys, P. and Rao, K. (2004). Allogenic stem cell transplantation. In: Pinkerton, R., Ploughman, P.N. and Pieters, R. (editors) *Paediatric Oncology*, 3rd edn. London: Arnold, pp. 513–537.

Voruganti, V., Klein, G., Lu, H., Thomas, S., Freeland-Graves, J. and Herndon, D. (2005) Impaired zinc and copper status in children with burn injuries: need to reassess nutritional requirements. *Burns* **31** (6), 711–716.

Wadler, S., Benson III, Al. B., Engelking, C., *et al.* (1998) Recommended Guidelines for the Treatment of Chemotherapy-Induced Diarrhea. *Journal of Clinical Oncology* **16** (9), 3169–3178.

Wagner, L.M., Billups, C.A., Furman, W.L., Rao, B.N. and Santana, V.M. (2004). Combined use of erythropoietin and granulocyte colony-stimulating factor does not decrease blood transfusion requirements during induction therapy for high-risk neuroblastoma: a randomized controlled trial. *Journal of Clinical Oncology* **22** (10), 1886–1893.

Walsh, T.J., Rolidies, E., Groll, A.H., Gonzalez, C. and Pizzo, P. (2006). Infectious complications in pediatric cancer patients. In: Pizzo, P.A. and Poplack, D.G. (editors) *Principles and Practice of Pediatric Oncology*, 5th edn. Philadelphia, USA: Lippincott Williams & Wilkins, pp. 1269–1329.

Ward, D.J. (2007) Hand adornment and infection control. *British Journal of Nursing* **16** (11), 654–656.

Watret, L. and Armitage, M. (2002) Making sense of wound cleaning. *Journal of Community Nursing* **16** (4). Available online at www.jcn.co.uk.

Watt, S. (2003) Safe administration of medicines. *Paediatric Nurse* **15** (5), 40–44.

Waugh, A. and Grant, A. (2006) *Ross and Wilson – Anatomy and Physiology in Health and Illness*, 10th edn. UK: Churchill Livingstone Elsevier.

Weetman, C. and Allison, W. (2006) Use of epidural analgesia in post operative management. *Nursing Standard* **20** (44), 54–64.

Weir, E. (2003) Congenital abdominal wall defects. *Canadian Medical Association Journal* **169** (8), 809–810.

Welch, S.B. and Nadel, S. (2003) Treatment of meningococcal infection. *Archives of Disease in Childhood* **88** (7), 608–614.

Wellings, T. (2001) Drawings by dying and bereaved children. *Paediatric Nursing* **13** (4), 30–36.

Wesdrop, R.I., Krause, R. and Van-Meyenfeldt, M. (1983). Cancer cachexia and its nutritional implications. *British Journal of Surgery* **70** (6), 352–355.

Whelan, J. and Morland, B. (2004) Bone tumours. In Pizzo, P.A. and Poplack, D.G. (editors) *Principles and Practice of Pediatric Oncology*, 3rd edn. USA: Lippincott – Raven Publishers, pp. 371–385.

White, M.C., Thornton, K. and Young, A.E. (2005) Early diagnosis and treatment of toxic shock syndrome in paediatric burns. *Burns* **31** (2), 193–197.

Whittingham, P.F. and Alonso, E.M. (2004) In Kelly, D.A. (editor) *Fulminant Hepatitis and Acute Liver Failure: Diseases of the Liver and Biliary System in Children*, 2nd edn. London: Blackwell Publishing.

Wilkes, G. (1999) Neurological disturbances. In: Yarbro, C., Frogge, M. and Goodman, M. (editors) *Cancer Symptom Management*, 2nd edn. Boston: Jones and Barlett, pp. 344–381.

Williams, V., Riley, A., Rayner R. and Richardson, K. (2006) Inhaled nitrous oxide during a painful procedure: a satisfaction survey. *Paediatric Nursing* **18** (8), 31–33.

Wilman, D. (1997) Neonatal transport: the effect on parents. *Journal of Neonatal Nursing* **3** (5), 16–22.

Wolf, A. (1999) Pain nociception and the developing infant. *Paediatric Anaesthesia* **9** (1), 7–17. Available online at www.dh.gov.uk.

Wolke, D. (1991) Annotation: supporting the development of low birth weight infants. *Journal of Child Psychology and Psychiatry* **32** (5), 723–741.

Wong, D. and Barker, C. (1988) Pain in children; comparison of assessment scales. *Pediatric Nursing* **14** (1), 9–17.

Woods Blake, W. and Murray, J.A. (2006) Heat balance. In Merenstein, G.B. and Gardner, S.L. (editors) *Handbook of Neonatal Intensive Care*, 6th edn. Philadelphia, USA: Mosby Elsevier.

World Health Organisation (1997) Thermal protection of the newborn [online]. Available at: www.who.int/reproductive-health/publications/ MSM_97_2_Thermal_protection

World Health Organisation (2001) *WHO Global Strategy for the Containment of Antimicrobial Resistance*. Geneva.

World Health Organisation (2003) *Infant and Young Child Feeding: A Tool for Assessing National Practices, Policies and Programmes*. Geneva.

Wright, E. (2004) Assessment and management of the child requiring haemodialysis. *Paediatric Nursing* **16** (7), 37–41.

Wright, J.D. (2000) Before the transport team arrives: neonatal stabilisation. *The Journal of Perinatal and Neonatal Nursing* **13** (4), 87–107.

Wright, M. (2006) The development, growth and context of high dependency care. In Sheppard, M. and Wright, M. (editors) *Principles and Practice of High Dependency Nursing*, 2nd edn. Edinburgh: Bailliere Tindall, pp. 3–20.

Wright, S. (2001) The meaning of love. *Nursing Standard* **25** (15), 23.

www.sickleandthal.org.uk/documents/stage1 appendix1.doc Newborn Bloodspot Screening Information Management System for England.

Yellow Alert Campaign from Children's Liver Disease Foundation. Available online at www.childliverdisease.org. Accessed July 2007.

Yoder, L. (1994) Comfort and consolation: a nursing perspective on parental bereavement. *Pediatric Nursing* **20** (5), 473–477.

Young, S. (2000) Comparing the use of Ketamine and Midazolam in emergency settings. *Emergency Nurse* **7** (8), 27–30.

Young, Y. (1999) Principles of chemotherapy. In Gibson, F. and Evans, M. (editors) *Paediatric Oncology. Acute Nursing Care*, Chapter 1. London: Whurr Publishers Ltd.

Zeigler, V.L. (2001) *Practical Management of Paediatric Cardiac Arrhythmias*. New York: Blackwell.

Zimmerman, J.L. (2004). Use of blood products in sepsis: an evidence-based review. *Critical Care Medicine* **32** (11 Suppl), 542–554.

USEFUL WEBSITES

Health Protection Agency (HPA) www.hpa.org.uk/
infections (epidemiological data and surveillance
information)
http://www.bnfc.nhs.uk/bnfc/
http://www.cafamily.org.uk/Direct/h17.html
http://www.ecoli-uk.com/
http://www.fsid.org.uk/reduce-risk.html
http://www.nephrotic.co.uk/
http://www.rcjournal.com/online_resources/cpgs/
soddnppcpg.html
http://www.vh.org/pediatric/provider/pediatrics/iowaneo-
natologyhandbook/general/commentsoxygen.html
Meningitis Research Trust – www.meningitis.org/
disease-info (general information)
Meningitis Trust – www.meninigitis-trust.org (general
information)

www.bhf.org.uk (British Heart Foundation)
www.brainandspine.org.uk (general information)
www.cardiomyopathy.org
www.ccad.org.uk/congenital
www.C-R-Y.org.uk – (Cardiac Risk in the Young)
www.dhg.org.uk (Downs Heart Group)
www.guch.org.uk (Grown Up Congenital Hearts)
www.heartstats.org
www.inmed.co.uk/resources (resources for healthcare
professionals)
www.kidney.org.uk (http://cnserverO.nkf.med.ualberta.ca/
nephkids/childhoodns.htm)
www.lhm.org.uk (Little Heart Matters)
www.patient.co.uk
www.sads.org.uk (Sudden Arrhythmic Death Syndrome)

INDEX